OCCUPATIONAL THERAPY

Principles and Practice

Second Edition

Alice J. Punwar, MS, OTR, FAOTA
Professor Emeritus
Therapeutic Science Program
Department of Kinesiology
University of Wisconsin-Madison
Madison, Wisconsin

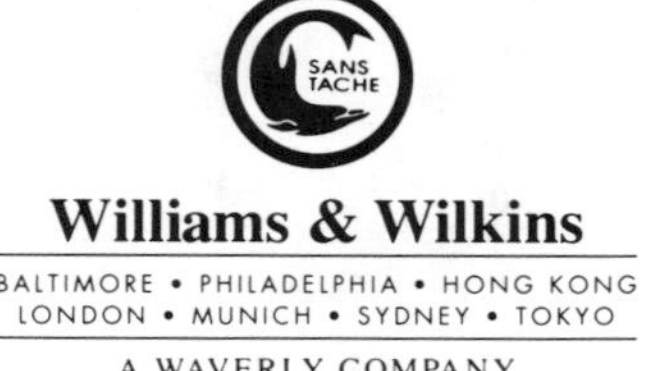

Williams & Wilkins
BALTIMORE • PHILADELPHIA • HONG KONG
LONDON • MUNICH • SYDNEY • TOKYO
A WAVERLY COMPANY

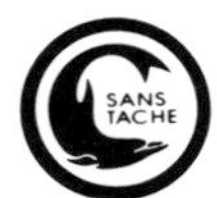

Editor: John P. Butler
Managing Editor: Linda S. Napora
Copy Editor: Klemie Bryte
Designer: Wilma E. Rosenberger
Illustration Planner: Lorraine Wrzosek
Production Coordinator: Charles E. Zeller

Williams & Wilkins
428 East Preston Street
Baltimore, Maryland 21202, USA

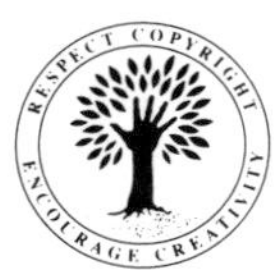

Printed in the United States of America

First Edition 1988

Library of Congress Cataloging-in-Publication Data

Punwar, Alice J.
Occupational therapy : principles and practices / Alice J. Punwar. —2nd ed.
p. cm.
Includes index.
ISBN 0-683-06975-6
1. Occupational therapy—Vocational guidance. 2. Occupational therapy—United States. 3. Occupational therapy—History.
I. Title.
[DNLM: 1. Occupational Therapy. 2. Occupational Therapy. WB 555 P984o]
RM735.4.P86 1994
615.8'515—dc20
DNLM/DLC
for Library of Congress

92-48838
CIP

93 94 95 96 97
1 2 3 4 5 6 7 8 9 10

Much have I learned from my teachers,
more from my colleagues, but
most from my students.

Talmud, Ta'anith, 7b

Preface

This book was written to introduce beginning students to the field of occupational therapy and the career opportunities it offers. It is directed at students in both technical and professional occupational therapy educational programs, since the author believes that beginning students have similar needs for basic information about the field. Throughout the book the contributions of both levels of personnel are discussed and the author hopes that students will recognize the complementary roles of the registered occupational therapist and the certified occupational therapy assistant and will learn how each supports the other in clinical practice. Nontechnical language has been used as much as possible, and where technical terms appear, they have been defined in the Glossary that is found at the end of the book.

The text is organized into four sections. Section I provides background information about the origins of the field, its basic concepts and philosophy, its education and certification patterns, and the practice functions of the registered occupational therapist and the certified occupational therapy assistant.

Section II looks at patterns of health care in the United States and how they developed (Chapter 7), discusses the team approach in health care delivery (Chapter 8), and gives an overview of the process of service delivery in occupational therapy (Chapter 9). Eight chapters look at practice within specialty areas of occupational therapy and identify practice issues and current trends.

Section III discusses professional organizations in occupational therapy (Chapter 18) and international occupational therapy (Chapter 19), and Chapter 20 identifies issues currently under discussion in the field and includes projections for the future of occupational therapy practice. The text is intended to provide a comprehensive review of the profession for students who are considering a career in occupational therapy. There is no attempt to discuss advanced theoretical concepts or practice techniques, as there are excellent texts available for this purpose.

In Section IV, the Appendices provide American Occupational Therapy Association standards, principles, guidelines, and sources of information as well as a comprehensive Glossary.

Because of space limitations, many topics are discussed only briefly in the text. For more detailed information, the reader is advised to use the lists of references and suggested readings that are provided at the end of each chapter. Instructors will no doubt wish to supplement the text with current articles from the professional literature. The discussion questions that follow each chapter are intended to stimulate students to think about the issues raised in the chapter and to generate further discussion of the topics presented.

Sexist language has been avoided as much as possible. The author has used the words "patient" and "client" interchangeably; however, in chapters with a historical content, "patient" has been used during the early periods, whereas "client" is used more frequently during later periods.

This second edition of *Occupational Therapy: Principles and Practice* includes a new chapter on the philosophy of occupational therapy and how that philosophy has been modified in accordance with social changes and changes in the health care environment. All of the chapters have been updated with current statistics and new information. Case studies have been condensed and rewritten in narrative style. New material has been added on ethics in education and practice, work programs, technology development and application, and emerging careers in occupational therapy. The Glossary and the Index have been expanded, and new documents have been added to the Appendices. The author hopes that these revisions accurately reflect the profession of occupational therapy today and the massive changes that are occurring in health care in the United States.

Each occupational therapist and therapy assistant is likely to have his or her own view of the field and the issues that confront it. This book represents the personal view of the author. Readers should recognize that there are differences of opinion on many of the topics presented. The perspectives given in this text represent the author's point of view and are not intended to represent the official views of the American Occupational Therapy Association or any other professional organization. If errors or omissions are found, the author hopes that students and colleagues will call them to her attention.

A.J.P.

Acknowledgments

This book could not have been completed without the help of many colleagues who provided material, read drafts of chapters, engaged in lively discussion of current issues in occupational therapy, gave both positive and negative feedback, and offered frequent encouragement throughout the writing process. I am grateful for their help and support. To those students who completed questionnaires about the book, my grateful thanks. Your suggestions were taken seriously.

Special thanks are due to those who made direct contributions of chapters or case material. Martha Stavros, senior clinical social worker at the University of Michigan Medical Center, and Daraleen C. Sitka, OTR, currently serving in the 34th General Hospital Unit in Germany, wrote Chapter 8 on the health care team.

Many clinicians contributed the original case studies. For this second edition, the following people reviewed and revised case study material: Pam Dallman, OTR; Amy Letourneau, OTR; Chris Sparrow, OTR; Joan Loeffelholz, OTR; Linda Speer, OTR; Patty Mader-Ebert, OTR; Bridget Connolly-Caflisch, OTR; and Cindy Wegrzyn Jernegan, OTR.

Recent materials were obtained from the American Occupational Therapy Association for inclusion in the text. I am particularly grateful to Jeanette Bair, Executive Director of AOTA, who supplied current data on the organization; Brena Manoly, Associate Executive Director of Professional Development, who provided materials on education, state regulation, and the most recent role delineation; Ira Silvergleit, Director of Research Information, who provided current statistics, charts, and graphs; Elouise Strand, who supplied material on the World Federation of Occupational Therapists; and Ann Rosenstein, Director of Publications, who gave permission to reproduce material previously published in AOTA publications. Suzanne Carlton of the AOTA Public Relations staff assisted with locating suitable photographs and gave permission for their reproduction.

Madelaine Gray, Executive Director of the American Occupational Therapy Certification Board, provided current data on the certification process for OTRs and COTAs. Professor Barbara Posthuma, Honorary Secretary of the World Federation of Occupational Therapists, made available current information on member organizations around the world. Barbara Joe aided in finding photographs of international occupational therapy.

The friendly staff of Odana Press helped with endless photocopying, and staff members at Econoprint prepared some of the charts for publication. I am grateful to John P. Butler, Executive Editor at Williams & Wilkins, for his encouragement and support; Linda Napora, Managing Editor, for her direct assistance with the manuscript; Klemie Bryte, who edited the copy; and Chuck Zeller, Production Coordinator, for his vigilant attention to all aspects of the production process. My husband, who suffered through the revision process with me, also deserves a special word of thanks.

Alice J. Punwar, MS, OTR, FAOTA
Professor Emeritus
Therapeutic Science Program
Department of Kinesiology
University of Wisconsin-Madison

Contents

SECTION I

OVERVIEW OF OCCUPATIONAL THERAPY

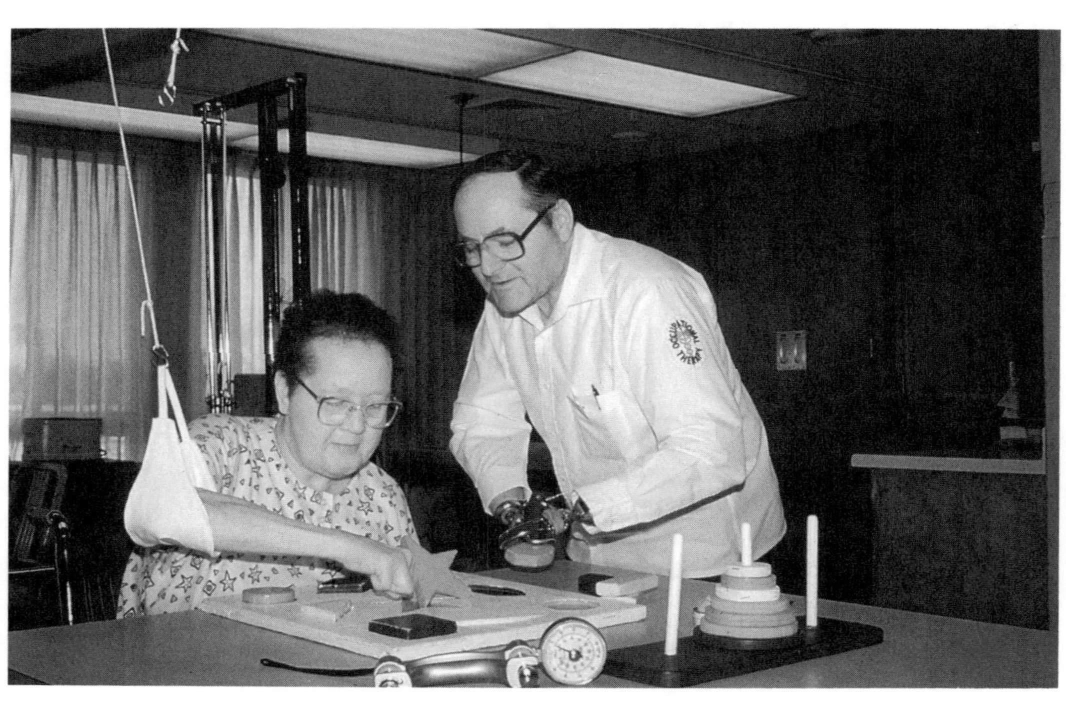

1 Defining Occupational Therapy

Passengers were boarding for a four-hour flight to San Francisco and a middle-aged businessman was searching for his seat. He found it and settled in beside a young woman. As the plane took off, he noticed that she was reading a magazine, apparently a trade journal of some kind. When the seat belt sign had been turned off, he introduced himself. "Hello! I'm Sam Hoffman. I'm a sales representative for an industrial equipment firm, and I'm on my way to a trade show in San Francisco. Are you flying for business or pleasure?" The young woman smiled and lowered her magazine. "Both," she admitted. "My name is Gerry White, and I'm on my way to a national occupational therapy conference there. I'm an occupational therapist at Hillside Rehabilitation Center in Chicago." Sam looked puzzled. "What do occupational therapists do?" he asked. "Oh wait, I know. You find jobs for disabled people." "No, not quite," Gerry corrected gently. "We work with people who have been injured or ill to help them regain their maximum function so they can pick up their lives again." Now Sam looked even more puzzled. "I thought physical therapists did that," he said. Gerry sighed. Then she resumed her efforts to explain occupational therapy in a way that would be meaningful to Sam.

Most occupational therapists have had this conversation countless times during their careers. *Occupational therapy* is not a household term, although many people have had family members or friends who have received occupational therapy services. According to a national Gallup survey conducted in 1989, 80% of other health professionals were familiar with occupational therapy, but only 40% of the general public were. Thirty-two percent of those responding were unable to differentiate between physical therapy and occupational therapy. Nine percent said that someone in their family had been treated by an occupational therapist (1). Because the field is a broad one and has undergone many changes since its beginnings, it is difficult to define simply and accurately. People often confuse occupational therapists with other health professionals, such as physical therapists, recreational therapists, workers in dance, music, or art therapy, craft instructors, and vocational rehabilitation personnel. Occupational therapy shares some interests with all of these fields, but its chief focus is different.

Occupation has been defined as the active or "doing" process of a person engaged in goal-directed, intrinsically gratifying, and culturally appropriate activity (2). Purposeful goal-directed activity is an essential part of any person's life. Occupational therapy is based on the belief that purposeful activity (occupation) may be used to prevent physical and psychosocial dysfunction and to restore function to more normal levels. *Occupations*, as used in this sense, are activities that are selected for their therapeutic value and that the occupational therapist uses to help the client regain abilities that have been lost or limited due to physical or psychological disturbances. Although an occupational therapist may utilize art, music, dance, or craft activities, the focus is always on the achievement of a therapeutic goal. Activities are not used as recreation or to fill in empty time but rather as a means to a therapeutic end. It is this goal directedness that characterizes the occupational therapist's use of activities. Each activity has a specific purpose and is used for a reason.

Definitions of occupational therapy have changed over the years. Early definitions emphasized the use of occupation as remedial activity to help restore the individual to an improved state of physical and mental health. It was viewed as a medically prescribed form of treatment and was usually conducted in a hospital, sanatorium, or community workshop. Arts and crafts activities were considered the primary tools of the occupational therapist during the formative years of the field, and the therapist was viewed as a specialist in the selection and application of planned programs of activity that were expected to directly improve the condition of the client. The goal of such programs was to help the individual resume as much of his or her normal pattern of living as possible. This included the work role as well as the daily home tasks of the client. Occupational therapy was regarded as a gradual preparation of the client to return to work responsibilities or, if that was impossible, to explore feasible vocational alternatives. The relationship of occupational therapy to the work roles of clients has caused people to confuse occupational therapists with vocational rehabilitation workers, who provide counseling and job training for individuals who are unable to return to their previous jobs.

As occupational therapy grew and expanded, it was used with clients who had many different kinds of limitations and who were being cared for in a variety of settings. Occupational therapists began to work in outpatient clinics, community mental health centers, public and private schools, nursing homes, home health care agencies, and private or group practices. Therapists were working with clients of all age levels and with a wide range of physical and psychosocial disorders. This diversity of practice made it difficult to define the field simply and yet comprehensively. The American Occupational Therapy Association, however, has provided definitions to reflect the growing scope of the field. A statement was published in 1981 when some states were beginning to adopt state licensure for occupational therapists. The following definition describes current occupational therapy practice and is one of several in general use today.

> *Occupational therapy is the use of purposeful activity with individuals who are limited by physical injury or illness, psychosocial dysfunction, developmental or learning disabilities, poverty and cultural differences, or the aging process in order to maximize independence, prevent disability, and maintain health. The practice encompasses evaluation, treatment, and consultation. Specific occupational therapy services include: teaching daily living skills; developing perceptual-motor skills and sensory integrative functioning; developing play skills and prevocational and leisure capacities; designing, fabricating, or applying selected orthotic and prosthetic devices or selective adaptive equipment; using specifically designed crafts and exercises to enhance functional performance; administering and interpreting tests such as manual muscle or range of motion tests; and adapting environments for the handicapped. These services are provided individually, in groups, or through social systems (3).*

This definition describes well the diverse practice and scope of occupational therapy today. There are several key phrases in the definition that are important to the understanding of occupational therapy. The concept of *purposeful activity* is a central one to the field. There is always a reason for the selection of a given client activity, and therapists draw on their scientific knowledge of their clients' conditions and needs as well as their repertoire of potential activities in making that selection.

The 1981 definition also clearly defines the populations with which occupational therapists work. With all clients, the end goals of occupational therapy intervention are "to maximize independence, prevent disability, and to maintain health" (3). This goes farther than earlier definitions in its inclusion of prevention and health maintenance as valid outcomes of occupational therapy. The specific services of occupational therapists are spelled out by the definition, as well as patterns of service delivery. Because of the increasing need for containment of health care costs, occupational therapy clients are being seen more often in groups today, although individual treatment still occurs. Occupational therapists are also becoming more involved in the legislative process and are serving as advocates for their client populations when health and social welfare issues are under consideration by legislative bodies.

This definition of occupational therapy accurately reflects the broad scope of the field today. We may well see further changes in the definition of occupational therapy as health care and services change to meet the needs of society. But let's get back to our in-flight conversation. Gerry is just finishing her explanation of occupational therapy to Sam by saying, "Although I myself work with the physically handicapped, other therapists are working with learning-disabled children, the mentally retarded, people who have psychological problems, or older people who need help in adapting to the changes caused by aging. Even though we work with so many different kinds of people, our goal is basically the same: to help people live as normally and as fully as possible within their own environment." "I see," said Sam enthusiastically, "you help people learn to help themselves." "That's it!" agreed Gerry, beaming, "Now you've got it!" Both settled back in their seats for the flight ahead.

Discussion Questions

1. What are some of the misconceptions about occupational therapy that you have heard?
2. When people ask you what occupational therapy is, how do you define it?
3. How did you learn about occupational therapy as a potential career?

References

1. Survey reveals awareness of O T. *O T Week* 3(21):2, 1989.
2. Evans AK: Nationally speaking: definition of occupation as the core concept of occupational therapy. *AJOT* 41(10):627–628, 1987.
3. Resolution Q: Definition of occupational therapy for licensure. Minutes of the 1981 AOTA Representative Assembly. *AJOT* 35:798–799, 1981.

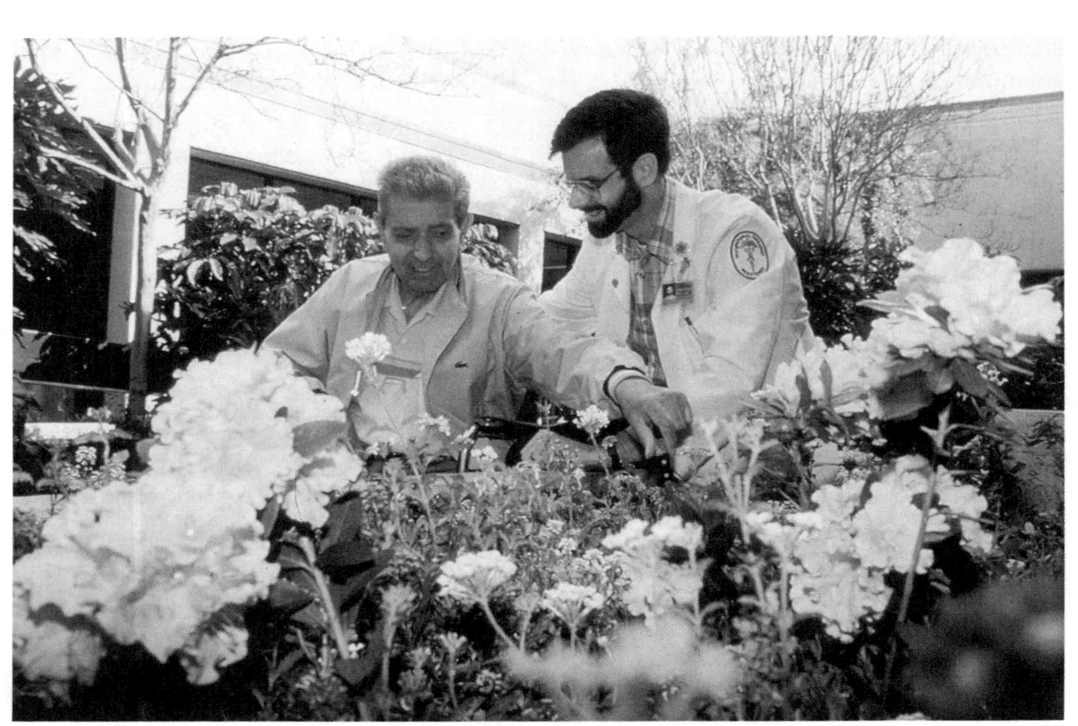

2 Philosophy of Occupational Therapy

Now that we've looked at some definitions of occupational therapy, we need to understand the philosophy of the field. A profession's philosophy includes the fundamental beliefs and values of the profession, analyzed in a critical way (1). In this chapter we review some of the concepts, ideas, and beliefs that have influenced the development of occupational therapy during its history. We will try to show how some occupational therapy beliefs have changed over time in accordance with changes in occupational therapy practice and with changing economic and social conditions. You will find that this chapter is closely related to Chapter 3, "Historical Development of the Field," and it may be helpful to read them in sequence to get a better idea of how occupational therapy philosophy evolved along with changes in the field.

MORAL TREATMENT: A PRECURSOR OF OCCUPATIONAL THERAPY

Before occupational therapy developed as a profession, there were treatment philosophies that were similar in nature and that influenced the founders of occupational therapy. During the latter part of the 18th century, a philosophy of moral treatment arose in the treatment of the mentally ill. Up till this time, persons with mental illness had been thought to be hopeless cases and beyond the scope of any known treatment approach. The mentally ill were usually segregated in ill-kept institutions, often housed in appalling conditions, and frequently mistreated by their caretakers. Dr. Philippe Pinel in France and William Tuke in England were among the first to suggest that a more humane approach might be worth exploring. Their experimentation evolved into a new treatment philosophy that became known as moral treatment. (The term "moral" was used in the sense of "psychological" or "emotional.") The methods they developed were intended to introduce order, active movement, and a diversity of daily occupation to inmates of mental institutions. Patients were to be treated with kindness and respect, and daily activities were organized that included manual labor, social functions, church services, and the ordinary activities of daily life. The philosophy was based on the idea that most mentally ill patients had the capacity to live an ordered and rational life.

Moral treatment programs offered a structured series of daily activities that were similar to those engaged in by healthy individuals. When such programs were instituted, many patients responded positively and moral treatment was thought to offer a new cure for mental illness. The approach was brought to the United States by a few enlightened physicians who had seen the value of such programs in European institutions. Moral treatment programs enjoyed a period of success in American institutions during the 19th century, but changing social patterns and a new concept of insanity led to the gradual decline of this treatment approach. In spite of their great promise, moral treatment programs were abandoned (2).

EARLY OCCUPATIONAL THERAPY CONCEPTS

The idea that activity could have therapeutic benefit was revived in the early years of the 20th century by people who were interested in working with the mentally ill and the physically disabled. The early practitioners of occupational therapy were a diverse group. Some came from medical backgrounds and brought with them the concepts and values of traditional medicine. Others were social workers, teachers, architects, and secretaries. They shared a mutual interest in seeking new tools and approaches in helping those with limited function to live a more satisfying life. They brought strong humanistic values to their work and were convinced that they could contribute to the improvement of the human condition. Most were well-educated, and they subscribed to some beliefs and values that became the heart of occupational therapy philosophy and that continue to have meaning for occupational therapists today.

HOLISTIC VIEW OF HUMAN BEINGS

Early supporters of occupational therapy viewed the human as a total integrated being. They saw no separation between the mind and the body, believing that both functioned together to produce action. In working with disabled individuals, there was no effort to isolate treatment to a specific body part or a specific mental function. Rather, the person was viewed as a complete being, and his or her physical, psychological, and spiritual needs were considered in the therapeutic program.

VALUE OF OCCUPATION AS A HEALING FORCE

The occupational therapists of the early 20th century were convinced that occupation or activity could exert a positive influence on health and well-being. Sometimes the activity took the form of work, but it could also be recreation, education, or various forms of creative expression. George Barton, an early proponent of occupational therapy, said that the goal of his therapy was "the making of a person," that is, a productive individual. In his view, occupation promoted physical development, clarified and strengthened the mind, and could become the basis for a new life after recovery (3). Dr. William Rush Dunton, Jr., a psychiatrist who was a strong advocate of the value of occupation in the treatment of mental illness, classified occupational work into three types: invalid occupations (intended to divert the patient during the acute phase of an illness), occupational therapy (prescribed occupation designed to restore function), and vocational training (intended to help the patient regain productive employment). Dr. Dunton went on to write a creed for occupational therapists that expressed his views on the value of occupation:

> *That occupation is as necessary to life as food and drink. That every human being should have both physical and mental occupation. That all have occupations that they enjoy . . . . That sick minds, sick bodies, sick souls may be healed through occupation. . . . (4)*

Susan Tracy, a nurse, emphasized the value of occupation as a healing force for the sick and saw occupational treatment as a continuum that began at the bedside and continued into the workshop. She and Dr. Dunton both stressed that it was the effect of occupation on the patient that was important, not the product that resulted from the work. Herbert Hall, in his work with neurasthenic patients, called occupational therapy "the science of prescribed work" and envisioned a continuum of restorative occupations. Occupation, then, was believed to have a normalizing effect on individuals and to be capable of making a strong contribution toward their recovery (5).

VALUE OF GOAL-DIRECTED ACTIVITY

Many of the occupational therapy pioneers emphasized that occupation alone was not enough. It must have a therapeutic goal or purpose. A given activity must be selected for logical reasons and was chosen to match the patient's physical or emotional needs. George Barton believed that certain activities could be specifically prescribed to meet occupational needs just as certain medications could be prescribed to act on specific symptoms. Each occupation was intended to meet a therapeutic goal and the occupational therapist was charged with the responsibility of selecting appropriate activities to meet the identified goals.

ACTIVE INVOLVEMENT OF THE PATIENT

Early occupational therapy practitioners strongly believed that the patient must take an active part in his or her own recovery. They encouraged patients to choose occupations that interested them and that they were motivated to participate in. The occupation selected needed to be meaningful to the patient and to fit into the patient's life-style. From the earliest days of occupational therapy practice, this idea that the patient was active in the treatment process was an important one. The therapist was seen as an enabler—one who offered opportunities for the patient to improve his or her physical or mental health.

Eleanor Clarke Slagle saw the occupational worker as a change agent who encouraged patients to regain control of their lives (6). Writing during a later period, Devereaux pointed out that "occupational therapy does not do to or for the patient, but instead does with." Throughout the treatment process, she said, it is the role of the therapist to facilitate the patient's doing for himself or herself (7). West, writing in 1984, reaffirmed the belief in the patient's active role during treatment and emphasized that "doing" experiences have always been thought to promote competence and independence (8).

DEVELOPMENT OF COMPETENCE

Occupational therapists have long believed that through mastery of physical and social skills individuals develop a sense of their own capability and competence. Feelings of self-esteem develop in part from many small successes that individuals achieve in dealing with the physical and human environments. Occupations offer opportunities to develop the needed skills and allow people to practice and refine them until they become part of their behavioral repertoire. Feelings of competence and self-worth are important benefits of occupational therapy.

VALUE OF HUMAN RELATIONSHIPS

From their earliest history, occupational therapists have recognized that part of their work involved helping their patients to build satisfying relationships with others and to learn to interact with others in positive ways. Dunton emphasized that occupational work should be carried out in groups whenever possible to offer opportunities for social interaction (6). Slagle felt that the relationship established between therapist and client was the single most crucial element in a successful outcome (6). During later periods, occupational therapists began to talk about "the use of self" as a therapeutic tool—using the personality and sensitivity of the therapist in guiding the patient into more constructive relationships. This idea of therapist-client interaction lies at the heart of most occupational therapy interventions and should be given equal weight with the more visible occupational therapy methods.

TOOLS OF OCCUPATIONAL THERAPY

In the eyes of its early practitioners, the proper tools of occupational therapy practice consisted of all forms of creative and manual skills as well as skills to be found in education, recreation, self-care, and work. Susan Johnson, a former teacher and an early occupational therapist, saw the re-educational function of occupation as an important element and stressed that occupational therapy was part medical and part educational in nature (6). In the early 1900s, industrialization was proceeding rapidly in the United States. The dollar, rather than pride in one's craft, was becoming the measure of success. The arts and crafts movement that developed in the United States around the turn of the century was an attempt to recapture the traditional values inherent in hand-crafted products made of natural materials. The use of crafts as treatment modalities in occupational therapy came largely from this influence, and many of the early therapists were classified as arts and crafts teachers (9).

The use of play activities was particularly important when working with children since play was their natural form of expression and led to the mastery of developmental skills. Educational activities formed an important part of the occupational therapy media when working with conditions that required long-term care: tuberculosis, medical and surgical conditions, chronic illnesses. Activities of self-expression (music, dance, art) were believed to be particularly beneficial when working with the mentally ill, as they offered opportunities for the free expression of emotions and were a form of nonverbal communication. Self-care activities were often the primary focus of attention when working with the physically disabled. Prevocational evaluation and work training were major areas of emphasis for the early occupational therapists, but these functions later became the domain of vocational evaluators. During the 1980s there was a resurgence of interest in work-related occupations, and occupational therapists again resumed their involvement in work preparation activities. It can be said, then, that in the early years of occupational therapy a wide range of media was used, and therapists needed an extensive knowledge of many forms of therapeutic occupation (8).

HEALTHY BALANCE OF OCCUPATIONS

Dr. Adolph Meyer, a psychiatrist and an early supporter of occupational therapy, proposed the idea that there was a rhythm of human life that helped to organize behavior and maintain health. He identified the elements of this rhythm as work, play, rest, and sleep and suggested that individuals required a balance of these elements in order to maintain health. He believed that part of the value of occupation lay in its ability to organize time so that the individual could create a satisfactory personal rhythm that suited his or her interests and needs. Dr. Meyer felt that the role of the occupational therapist was to provide opportunities for work, recreation, creative activity, and learning to use materials. "Man learns to use time," he said, "and he does it in terms of doing things. . . . We call it work and occupation. . . ." (10). Occupation, Meyer believed, had value as an organizing and regulating factor in human life.

CHANGING CONDITIONS AND CHANGING PHILOSOPHY

These early beliefs about the value of occupation as a therapeutic tool continued to be held throughout the 1920s and 1930s. With the impact of World War II on American society, priorities shifted sharply. The patient population that occupational therapists worked with was changing. The increasing number of returning veterans that were severely disabled led to an increasing emphasis on physical rehabilitation in occupational therapy. Occupational therapy remained closely allied to medicine; this had both advantages and disadvantages. One advantage was that occupational therapy gained new prestige as part of the rehabilitation movement. New services and treatment facilities were required to meet the needs of disabled veterans, and rehabilitation became a branch of organized medicine. Physicians who specialized in this new treatment area were called physiatrists, and in the period following the war a small group of them attempted to gain control of occupational therapy education and the registration process of occupational therapists, feeling that these should be directly supervised by physicians. Occupational therapy educators and clinicians successfully resisted this attempt to take over their profession and were able to retain their professional independence. They were determined to maintain the diversity of practice in the field and continued to educate students for mental health practice as well as for work with physical disabilities (11).

The media used by occupational therapists was also undergoing rapid change. The widespread use of handicrafts, games, recreation, and work activities had given way to more specialized, technical methods. Training patients in self-care procedures was being emphasized as well as work simplification techniques. New types of adaptive equipment were being developed, and complex prosthetic and orthotic devices had been invented.

The biomedical model of practice tended to dominate occupational therapy practice with adults while a developmental model was commonly used by those who treated children. Medicine had given up its holistic approach to patient care and had adopted a scientific, reductionistic model in its place. Occupational therapists were being urged to adopt a more scientific model of practice as well and gradually did so. This led to a de-emphasis on the holistic view of humanity in occupational therapy as therapists turned their focus to ever-smaller elements of function. Some saw this as a betrayal of occupational therapy's long-held belief in working with the whole person and feared that fragmentation of the profession would result.

During the 1950s and 1960s, sensorimotor treatment methods that had originally been used by physical therapists gained widespread acceptance by occupational therapists. Occupational therapy practice was changing rapidly, and there was considerable conflict between traditional values and the need to adapt to changing social conditions and a changing health care environment. One way to study the changing philosophy of occupational therapy during this and later eras is to review statements made by acknowledged leaders in the field. Beginning in 1954, the American Occupational Therapy Association had established the Eleanor Clarke Slagle Lectureship to be awarded annually to an outstanding member of the profession who had actively contributed to the body of knowledge of the field. Slagle lecturers delivered their addresses to their colleagues at the annual meeting of the association, and some of these lectures provide us with a view of the changing concepts and philosophies from 1955 onward.

PHILOSOPHY OF THE 1960s AND 1970s

Although occupational therapy was becoming more technical and complex, some of its leaders were eloquent defenders of the holistic point of view of its founders. In a much-quoted 1961 Slagle lecture entitled "Occupational Therapy Can Be One of the Great Ideas of Twentieth Century Medicine," Mary Reilly said:

> *The logic of occupational therapy rests upon the principle that man has a need to master his environment, to alter and improve it. When this need is blocked by disease or injury, severe dysfunction and unhappiness results. Man must develop and exercise the powers of his central nervous system through open encounter with life around him. Failure to spend and use what he has in the performance of tasks that belong to his role in life makes him less human than he could be.*

Reilly ended her lecture with the ringing assertion that "man, through the use of his hands, as they are energized by mind and will, can influence the state of his own health" (12). This restatement of traditional occupational therapy values was a strong reminder that those values had not been forgotten.

During the 1960s and 1970s, occupational therapists were questioning some of the basic premises of their profession. Occupational therapy media were beginning to include exercise, biofeedback, massage, joint manipulation, and other physical agents. Therapists were working more frequently with patients who were in the acute phase of their illness or disability, and changes in health care and its reimbursement system were strongly influencing what occupational therapists did and how they did it. New opportunities were being explored in the areas of prevention and health maintenance. There was increasing pressure for research into occupational therapy methods and their effectiveness. Therapists were expressing increasing dissatisfaction with the medical model, and new practice models were being explored.

Lorna Jean King in her 1978 Slagle lecture proposed that a science of occupation be constructed. She noted that the profession badly needed a unifying concept that would clearly distinguish occupational therapy theory and techniques from those of other professions and that would organize the profession's beliefs into propositions that could be scientifically tested and validated. King proposed that adaptation be considered the central core of occupational therapy. Adaptation, she held, demands positive action on the part of the individual and is the result of environmental demands. It is an integrated, total-body response that is often organized at the cortical level. It is self-reinforcing. It is goal-directed and results in purposeful behavior. The main goal of occupational therapy, King believed, was to develop the adaptive responses that would enable an individual to develop the necessary skills to meet his or her life goals. She challenged her fellow occupational therapists to develop a science of adaptive responses as a model for their professional practice (13, 14).

In 1979 the American Occupational Therapy Association had formulated a statement on the philosophical base of occupational therapy. It said:

> *Man is an active being whose development is influenced by the use of purposeful activity. Using their capacity for intrinsic motivation, human beings are able to influence their physical and mental health and their social and physical environment through purposeful activity. Human life includes a process of continuous adaptation. Adaptation is a change in function that promotes survival and self-actualization. Biological, psychological, and environmental factors may interrupt the adaptation process at any time throughout the life cycle. Dysfunction may occur when adaptation is impaired. Purposeful activity facilitates the adaptive process.*
>
> *Occupational therapy is based on the belief that purposeful activity (occupation), including its interpersonal and environmental components, may be used to prevent and mediate dysfunction and to elicit maximum adaptation. Activity as used by the Occupational Therapist includes both an intrinsic and a therapeutic purpose. (15)*

With this statement, the AOTA reaffirmed its belief in purposeful activity as an influence on health and identified adaptation as the process by which positive change takes place.

During the 1960s and 1970s, other theoretical models had been proposed. In 1979 Clark had reviewed some of the current models of occupational therapy practice. Fidler and Mosey had suggested an adaptive performance model that was based on the psychodynamic concepts then current in mental health practice. A biodevelopmental approach was advocated by Reilly, and many of the practice models then in use seemed to fit well into this philosophy. Llorens had proposed a growth and development model in which the therapist's role was that of a change agent, facilitating the growth and development of the client. Reilly had in 1966 proposed a return to the philosophy of Dr. Adolph Meyer who had divided human occupation into the elements of work, play, rest, and sleep and had suggested that an optimum balance between these elements led to health and well-being. Later some of Reilly's students carried this idea further and proposed a model of occupational behavior based on the acquisition and performance of "human activities that occupy time, energy, interest, and attention." In this model, clients were encouraged to explore their competence in relation to their occupational role requirements (16).

Clark went on to further delineate this conceptual model, now called the model of human development through occupation. Its proponents viewed humans as able to influence their own world of self, culture, and environment. Humans, they said, spend their time occupied by purposeful activities including self-maintenance, play, and work. They maintain health through a flexible balance of these activities, and the balance varies during different developmental periods. Role performance is influenced by a person's basic biological endowment, maturation of skills, the cultural, spatial, and temporal requirements of the environment, and the individual's personal requirements. In this model, occupational therapy was viewed as a health profession that was concerned with the quality and satisfaction of daily life for an individual from birth to death. The therapist's role was thought to be that of assisting with the adaptation processes necessary for the client to build a productive and satisfying life-style. Figure 2.1 presents a graphic representation of this model (17).

The model of human development through occupation captured the imagination of many occupational therapists since it was sufficiently broad to include the whole spectrum of occupational therapy practice and appeared to reinforce traditional beliefs about occupation as the core of the profession.

OCCUPATIONAL THERAPY PHILOSOPHY: 1970s and 1980s

In 1985 Kielhofner and his associates expanded upon the model in a publication entitled *A Model of Human Occupation: Theory and Application* (18). They described the human being as an open system, influenced by many biological determinants but able to override them when necessary. Three subsystems were hypothesized to underlie occupational behavior. A volitional system was thought to regulate overall operations and to select and initiate occupational behavior; a habitual system was believed to organize behavior into patterns or routines; a performance system then produced the complete occupational behavior. Each person was seen as having occupational goals and personal standards that determined how occupational performance would be carried out. The occupational roles that each individual was expected to fulfill based on personal and social expectations were given major importance in the model, and an appropriate balance of roles was believed to result in comfort and satisfaction. Occupation was thought to require constant interaction with the environment. When dysfunctions in occupational behavior occurred, it was the job of the occupational therapist to intervene and provide opportunities for the individual to change and improve his or her occupational performance. The occupational therapist might do this either by changing the entire cycle of occupational behavior or by reorganizing components of the system. This theoretical model took a holistic view and offered a new way of thinking about human occupation and performance. It was less concerned with diagnostic categories than with overall occupational performance and could be applied to many different client groups. The model of human occupation attracted a wide following among occupational therapists, and it continues to exert a strong influence on practitioners today (18).

During the 1980s occupational therapists began to voice a need to return to the humanistic values of the founders of the profession. Gilfoyle, in a 1980 address to members of the American Occupational Therapy Association, noted that research was beginning to lead toward a science of occupational therapy but urged that the art of therapy not be neglected. She stressed that caring had always been a basic concept in occupational therapy practice and that the caring attitude was then needed more than ever (19). Devereaux, writing in 1984, agreed and pointed out that the caring relationship between therapist and patient reinforces the holistic approach of occupational therapy. She stated that caring was "a counterbalance to the high-tech world . . . and the depersonalization of the individual" (7).

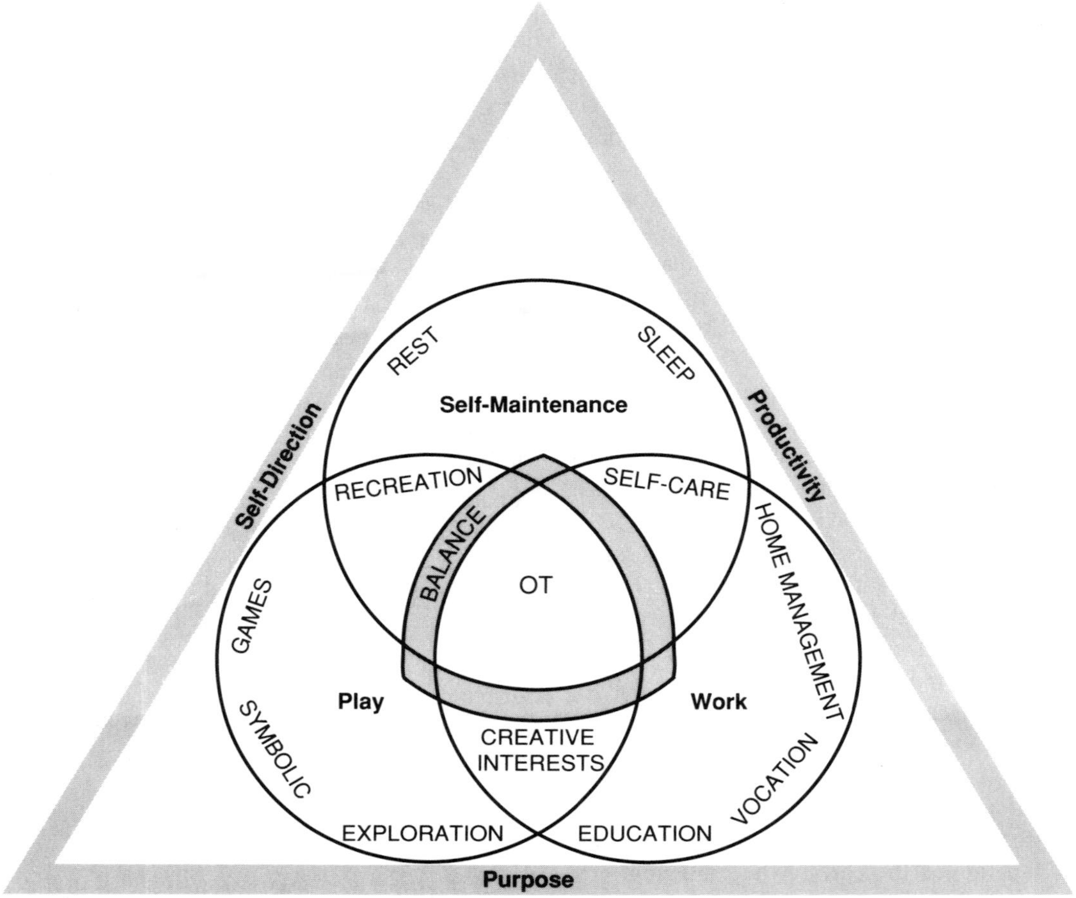

Figure 2.1. Model of human development.

Johnson, in a 1981 paper, reviewed traditional occupational therapy values and beliefs and examined them in the light of current practice. She saw the profession as being in a period of transition and urged her colleagues to recognize the conflict between traditional values and the values of science and research. She suggested that a new sense of direction was needed for the profession. Occupational therapists should acknowledge the validity of their traditional beliefs, Johnson said, and should not discard them to meet short-term needs (20).

In 1983 the American Occupational Therapy Association, needing to redefine purposeful activity, issued a position paper regarding the use of purposeful activity (21). Rogers, in a 1984 paper, pointed out that, although functional independence was the chief goal of occupational therapy, this concept rested upon some basic assumptions about human beings. Occupational therapists tended to view individuals as being competent and autonomous. Rogers wondered whether a skills approach or a subskills approach was more effective in developing functional independence and suggested that occupational therapy required a philosophy that had room for both approaches. Both the physical and the psychosocial elements of occupation needed to be considered in any comprehensive theory, Rogers believed (22).

Robert Bing, when he assumed the presidency of the American Occupational Therapy Association in 1983, stated that "the grand tasks of occupational therapy are to attend to the multiple, complex, interrelated, and critical human activities of not just living but living well." He proposed that occupational therapists help their clients to regain the functions that ensure survival, those characteristics that promote balanced growth and development, and to attain a purposeful, fulfilled life (23).

West, in a 1984 paper, looked at the conflicts between traditional occupational therapy beliefs and current practice realities and suggested that changing social conditions and the high-tech world of the future would require a broader approach to practice. She urged that occupational therapists agree that their mission was to serve a person's occupational needs. Performance dysfunction rather than specific diagnostic groups should be the focus of treatment, West said. The mind-body unity stressed by early practitioners of occupational therapy should again be emphasized (8).

Elnora Gilfoyle, in her Slagle lecture of 1984, described occupational therapy in the 1980s as being "in a period of transformation: a shift in thinking about old concepts." She identified three major factors that were influencing this change:

A shift in professional values, dimensions of practice, and educational focus,
Declining allegiance to the medical model, and
Decline of patriarchy in society.

Gilfoyle discussed the emerging science of occupation and noted that, although occupational therapy had not abandoned its past, it had not fully accepted the future. In the mid-1980s the profession was at a turning point. Although new theoretical models had been proposed, Gilfoyle noted that "in the science of occupation no concept or belief can be considered final" (24).

Throughout the 1980s the debate about a theoretical base for occupational therapy continued. Anne Mosey gave the Slagle lecture in 1985 and noted that the theories thus far proposed had represented a monistic approach. Monism is the belief that one basic principle can be used to explain reality. Each of the theories thus far proposed had focussed on a single element within occupational therapy, Mosey claimed. She suggested that no single theory could be comprehensive enough to include the great variety within the field and proposed instead that a pluralistic approach be considered. In this way, a number of theories could be accepted and organized loosely into a taxonomy. A variety of theories could be explored, tested, and analyzed. This approach would have the advantage of flexibility and would allow the profession to continue to add new theories as the field progressed and evolved (25).

In the 1988 Slagle lecture, Anne Henderson identified three kinds of knowledge that were specific to occupational therapy: professional philosophy, scientific knowledge, and technology. She stressed that all three kinds of knowledge were important as a basis for practice but warned that occupational therapists might be emphasizing philosophy and scientific knowledge at the expense of technology. Technology, she noted, is the knowledge that tells occupational therapists how to use purposeful activity with their clients. It includes the products and methods of practice. This is a valid kind of knowledge, Henderson said, and should not be disparaged. Philosophical beliefs and values are enduring, she stated, but scientific knowledge and technology are ever-changing. Henderson suggested that both the research-first and the theory-first model-building approaches were needed in occupational therapy and both should be given equal emphasis (26).

Grossman, writing in 1991, asserted that occupational therapy lacked a theoretical model for prevention services in its practice. She believed that adherence to the medical model restricted occupational therapists' ability to engage in prevention programs and suggested that the holistic and occupational performance models seemed to offer the best options. Role theory, she noted, is important to occupational therapy practice and lends itself to a preventive approach. An occupational therapy theoretical model should focus on health and wellness rather than on disability and illness, Grossman believed. She urged occupational therapists to begin to build and test prevention models for their client populations (27).

In another 1991 article, Vogel identified three major problems that were of concern to occupational therapists:

Continuing debate over occupation as the profession's philosophical base,
Fragmentation of the profession into loosely related technical specialties because of a lack of agreement on a generic basis of knowledge and practice, and
Differences between groups of therapists in their perceptions of the status of the profession and little agreement on how it can be reached.

Vogel conducted a survey to determine respondents' degree of agreement or disagreement with a series of statements about occupational therapy and practitioners' roles. She found little disagreement among groups of educators, students, and clinicians on most items but did find that students and educators tended to favor traditional occupational therapy media, whereas practitioners appeared to be more open minded about nontraditional methods (28).

In 1991 occupational therapists were beginning to read and hear about a new academic discipline called occupational science. Clark and her colleagues from the University of Southern California wrote a comprehensive description and defined occupational science as a new scientific discipline that was engaged in the systematic study of the human as an occupational being. Clark and her colleagues said, "We have come to call the ordinary and familiar things that people do every day 'occupations' and we believe that humans are most true to their humanity when they are engaged in occupations" (29). They urged occupational therapists to begin the construction of theories about why people select one activity over another and to identify the factors that influence how people decide to live their lives.

The model of occupational science takes into account the subsystems of the physical body, its biological substrates, the information processing systems, the sociocultural environment, the symbolic systems of language and communication, and the transcendental system that is concerned with the meaning of experiences to the individual. Because of this broad area of focus, occupational science is believed to be interdisciplinary in nature. These authors suggest that social science research methods may offer the most promise for scientifically testing the concepts of human occupation. Clark and her colleagues stress that the main focus of occupational science is not immediate application to the practice of occupational therapy but rather identification of the basic principles and concepts of occupation. They believe that occupational science will benefit occupational therapy in three ways:

By preparing doctoral scholars in their own discipline rather than in a related field,
By the proliferation of basic science research in the field, and
By providing sound justifications and enhancements to occupational therapy practice.

Occupational science attempts to address the entire range of behavior and phenomena around human occupation and looks at the ways that people adapt over the life span through the use of occupations. The establishment of a formal discipline of occupational science may lay the foundation for a new respect and recognition of the basic concepts that underlie occupational therapy and may allow it to develop into a true social science (29).

As occupational therapists seek to build a science of human occupation in the 1990s, some practitioners continue to remind their colleagues not to neglect the art of occupational therapy. Peloquin eloquently made the case for retaining the art of practice, which throughout the history of the field has provided so much of the foundation for intervention. The art of practice is concerned with human values rather than with treatment procedures. The therapist-client relationship is a key element in the art of practice and the ability of the therapist to establish rapport, to empathize, and to accept the feelings of the client is as important as the application of physical procedures. As new theoretical models are developed, occupational therapists will need to utilize both the art and the science of their profession in their daily client interactions (30).

SUMMARY

We have reviewed some of the traditional beliefs of occupational therapy that were stated during its early years and have seen how these beliefs were questioned and altered along with changing social conditions and a changing practice environment. Traditional values continue to form an important part of occupational therapy philosophy and were revived and re-examined during the 1980s and 1990s. Occupational therapists will continue to seek theoretical models that can explain and clarify the value of occupation to the healthy individual and to the person with functional limitations. Some models may be discarded if they fail to meet the test of scientific inquiry, but others will endure. It remains to be seen whether a single theoretical model can be accepted by all occupational therapists; however, the process of study and investigation will continue as practitioners search for the answers to many questions about occupation and the role it plays in our daily lives.

Discussion Questions

1. Does modern medical practice encourage a holistic view of human beings? Why do you think that it does or does not?
2. Compare occupational therapy's view of the patient's role in the treatment process with that of the medical profession's view. Are they different? How?
3. Do you think that a single theory can be broad enough to explain the whole range of occupational therapy practice? Why or why not?
4. Should occupational therapy retain its close ties with medicine or broaden its professional base? Why?
5. Are the traditional beliefs of occupational therapy a help or a hindrance as the profession moves forward into the 21st century?
6. Is health care an art or a science? Why do you think so?

References

1. Morris W (ed): *American Heritage Dictionary of the English Language*, New College Edition. Boston, Houghton Mifflin, 1981.
2. Peloquin SM: Moral treatment, contexts considered. *AJOT* 43(8):537–544, 1989.
3. Peloquin SM: Occupational therapy service: individual and collective understandings of the founders, part 1. *AJOT* 45(4):352–360, 1991.
4. Dunton WR: *Reconstruction Therapy*. Philadelphia, WB Saunders, 1919.
5. Hall HJ: Forward steps in occupational therapy during 1920. *Modern Hospital* 16:245–247, 1921.
6. Peloquin SM: Occupational therapy service: individual and collective understanding of the founders, part 2. *AJOT* 45(8):733–744, 1991.
7. Devereaux EB: Occupational therapy's challenge: the caring relationship. *AJOT* 38(12):791–798, 1984.
8. West W: A reaffirmed philosophy and practice of occupational therapy for the 1980s. *AJOT* 38(1):15–23, 1984.
9. Levine RE: The influence of the arts and crafts movement on the professional status of occupational therapy. *AJOT* 41(4):248–254, 1987.
10. Meyer A: The philosophy of occupation therapy. *Arch Occup Ther* I:1–10, 1922.
11. Colman W: Maintaining autonomy: the struggle between occupational therapy and physical medicine. *AJOT* 46(1):63–71, 1992.
12. Reilly M: Occupational therapy can be one of the great ideas of twentieth century medicine. *AJOT* 26:1, 1962.
13. King L: Toward a science of adaptive responses. *AJOT* 32(7):429–437, 1978.
14. Klienman BL, Bulkley, BL: Some implications of a science of adaptive responses. *AJOT* 36(1):15–19, 1982.

15. The philosophical base of occupational therapy. Minutes of the 1979 AOTA Representative Assembly. *AJOT* 33:785, 1979.
16. Clark PN: Human development through occupation: theoretical frameworks in contemporary occupational therapy practice, part 1. *AJOT* 33(8):505–514, 1979.
17. Clark PN: Human development through occupation: a philosophy and conceptual model for practice, part 2. *AJOT* 33(9):577–585, 1979.
18. Kielhofner G: *A Model of Human Occupation: Theory and Application*. Baltimore, Williams & Wilkins, 1985.
19. Gilfoyle EM: Caring: a philosophy for practice. *AJOT* 34(8):517–521, 1980.
20. Johnson J: Old values–new directions: competence, adaptation, integration. *AJOT* 35(9):589–598, 1981.
21. AOTA: Purposeful activities. *AJOT* 37(12):805–806, 1983.
22. Rogers JC: Spirit of independence: the evolution of a philosophy. *AJOT* 36(11):709–715, 1982.
23. Bing R: Nationally speaking: beliefs at a new beginning. *AJOT* 37(6):375–379, 1983.
24. Gilfoyle EM: 1984: the transformation of a profession. *AJOT* 38(9):575–584, 1984.
25. Mosey A: A monistic or a pluralistic approach to professional identity? *AJOT* 39(8):504–509, 1985.
26. Henderson A: Occupational therapy knowledge: from practice to theory. *AJOT* 42(9):567–576, 1988.
27. Grossman J: A prevention model for occupational therapy. *AJOT* 45(1):33–39, 1991.
28. Vogel KA: Perceptions of practitioners, educators, and students concerning the role of the occupational therapy practitioner. *AJOT* 45(2):130–136, 1991.
29. Clark F, Parham D, Carlson M, Frank G, Jackson J, Pierce D, Wolfe R, Zemke R: Occupational science: academic innovation in the service of occupational therapy's future. *AJOT* 43(4):300–310, 1991.
30. Peloquin SM: Sustaining the art of practice in occupational therapy. *AJOT* 43(4):219–226, 1989.

Suggested Readings

Bing RK: To survive, to become: our way of life. *AJOT* 38(12)785–790, 1984.

Breines E: Pragmatism as a foundation for occupational therapy curricula. *AJOT* 41(8):522–525, 1987.

Fidler GS: From crafts to competence. *AJOT* 35(9):567–573, 1981.

Katz N: Occupational therapy's domain of concern: reconsidered. *AJOT* 39(8):518–524, 1985.

Kielhofner G: *Conceptual Foundations of Occupational Therapy*. Philadelphia, FA Davis, 1992.

Reed KL: Tools of practice: heritage or baggage? *AJOT* 40(9):597–605, 1986.

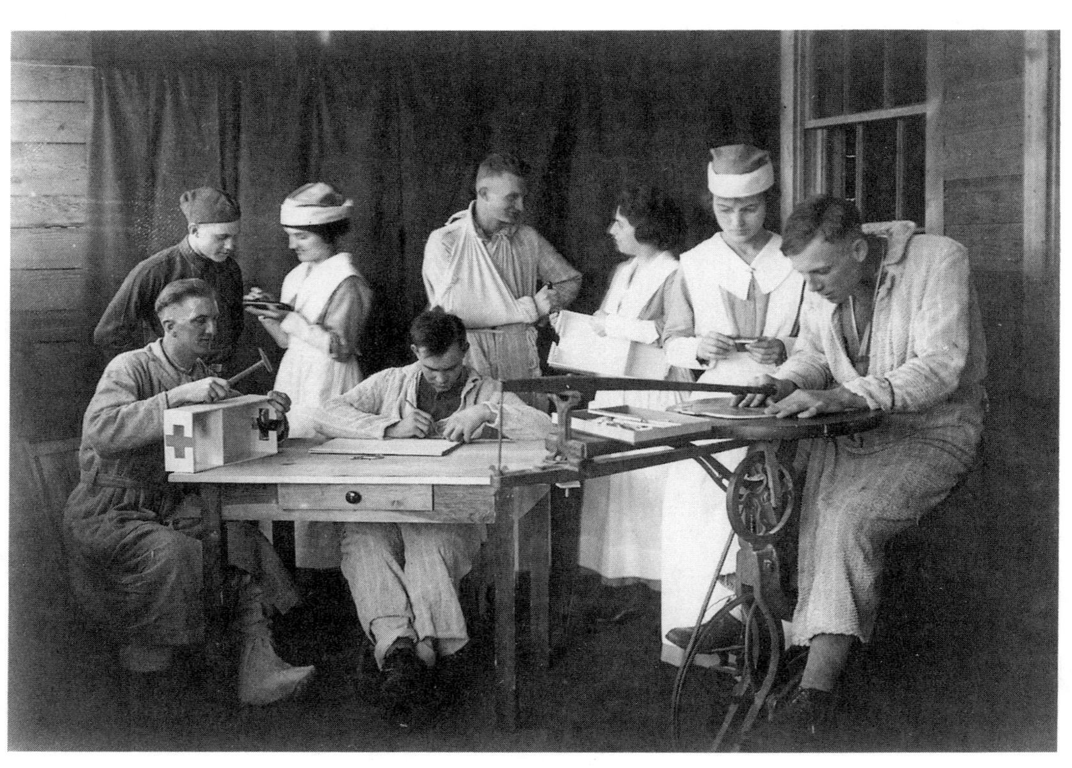

3 Historical Development of the Field

EARLY FORERUNNERS OF OCCUPATIONAL THERAPY

Although occupational therapy is a relatively new field, beliefs concerning the curative value of occupation are found in the records of many civilizations. Dr. Sidney Licht, in his *Occupational Therapy Source Book*, quotes from the writings of Asclepiades, the early Greek physician who advocated the use of music, exercise, and occupation for the treatment of mental illness (1). There are references in Egyptian records from 200 BC describing large temples dedicated to Saturn to which people afflicted with melancholia were brought in search of a cure. Groves and gardens were cultivated in which they could exercise, and boating excursions on the Nile and other pleasurable activities were arranged to distract individuals from their troubles and offer them alternative occupations (2).

It is generally agreed that the progressive ideas of Dr. Philippe Pinel, who was medical director of the Bicêtre Hospital in Paris in the late 18th century, provided inspiration for the use of organized programs of activity and occupation in institutions for the mentally ill in Europe and in America. Pinel could not accept the neglect and cruelty commonly found in asylums for the insane at that time and shocked many of his contemporaries by releasing 50 "maniacs" from their chains at his institution in 1792. He experimented by replacing physical restraint with physical exercise and manual occupations with these inmates, and in 1801 he described his results in a book. Pinel recommended the use of such activities in all mental hospitals "as a means of securing good morale and discipline" (1). Johann Reil in Germany agreed and in a paper published in 1803 added his own verification of the effectiveness of such methods (1). Other enlightened thinkers in Europe had begun to make similar efforts.

In England, William Tuke, an English Quaker, established an asylum for the insane at York and began to implement a new philosophical approach to the problems of mental illness. Tuke described his approach as "moral treatment" and reasoned that natural methods should be used to remedy diseases of the mind. At the York Retreat, inmates were encouraged to participate in the ordinary activities of daily life. Such activities as gardening, sewing, knitting, and helping with the work of the institutional farm were actively encouraged. Tuke believed that occupation for the mentally disturbed helped the individual achieve better self-control and provided habit training, which had a normalizing effect. No physical restraint or coercion was used, although quiet seclusion of manic patients was sometimes employed. Special events and entertainments, at which normal behavior was expected, were organized for the patients. Patients, staff, and visitors mingled at teas, church services, and outings. Every kind of "rational and innocent employment" was encouraged, and visitors were impressed to see the effectiveness of this program in action. Tuke's work was much admired by several American visitors who came to observe the new methods.

OCCUPATION THERAPY IN THE UNITED STATES

Thomas Scattergood, a Quaker minister, became convinced of the value of Tuke's approach after a visit to the York Retreat, and on his return to Philadelphia in 1800 he actively worked to establish a similar institution there. Thomas Eddy, another Quaker, pressed for the introduction of moral treatment methods in the Lunatic Asylum of New York Hospital in 1815. The first American physician to endorse and supervise a program of planned occupation for mental patients was probably Dr. Rufus Wymann, who in 1818 opened the McLean Asylum near Boston. Wymann wrote:

> *The treatment of insanity chiefly depends upon the connection between the mind and the body. If there be inflammation of the brain or its membranes, it is to be treated as an inflammation of those parts. But in mental disorders without symptoms of organic disease, a judicious moral management is more successful. It should afford agreeable occupation . . . engaging the mind and exercising the body. (1)*

During the second quarter of the 19th century, in Europe there was growing acceptance of the use of occupation as a treatment method for the mentally ill, but there was much less interest in the United States. Some American physicians claimed that American citizens equated "occupation" with paid employment and that American patients would refuse to participate in "work therapy" programs unless they were paid. Whether this was the real reason or not, American physicians did not press for large-scale occupation programs in their mental hospitals. One notable exception was the Asylum at Utica, New York, at which full-time instructors were hired to teach the patients academic subjects and to organize a wide variety of recreational and work activities for them. A hospital newspaper was published, and "occupation therapy" flourished under the direction of Dr. Aramiah Brigham.

Another early supporter of occupational therapy was Dr. Thomas Kirkbride, superintendent of the Pennsylvania Hospital for the Insane during the 1840s. Kirkbride had visited asylums in England and the United States to acquaint himself with the methods currently in use and became a strong advocate of "activity treatment." He introduced a planned program of patient occupations at the Pennsylvania institution between 1840 and 1842 and wrote:

> *The value of employment in the treatment of insanity is now so universally conceded that no arguments are required in its favor. Its value cannot be reckoned in dollars and cents. The object is to restore mental health and tranquilize the restlessness and mitigate the sorrows of disease. (1)*

Kirkbride later helped to form an association of asylum medical superintendents that eventually became the American Psychiatric Association. For the rest of his life, Kirkbride actively supported the concepts of patient occupation in the treatment of mental disease.

The final quarter of the 19th century was not an auspicious period for occupational therapy. Successive waves of immigrants from Europe had swelled the population in mental hospitals with people who spoke little or no English and whose values and customs seemed strange and different from those of the native-born population. As hospitals became larger and more crowded, programs of therapeutic occupation grew less practical to organize and run. Widespread prejudice against the newly arrived immigrants provided additional rationalizations for neglect of such persons who became mentally disturbed. A more important factor that influenced change in the treatment of mental illness, however, was that medical concepts about the causes of mental illness were changing. Medicine had embraced the scientific method employed by the physical sciences and had applied it to the study of disease. This method tended to reduce everything to its lowest common denominator for purposes of study. Thus the brain was viewed in terms of cellular structure and pathology. Physical pathology of the brain was believed to be the basis for mental illness, and since there was no known cure or remedy for brain pathology, the mentally ill were considered hopelessly incurable and any form of treatment to be useless. A period of pessimism and neglect set in, and mental institutions reverted to their former status of custodial facilities. The activity programs so enthusiastically begun were largely abandoned during this era (4).

Early in the 20th century, however, reformers began to agitate for improvements in conditions in mental hospitals and for active treatment of mental disorders. Dorothea Dix and Clifford Beers publicized the poor conditions that prevailed in many asylums and documented the mistreatment of patients confined to them. Public sentiment for improvements was aroused and some institutions began to make changes.

OCCUPATIONAL THERAPY PIONEERS

In 1906 a progressive physician, Dr. Herbert Hall, was awarded a grant by Harvard University to study "the treatment of neurasthenia through progressive and graded manual occupation" (1). Hall patterned his experimental program after one he had observed in Switzerland and set up a workshop for industrial therapeutics. Craftspeople were hired to work side by side with neurotic patients to improve their adjustment and ability to function in daily life. After four years of operation, Hall reported that the manual and intellectual work his patients had participated in had indeed had a normalizing effect on their behavior (1).

At about the same time, Susan Tracy, a nurse who taught nursing students at the Adams Nervine Hospital in Boston, began teaching a course in "invalid occupations" to her students. Tracy is often considered the first "occupational therapist," since she had observed as a nurse the positive effects that occupation could have on bedridden hospitalized patients. She emphasized to her students that the goal of patient occupation was to improve the patient's condition, not to produce beautiful handiwork. In 1910 her lectures were published in book form and were available to hospital nurses as a guide to patient activities (1).

In the spring of 1911, a course in occupation treatment was offered for nurses at the Massachusetts General Hospital. At about the same time, Dr. William Rush Dunton, Jr., was teaching a course in patient occupation for nurses at the Sheppard and Enoch Pratt Hospital in Towson, Maryland. Dunton's lectures were also published in book form and included guidelines on how occupational therapy should be prescribed and utilized. Dunton believed that nurses were the best qualified to carry out occupational work with patients. He strongly supported the employment of occupational workers in army field hospitals in 1918 and articulated many of the early concepts of occupational therapy (5).

Dr. Adolph Meyer, a Professor of Psychiatry at Johns Hopkins University in Baltimore, was another early promoter of the use of occupation for the mentally ill. Meyer viewed mental illness as a manifestation of problems in living and believed that "systematic engagement of interest and concern about the use of time and work was an obligation and a necessity" in the treatment of mental disorders (6). He pointed out that human beings operate on the basis of rhythmic cycles of work, play, rest, and sleep. For the individual to function well, Meyer suggested that a balance was required between these different activity states. He proposed organizing patients' activities in a balanced daily schedule of work, play, and rest. Meyer stressed that opportunities must be created for mentally ill persons to engage in learning activities, manual occupations, and creative pastimes to regain their ability to function as integrated individuals in their environment (6).

Another person much interested in the therapeutic uses of occupation was George Barton. Barton was an architect who developed tuberculosis and underwent several hospitalizations for this disease. He later had a gangrenous foot amputated and developed a left hemiplegia. During his long convalescence, he discovered the value of activity in helping him to overcome his feelings of depression and taught himself to garden and do structural work within his physical limitations. He became a keen advocate of "occupation therapy." In 1914 Barton organized Consolation House, a school and workshop for convalescents in Clifton Springs, New York. Its program emphasized adjustment to disability and the use of occupations to train the disabled for a productive life.

To develop his program, Barton initiated a correspondence with other people who were also using occupation as a form of treatment. He contacted Dunton and Tracy, whose work we have already described. Another contact was with Eleanor Clarke Slagle. Slagle had completed one of the early courses in curative occupations at the Chicago School of Civics and Philanthropy. She then worked in the field of psychiatry and in 1913 became Director of Occupational Therapy in the Henry Phipps Psychiatric Clinic in Baltimore under the supervision of Dr. Adolph Meyer. Later she served as director of the Chicago school (now called the Henry Favill School of Occupations) from 1918 to 1922. Barton also corresponded with Susan Johnson, an arts and crafts teacher who was one of the early educators and practitioners of occupational therapy. Thomas Kidner was another person whom Barton got in touch with to discuss occupation therapy. Kidner was an English architect who had organized a system of vocational rehabilitation for the disabled veterans of Canada during World War I and later served as a consultant to the United States government when the United States wished to establish reconstructive services for their own veterans of the war (5, 7).

In 1917 Barton invited these six persons to meet with him in Clifton Springs to discuss forming an organization to promote and publicize this new field of occupation therapy. Slagle, Johnson, Kidner, Dunton, Barton, and his secretary, Isabel Newton, met and agreed to develop such an organization. The fledgling group was called the National Society for the Promotion of Occupational Therapy, and Barton agreed to serve as its first president. In 1921 the group changed its name to the American Occupational Therapy Association and continues to function under that title today (1, 7).

During the early periods of development of occupational therapy, this new form of treatment was called by many different names. *Activity therapy, moral treatment, the work cure*, and *ergotherapy* were all terms used to identify the new approach. Dunton is credited with originating the term *occupation therapy*, which was later modified by Barton to *occupational therapy*. This became the generally accepted term, although there have been periodic movements to change the name of the field to something more readily recognizable.

IMPACT OF WORLD WAR I

World War I provided a major impetus to the development of the young field. As the United States mobilized for war, the military organized field hospitals near the battle lines for the treatment of casualties. Dr. Frankwood Williams was an army psychiatrist who was responsible for organizing Base Hospital 117. He was familiar with the use of occupation with mentally disturbed patients and asked his superiors for occupational workers to accompany his hospital unit to France. His pleas fell on deaf ears, since his request was interpreted as a request for workers to provide vocational training and this was believed inappropriate. Williams was undeterred, however, and convinced a small group of women who had some training in crafts to join the hospital unit under the unglamorous job title of "scrubwomen," as there was no suitable army classification for their service.

The women were classified as civilian aides, with no military rank or uniform and very minimal pay. Their training consisted of three lectures in neuropsychiatry. These intrepid women sailed on a troopship for France, bringing their own tools and such minimal supplies as they could collect on short notice to outfit their workshops. Upon landing in Le Havre, they traveled by train to the location of Base Hospital 117 at LaFauche, France, near the front lines.

They were assigned to a drafty, unused barracks in which the hospital barber, the carpenter, and a gardener were already installed. The women rolled up their sleeves and went to work, cleaning up the area as well as they could and wangling usable items of furniture from sympathetic officers. Makeshift workbenches were constructed from old hospital beds, and large tin cans from the kitchen were transformed into charcoal furnaces for the heating of soldering irons. The kitchen dump proved to be a treasure trove of discarded tin cans that, when cleaned, became the raw material for many craft projects. Soon the workshop was a reality, and soldiers flocked to it, out of curiosity at first and then out of interest in the craft work that was available. Metal work, woodworking, weaving, block printing, wood carving, and toy making were among the crafts used. Later the Red Cross assisted by supplying the needed raw materials and provided a more suitable building to house the workshops.

Visiting medical officers were impressed with the effect of constructive activities on the neuropsychiatric patients who participated and began to make urgent requests of Washington for similar workers for their own field hospitals. By 1918 there were 116 reconstruction aides, as they were now called, and they had become a recognized category of hospital worker. After the armistice, these workers returned home to find that their wartime work had been much publicized in the civilian press. To their surprise, they found themselves in demand by civilian hospitals. Cordelia Meyers, who led the initial group of reconstruction aides to France, later established a therapeutic workshop in the Panama Canal Zone at the request of Dr. Williams and trained workers to staff it (8–10).

Canada was the first country to organize occupational therapy in its military hospitals. Two early graduates of the Chicago school were among those who served in Canadian military hospitals. When the United States entered the war, it sought the assistance of Thomas Kidner, who had helped to organize the Canadian reconstruction program for its wounded veterans. Several emergency training programs were hastily established during the war years to train reconstruction aides for army hospitals. Most of the emergency training programs were of four-month duration and included both medical background and hospital practice. There was at that time a perception that occupational therapy was womens' work and all of the reconstruction aides were women. The craft emphasis in army hospitals gradually led to a shift in the thinking that occupational workers should come from the ranks of nurses. It was seen that people with only a basic medical background could successfully carry out occupational work, and during the postwar period, most recruits to the new field were from nonmedical backgrounds.

The war also caused a shift in the population that occupational therapists worked with. Prior to World War I, occupation had been used chiefly with the mentally ill. Afterward, however, the emphasis was more on patients with physical limitations. The wartime experience with occupation used to restore physical function opened a new area of practice to the early practitioners in the field (9).

1920–1940

In 1922 the American Occupational Therapy Association voted to hold annual meetings in conjunction with the American Hospital Association and to publish an official journal. The new journal was titled *Archives of Occupational Therapy* and was published from 1922 to 1924. In 1925 its name was changed to *Occupational Therapy and Rehabilitation*, a title felt to be more in keeping with the broad scope of the field. The journal had by now become one of the membership benefits of the organization. Eleanor Clarke Slagle accepted the position of Executive Secretary of the Association in 1923 and provided strong leadership to the growing organization. Slagle was instrumental in starting a national registry of qualified occupational therapists, thus assuring employers of a reliable listing of trained workers who held a professional standing comparable to that of registered nurses.

In an editorial that appeared in a 1922 issue of the *Archives of Occupational Therapy*, Thomas Kidner (then president of the Association) noted that 67 hospitals had sent exhibits of occupational therapy work to the 1921 meeting of the organization. Over half of these were tuberculosis hospitals, followed by a number of hospitals for nervous and mental diseases. Orthopedic and general hospitals were less well represented, and Kidner urged that therapists make more effort to promote occupational therapy in these types of institutions. He advised occupational therapists to follow the lead of political reformers whose motto was "organize, agitate, and educate" in order to further the goals of the new profession (11). Members of the association must have done so, for during the 1920s and 1930s occupational therapy gradually expanded from its initial focus on mental and nervous diseases to orthopedic and general hospitals and even to private practice.

The period from 1910 to 1929 was one of significant medical advance. The war, a serious polio epidemic in 1916, and increasing numbers of industrial and automobile accidents resulted in larger numbers of chronically disabled people who required long-term care and rehabilitation. Conditions in hospitals were improving, making them safer places for patients to recover. Freud's psychoanalytic theory was revolutionizing many physicians' ideas about the roots of mental disturbances and was providing new tools for treatment. Behaviorist theory was developing and offered an alternative explanation and treatment approach for aberrant behavior. The concept of occupational therapy as a way of reactivating the minds and motivation of the mentally ill and of restoring function to the physically disabled was gaining momentum. The literature of this period reflects much concern over craft modalities to be used for specific types of disabilities and a strong work orientation. The goal of occupational therapy was seen as a return to productive employment, and the craft activities employed were viewed as tools to help the patient advance step by step toward that goal (12).

The 1920s and 1930s saw a steady growth of educational programs preparing registered occupational therapists. It was also a time in which some of the enduring traditions of the field were established. Because many of its early practitioners were nurses, teachers, and social workers, occupational therapy developed as a female profession. Nurturing attitudes, then felt to be largely a female characteristic, were believed to be essential in working with the sick and the mentally ill. Early training programs in the field were open only to women, and this set a pattern that was modified very slowly. In the 1920s and 1930s more women began to enter the work force, and occupational therapy, along with teaching and nursing, was considered a respectable field for a woman to enter. This tradition of female dominance has engendered much concern and discussion in recent years; salary levels in this field and opportunities for independent decision making have been viewed by some occupational therapists as lagging behind other fields that are less female oriented.

Another tradition established during this period was that of close association and identification with organized medicine. Much of the early progress in the field was due to dedicated physicians who recognized the limitations of currently used medications and technology to improve the condition of patients with long-term disease or disability. The support they provided for occupational therapy as a new approach to improving mental and physical abilities was crucial in gaining acceptance by the conservative medical establishment of the time. When the American Occupational Therapy Association joined forces with the American Medical Association in 1935 to accredit educational programs for the registered occupational therapist, close links were forged that firmly connected occupational therapy with organized medicine. This alliance has been questioned seriously in recent years, and the debate continues as occupational therapy moves through the 1990s.

By 1930, occupational therapy was becoming known as a field. It had established a viable professional organization and was increasingly recognized as a contributor to medical care of the sick and injured. Because of its ties with medicine, occupational therapy was beginning to accept the need for a more scientific approach to the problems presented by the mentally ill and the physically disabled. Increasingly, occupational therapy practice focused on the subcomponents of functional performance—muscular function, neurophysiology, biomechanical principles, and specific abnormal behaviors—rather than the holistic view of the individual that had been prevalent in the earliest years of the field.

The professional progress of occupational therapy in the 1930s was severely limited by the great economic depression that affected the United States from 1929 to 1941. Health care suffered massive setbacks during this period, and occupational therapy was directly affected along with other health care fields. Spending on medical care dropped 33% from 1929 to 1933, even though physicians and hospitals lowered their fees. Many hospitals refused to accept patients unless payment of the bill was guaranteed. The American Medical Association acted to protect the financial interests of its members by reducing the number of medical schools, limiting admissions, and tightening up licensure provisions. It was a period of no growth for medical education or medical services. Many hospital occupational therapy clinics were forced to close during this period, and those that survived were inspired to new heights of creativity in the use of scrap materials and donations.

Rerek (13), in her review of the effect of this period on the development of occupational therapy, lists three major influences. First, future leaders of the field, who were growing up during this period, were strongly influenced toward caution and conservatism because of their experiences with economic uncertainty. Second, the federal government entered the health care arena during this period, and its influence on funding mechanisms and regulation of health care took root and became a major factor in the delivery of health services. Third, the public developed a pervasive attitude of suspicion and skepticism toward elected officials and the federal government; this suspicion would last for decades. No longer would the population give its leaders the unquestioned support and trust that predepression leaders had enjoyed.

WORLD WAR II AND THE REHABILITATION MOVEMENT

The United States was rescued from the economic depression by new government policies and by the outbreak of a second world war. Again the military sought occupational therapists to organize and run restorative programs for wounded and disabled veterans. Emergency training courses were again developed to meet the urgent need for occupational therapists. As ever larger numbers of veterans with severe physical disabilities and mental impairments were returned home, it was increasingly apparent that services to meet their needs were totally inadequate. Although many new medical techniques had been developed to save the lives of wartime casualties, few facilities were available for the rehabilitation and long-term care of wounded veterans. Families had become more mobile during the war years, and housing was in short supply. Most families were unable to provide the kind of care needed by the disabled veterans. Educational institutions were not prepared to deal with the needs of war veterans for job training and reintegration into civilian life. The medical establishment was more concerned with the treatment of acute illness and injury and was unconvinced of its role in long-term care. Families and veterans' groups pressed hard for services, and their needs could no longer be denied. Government support was made available for the construction and operation of rehabilitation facilities, staff training, and research. Organized medicine reluctantly accepted rehabilitation as a legitimate medical responsibility but never awarded it the kind of prestige that some of the other medical specialties enjoyed (13).

The era from 1942 to 1960 is often referred to as the period of the rehabilitation movement. During this time the needs of the disabled population were increasingly recognized and new facilities and methods for improving functional abilities were developed. Occupational therapy took its place as a rehabilitation field and therapists became involved in such areas as training patients in the use of prosthetics, developing orthotic devices, training patients in activities of daily living, using progressive resistive exercise to increase muscle strength, evaluating patients' vocational aptitudes and abilities, and using neuromuscular facilitation and inhibition. The use of antibiotics increased the survival rate of patients with serious illnesses and resulted in greater numbers of disabled adults. In psychiatric settings, therapists were involved with exploring the therapeutic use of self, dealing with patients' subconscious needs, analyzing patients' artwork in psychodynamic terms, and using group techniques to improve self-awareness and interpersonal communication. Occupational therapists continued to practice primarily on a technical level. There was little attempt during this period to relate treatment approaches to a theoretical framework or to seek the underlying principles of treatment. Therapists tended to work with specific diagnostic categories and were becoming more specialized. Educational programs preparing the registered occupational therapist were including more medical content in their curricula, and programs were becoming more comprehensive.

During the 1950s another occupational therapy staff member emerged: the certified occupational therapy assistant (COTA). During the postwar period, a critical staff shortage had developed in occupational therapy. At the same time, occupational therapists were broadening their role in the rehabilitation process. A plan for educating occupational therapy assistants had been proposed as early as 1949, but little was done until 1953 when the AOTA House of Delegates passed a resolution requesting a study of the feasibility of training nonregistered personnel to assist registered occupational therapists. In October of 1958, a three-month educational program was begun to educate assistants for mental health practice and that same year the AOTA began approving such educational programs. By 1960, assistants were being educated to assist with general practice as well. The first assistant training programs were hospital-based, but later were relocated in technical and community colleges. In 1961, the first directory of certified occupational therapy assistants appeared. The COTAs were employed to supplement and expand occupational therapy services and provide additional personnel for existing programs. By 1960, a number of schools had been established to prepare COTAs, and their contributions to the practice of occupational therapy were increasingly recognized. The development of the COTA level of personnel represented an important step in the growth of the profession and reflected the fact that the field had grown so complex that more than one level of practitioner was needed (14, 15).

1960–1980

The 1960s ushered in a turbulent period in the United States. Politically and socially it was a time of great change. The country's intervention in Viet Nam and other unstable governments gave rise to widespread political unrest and the polarization of attitudes concerning the country's role in international affairs. Economic inflation made for a growing gap between the "haves" and the "have-nots" of society. Traditional values and institutions were being challenged. The traditional family structure was weakening, and many experimented with alternative family arrangements and life-styles. Early retirement was encouraged, and the elderly were becoming a larger proportion of the population. Technology was forcing many workers from their jobs, and ideas about what competencies were necessary to exist in society were rapidly changing. Enrollments in colleges and technical schools boomed, as students tried to prepare for the changing job market. The incidence of drug and alcohol abuse, crime, and suicide rose sharply. On the positive side, progressive civil-rights legislation was enacted and enforced, the problems of poverty were discussed and solutions proposed, and there was greater recognition of personal responsibility in matters of health and disease prevention. People were paying more attention to diet, exercise, methods of reducing stress, and constructive use of leisure time. There was a new search for spiritual values among the younger generation, and religious groups attracted many new members.

The technological advances seen in society as a whole were reflected in health care and in occupational therapy practice. Medicine was becoming highly specialized, since new information was proliferating so rapidly that no one could hope to remain current with broad areas of medical practice. The same trend was seen in occupational therapy, with some therapists now identifying themselves as "hand therapists" or specialists in sensory integration, spinal cord injury, or burns. The kinds of medical conditions that occupational therapists were treating had changed since the 1940s and 1950s. Devastating epidemic diseases, such as poliomyelitis, were now things of the past, thanks to the development of effective vaccines. Tuberculosis was no longer common, as preventive measures and effective drug treatment controlled its incidence. On the other hand, stress-related diseases and dysfunctions were on the increase. Drug and alcohol abuse had become a national problem, as had the incidence of some forms of cancer. The growing population of elderly persons brought about a recognition that new services were needed to maintain their health and provide for a reasonable quality of life. Because of improvements in prenatal care and delivery, more disabled children were surviving with more severe handicapping conditions.

The medical community was seeing the need to educate the public about disease and injury prevention and was advocating the use of methods and technology to safeguard the public's health. Occupational therapy also was reviewing its role in health care and was becoming more involved in education, prevention, screening programs, and health maintenance efforts. Therapists were seeking new ways of delivering their services to meet these needs and were entering new markets, such as public school programs for handicapped children, community mental health centers, agencies promoting independent living for the elderly and the disabled, hospital outreach programs, and private practice (16).

Traditional medical institutions were undergoing major changes as they moved into the 1970s and 1980s. Many mental hospitals and residential institutions for the mentally retarded were closed across the country as the concepts of deinstitutionalization gained acceptance. It was believed that patients in such institutions could live more normal and more productive lives in community settings than in large state and private residential institutions where they had traditionally received care. There was growing concern over protection of civil rights for such individuals and a belief that the civil rights of many may have been violated by long-term confinement to an institution. As a result, large numbers of mental patients and mentally retarded persons were discharged or transferred from institutional to community facilities. Unfortunately the development of adequate community programs lagged far behind the need for such facilities, and many chronically mentally ill and retarded persons were reduced to life on the streets or in slum housing with no adequate resources to maintain health and prevent serious deterioration. Steps were taken to correct the situation, but its effects remain to haunt us today.

Along with the closing of custodial institutions, health care in general was moving from a hospital base to a community base. By the 1980s, hospital costs were so high that hospitalization was feasible only for severe illnesses and injuries. Routine medical care continued to be delivered by private physicians but also by new forms of medical practice, such as community health centers and outpatient surgical facilities. Occupational therapy was part of this trend, with increasing numbers of therapists and therapy assistants employed in public and private schools, outreach programs, community service agencies, and private or group practices.

In the late 1970s and early 1980s many occupational therapists were voicing concern over their traditional role as an associate or an assistant to the physician. There was a growing opinion that the medical model no longer served occupational therapy well. Many therapists were now convinced that they had a role to play in the prevention of disability and the maintenance of health as well as fulfilling their traditional role in treating existing limitations of function. Occupational therapists were beginning to see themselves as fitting better into an educational or a social model of practice, rather than a model that emphasized pathology and illness (16, 17).

Graduate programs had begun in occupational therapy education in the 1960s, but the 1970s and 1980s saw a steady growth in the number of graduate programs available. With knowledge expanding at an ever increasing rate, advanced education was becoming more and more necessary for the occupational therapy practitioner. The need for research in occupational therapy had long been recognized, but in the 1970s it became a major issue for the field. There was an urgent need to test basic occupational therapy concepts, to explore the value of assessment and treatment techniques, and to determine whether occupational therapy was cost-effective. A sound theoretical base was believed to be needed to explain why occupational therapy worked and to provide unifying concepts for occupational therapy practice. During this period the *American Journal of Occupational Therapy* changed its focus from that of occupational therapy practice to research. It was now publishing more scientific investigations into aspects of occupational therapy; several other new journals were also contributing to the research literature in the field.

The 1970s and 1980s saw greater involvement of occupational therapists and their professional organization in legislative activities. It was recognized that the profession and its clients must be represented when health care legislation was being proposed, and lobbying activities and testimony to various legislative bodies became an important priority for the profession during this era. State licensure had also become an important issue during this period. By 1991 the AOTA reported that 38 states plus the District of Columbia and Puerto Rico had enacted licensure laws regulating occupational therapy practice. Three states had registration regulations, four had state certification laws, and two had trademark laws (18). In 1993 only Colorado lacked some type of state statute regulating occupational therapy practice. State licensure has enabled legal recognition of occupational therapy services in states that regulate occupational therapy practice and provides legal recourse when abuses occur by unqualified practitioners.

1990s AND BEYOND

In the mid-1980s the health care system in the United States was undergoing a great deal of change in an attempt to contain health care costs while still maintaining quality services. As occupational therapy practitioners entered the 1990s, many factors were influencing occupational therapy practice. Acquired immune deficiency syndrome (AIDS) was a new disease entity that was affecting large segments of the United States population and no effective treatment was known. Research efforts were begun, but the devastating impact of this disease caused health care workers to question the adequacy of traditional health care facilities in dealing with the needs of this patient population. Ethical dilemmas were becoming more commonplace in occupational therapy practice. How should health care resources be allocated? Should the patient's wishes prevail over the opinions of a health professional? How could an occupational therapist know that a given treatment approach would be the most successful method for an individual patient? In 1984 the AOTA had developed a position paper entitled "Principles of Occupational Therapy Ethics," and in 1988 an entire issue of the *American Journal of Occupational Therapy* was devoted to papers focusing on various aspects of ethical practice.

During the 1980s and 1990s, "quality of life" was becoming increasingly accepted as a valid goal of occupational therapy intervention. Enabling a client to live with dignity, even though terminally ill, was now being seen as an important aspect of health care. Occupational therapy scholars were beginning to study the clinical reasoning process by which therapists made critical decisions concerning their treatment programs for clients. It was becoming more and more important to be able to utilize theory in analyzing client problems and selecting treatment approaches.

The rapidly increasing cultural diversity of the population of the United States was posing challenges for OTRs and COTAs during the 1990s. They were working with African-Americans, displaced Asians, people of Hispanic origin, and refugees from Tibet, the Middle East, and the former Soviet Union. All of these groups had unique cultural backgrounds that it was necessary to understand and respect in order to work effectively with them. It was essential that OTRs and COTAs become sensitized to the real cultural differences that existed among their clients and be able to bring clients' values and traditions into the therapeutic process.

Some communicable diseases that had been well-controlled for decades were making a comeback in the 1990s. Rheumatic fever was again on the increase in the United States. Even more alarming was the reappearance of tuberculosis. Although virtually eradicated through preventive measures and drug therapy, the incidence of tuberculosis began to rise along with the AIDS epidemic in the mid-1980s. It seemed resistant to the drugs that had previously been used to treat it and began to make inroads into the population. Victims were typically young and often homeless; many were alcoholics or drug addicts who had no source of regular medical care. Physicians were also finding that few lower income parents were immunizing their children against common childhood communicable diseases. Outbreaks of measles, rubella, and whooping cough were frequently seen and spread rapidly through the child population.

Occupational therapists were facing increasing constraints in their practice from the reimbursement systems that paid for health care in the 1990s. The traditional fee-for-service system was giving way to a managed care system in which a third party payer (a health insurance company) determined which services would be covered and to what degree. As health care was increasingly administered on a business basis, there was strong pressure to decrease costs; at the same time, patients were demanding higher quality care. These conflicting pressures were directly impacting upon occupational therapists and their practice. The idea of national health care insurance was revived during the early 1990s, and in 1992 there were a number of proposals for new funding mechanisms for health care to insure that low-income persons would have access to health services. As we progress through the 1990s we will continue to see rapid change in health care delivery and funding. These trends will be discussed more fully in Chapter 20 as we look toward future developments in occupational therapy.

SUMMARY

Would the founders of occupational therapy recognize the field today? One wonders what they would make of biofeedback training, the use of computer programs for cognitive retraining, or electronic equipment for the severely handicapped. In a 1977 paper reviewing the evolution of occupational therapy, Kielhofner and Burke (19) pointed out that early occupational therapy was based on a humanistic philosophy that reflected beliefs about the nature of people in the 18th and 19th centuries. Moral treatment, and subsequently occupational therapy, arose out of a holistic view of individuals in the context of their environment. Later a competing scientific school of thought gained dominance in medicine and in occupational therapy. This viewpoint focused on pathology and the study of function and dysfunction at the cellular level. This became the medical model that continues to dominate organized medicine today. Kielhofner and Burke suggested that by accepting the medical model, occupational therapy became fragmented and less cohesive. Therapists under this model tended to focus on muscles, psychic mechanisms, or sensorimotor interactions rather than taking a broad view of the individual. In doing so, these authors claimed, occupational therapy became scientifically respectable but lost its original broad concepts of occupation and its contributions to health and well-being. These authors and others have proposed an occupational behavior frame of reference for the field that would recapture some of the founders' original concepts of occupation and its contributions to health. They suggest retaining the technology that has been developed within the medical model, but reorganizing occupational knowledge under its original philosophy of occupation.

George Barton, Dr. William Rush Dunton, Eleanor Clarke Slagle, and the other pioneers of the field might marvel at some of the techniques used today in occupational therapy and at the broad scope of practice, but they would also recognize that humanistic values continue to guide the practice of occupational therapy. The field has come a long way from its early beginnings and from the concepts so well-stated by its pioneers. Its future depends to a great extent on the decisions that the profession and its organization make in the 1990s.

Discussion Questions

1. Do you think that occupational therapy's close relationship with organized medicine helped or hindered the development of the profession?
2. COTAs were originally educated to be support staff for registered occupational therapists. Is that role still realistic in the health care environment of the 1990s?
3. How did political and social conditions influence the nature of occupational therapy practice during different periods of history?
4. Has the client population of occupational therapy changed over the last 50 years? How?
5. Why do more women than men enter occupational therapy today?
6. Are the humanistic values of occupational therapy compatible with the modern view of health care as a business or industry? Why or why not?
7. Invite a retired occupational therapist to visit your class and share his or her experiences. What was their education like? What changes did they see and experience during their career in occupational therapy?

References

1. Licht S: *Occupational Therapy Source Book*. Baltimore, Williams & Wilkins, 1948, pp. 1–17, 41–56.
2. Slagle EC, Robeson HA: *Syllabus for Training of Nurses in Occupational Therapy*, ed. 2. Utica, New York State Department of Mental Hygiene, 1941, pp. 3–75.
3. Bockoven JS: The legacy of moral treatment. *AJOT* XXV:223–225, 1971.

4. Peloquin SM: Moral treatment: contexts reconsidered. *AJOT* 43(8):537–544, 1989.
5. Peloquin SM: Occupational therapy service: individual and collective understandings of the founders, part 1. *AJOT* 45(4):352–360, 1991.
6. Meyer A: Philosophy of occupation therapy. *Arch Occup Ther* I:1–10, 1922.
7. Licht S: The founding and founders of the American Occupational Therapy Association. *AJOT* XXI:268–277, 1967.
8. Low J: The reconstruction aides. *AJOT* 46(1):38–43,1992.
9. Peloquin SM: Occupational therapy service: individual and collective understandings of the founders, part 2. *AJOT* 45(8):733–744, 1991.
10. Meyers C: Pioneer occupational therapists in world war I. *AJOT* II:208–215, 1948.
11. Kidner TB: Editorial. *Arch Occup Ther* I:499–501, 1922.
12. Woodside H: The development of occupational therapy, 1910–1929. *AJOT* XXV:226–230, 1971.
13. Rerek M: The depression years—1929–1941. *AJOT* XXV:231–233, 1971.
14. *O.T. News*. AOTA at 70: the growth of a dynamic profession. 41(7):6, 1987.
15. Mosey A: Involvement in the rehabilitation movement—1942–1960. *AJOT* XXV:234–236, 1971.
16. Diasio K: The modern era—1960–1970. *AJOT* XXV:237–243, 1971.
17. Reilly M: The modernization of occupational therapy. *AJOT* XXV:243–246, 1971.
18. AOTA state regulatory update, Professional Development Section, June 21, 1991.
19. Kielhofner G, Burke J: Occupational therapy after 60 years: an account of changing identity and knowledge. *AJOT* 31:675–690, 1977.

SUGGESTED READINGS

Christensen E: *A Proud Heritage: The American Occupational Therapy Association at 75*. Rockville, MD, AOTA Inc, 1991.

Gilfoyle EM: 1984: Transformation of a profession. *AJOT* 38(9):575–584, 1984.

Levine RE: The influence of the arts-and-crafts movement on the professional status of occupational therapy. *AJOT* 41(4):248–254,1987.

Reed KL: Tools of practice: heritage or baggage? *AJOT* 40(9):597–605, 1986.

Special 75th anniversary issue. *AJOT* 46:1, 1992. Contains a variety of articles on aspects of occupational therapy history.

West WL: A reaffirmed philosophy and practice of occupational therapy for the 1980s. *AJOT* 38(1):15–23, 1984.

Yerxa EJ: Some implications of occupational therapy's history for its epistemology, values, and relation to medicine. *AJOT* 46(1):79–83, 1992.

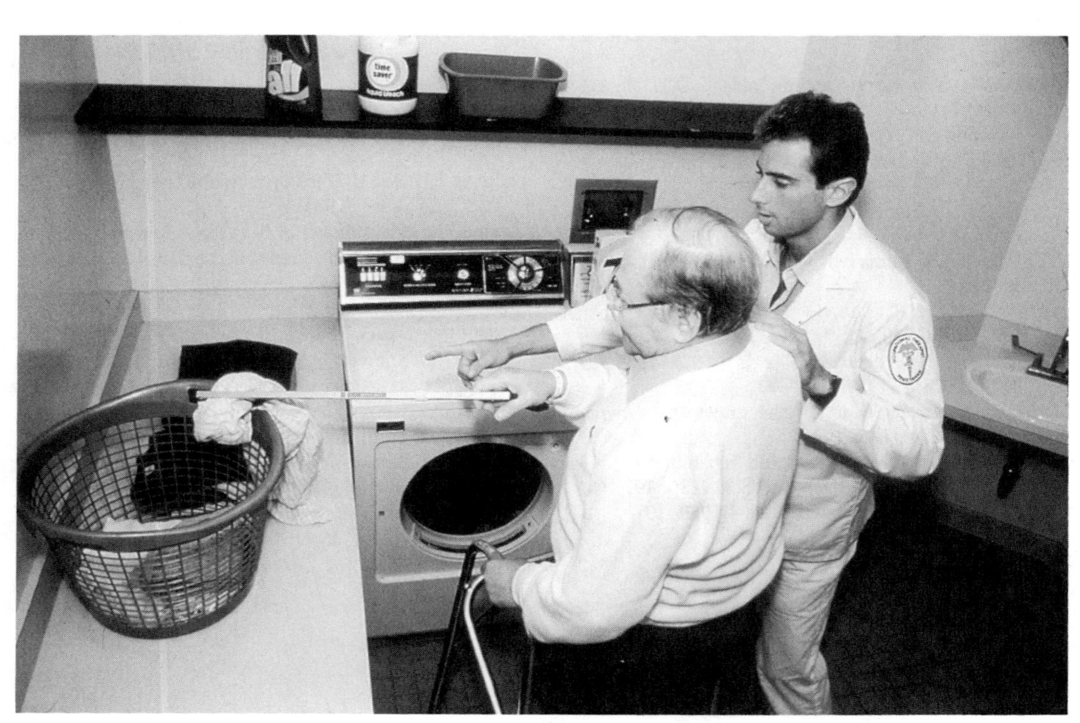
all
time saver
liquid bleach

4 Use of Activity as a Therapeutic Tool

Occupational therapy uses purposeful activity as its medium to help clients accomplish their desired goals. Occupational therapists and therapy assistants are activity specialists; their primary role is to draw on their knowledge of activities and select and apply those that are most likely to meet the needs of their clients. This chapter discusses how occupational therapists and certified occupational therapy assistants use activities to promote and maintain health, prevent injury or disability, and help their clients develop or redevelop needed abilities and skills.

When occupational therapists discuss their field, they are careful to describe their methods as *purposeful activity*, a term that the American Occupational Therapy Association has defined.

> *Individuals engage in purposeful activity as part of their daily life routine. Purposeful activity, in this natural context, can be defined as tasks or experiences in which the individual actively participates. Engagement in purposeful activity requires and elicits coordination between one's physical, emotional, and cognitive systems. An individual who is involved in purposeful activity directs attention to the task itself, rather than to the internal processes required for achievement of the task. Activities may yield immediate results or may require sustained effort and multiple repetition. They may represent novel and singular responses or be part of complex, long-standing patterns of behavior. Purposeful activities, influenced by the individual's life roles, have unique meaning to each person (1).*

When we look at healthy people, we see that activity is part of the normal pattern of life. We all engage in many different activities each day and often complete them with little conscious thought or effort. The routine self-care tasks of getting up in the morning, i.e.,bathing, dressing, combing our hair, shaving or putting on makeup, eating breakfast, and getting ourselves off to work or school, do not take up much of our attention; yet they are essential parts of our daily life. It is only when some circumstance—an injury, an illness, or psychological stress—interferes with our ability to perform these tasks in the ordinary way that we begin to be concerned and realize how much we have taken for granted.

Each individual has his or her own pattern of daily activities. The pattern may be influenced by the individual's environment, age or developmental level, socioeconomic status, life-style, family and friends, and culture. As individuals grow and develop, their activity pattern changes as their life roles and societal expectations change. Play forms an important part of the young child's pattern of daily activities. Through play, the child learns how to interact with the environment, to master gross and fine motor skills, to communicate, and to relate to people. Rest or sleep is another large part of the child's daily activity schedule. Work activities are present only in the form of play, as new skills are practiced and refined. When the child begins school, learning activities become the "work." For the middle-aged person, work takes up a very large proportion of the daily activity pattern. Leisure hours may be few, since work may be taken home in the evening or thought about even though it was left at the workplace. The weekend is anticipated with pleasure, since it means a welcome break from the daily demands of a job. Sleep and rest take up a moderate amount of time, but often the amount of rest is considered insufficient. The daily activity pattern is dramatically different for these two individuals, but each is typical for the period of life represented. Cynkin (2) has written about how normal individuals use activity in their daily lives: "Health is manifested in the ability of an individual to participate in socioculturally delineated and prescribed activities with satisfaction and comfort." In other words, participation in the activities sanctioned by the culture is a mark of physical and psychological health.

When the ability to function in daily life is impaired because of injury, illness, psychological stress, changing developmental or environmental demands, or lack of skill, the individual becomes a candidate for occupational therapy services. The occupational therapist will evaluate the client's present performance abilities and, based on those findings, will develop a program of activities to help meet the client's needs. Activity experiences will be designed to offer the client opportunities to learn and practice needed skills so that much or all of the client's personal pattern of daily activities may be resumed. If the injury or disorder is complex, a remedial activity may be broken down into very small steps so that the client can work on each step sequentially. The end goal is accomplishment of the total task. In situations where the disability is permanent, the occupational therapist may decide to help the client adapt to the limitations by teaching different ways of performing needed tasks or by providing special pieces of equipment that will enable the client to function. In this way, the disability is compensated for and the client may continue to perform the desired activity.

Occupational therapy treatment activities must usually be individually planned for each client. Although two people may have similar disabilities, their attitudes, interests, goals, and life circumstances may be quite different. Occupational therapy attempts to meet these individual needs by designing activity programs that will provide the specific support and assistance needed by each client. Although occupational therapy does make use of group treatment approaches, individual client goals are never lost sight of. The group may be a vehicle for the achievement of some of those goals. Occupational therapy treatment activities cannot be routinely prescribed and applied. There are no "recipes" for the use of activity as a therapeutic tool.

OCCUPATIONAL PERFORMANCE AND PERFORMANCE COMPONENTS

One way to view the therapeutic use of activity is to look at the domain of occupational therapy. Mosey (3) has said that the domain of occupational therapy consists of "performance components within the context of age, occupational performance, and an individual's environment."

The term *occupational performance* refers to the individual's total life pattern, including activities of daily living, work, recreation or leisure, and the ability to organize one's time to meet one's roles and responsibilities (temporal adaptation). Occupational performance is the big picture of how the individual functions within the context of his or her environment. To function effectively, the individual must have a variety of subskills that contribute to total performance. These microabilities or performance components are the building blocks that support occupational performance and are necessary for normal functioning. Sensory-motor functions refer to one group of performance components that focus on the ability of the central nervous system to organize and use sensory stimuli for planned interaction with the external environment. Neuromuscular functions are another component of performance and refer to the ability to use one's body to move and respond effectively. Motor functions relate to the abilities necessary for the physical performance of tasks.

Cognitive function refers to the ability of the brain to learn, remember, understand, conceptualize, and solve problems. Psychosocial performance components include the ability to perceive oneself and others realistically and to express one's feelings and understand those of others. They include being able to relate to others in meaningful ways and to function in group situations. As occupational performance describes the global picture of the individual's ability to function in his or her environment, performance components describe the subskills that, when combined effectively, allow participation in a full range of daily activities. Figure 4.1 illustrates the relationships between occupational performance, performance components, and the environment.

Looking at the domain of occupational therapy in this way helps us to understand how activities are used as therapy in clinical occupational therapy programs. Table 4.1 lists the occupational therapy performance areas that are of concern to occupational therapy personnel when a client is referred for services. The occupational therapist or therapy assistant tries to identify the performance areas in which problems are occurring. These functional performance areas are what the client needs to work on in order to resume their normal pattern of life. There may be specific reasons why a client cannot perform activities of daily living. Does the client have deficiencies in sensory functions? Does he or she lack the range of motion needed to dress him- or herself? Is coordination impaired? These subskills are called performance components, and often they must be worked on and improved before a client can be expected to attain performance of daily living skills or other occupational performance areas. Table 4.2 lists the specific performance components that can interfere with function and that occupational therapists may need to treat before improvements in performance can occur. Some of these

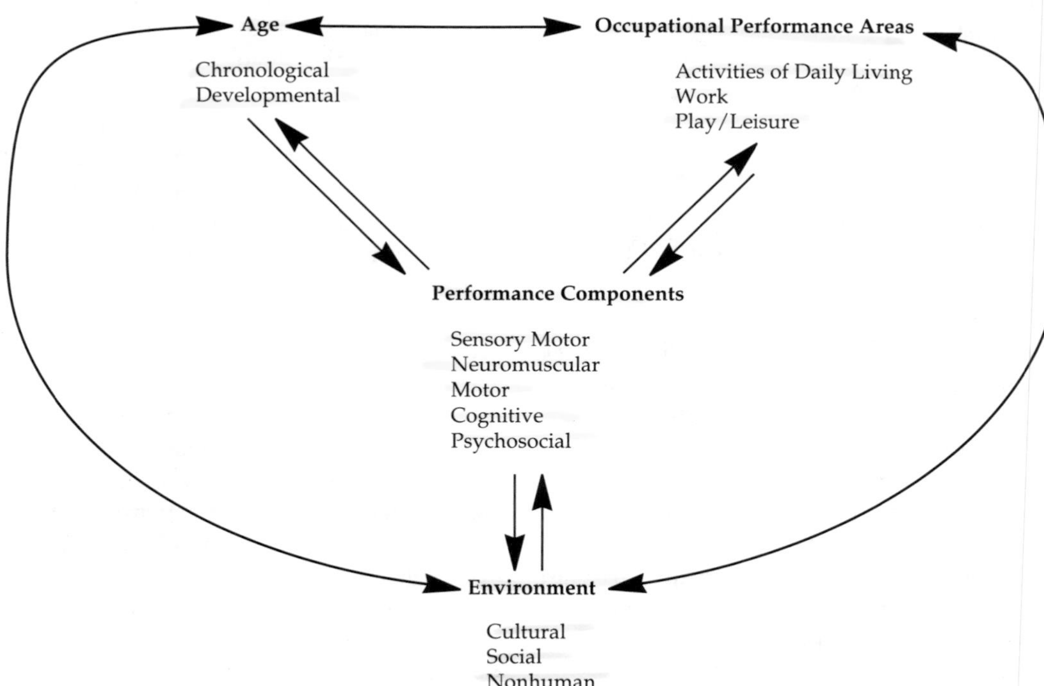

Figure 4.1. Domain of concern for occupational therapy.

Table 4.1. Occupational Therapy Performance Areas

Activities of daily living
Grooming
Oral hygiene
Bathing
Toilet hygiene
Dressing
Feeding and eating
Medication routine
Socialization
Functional communication
Functional mobility
Sexual expression
Work Activities
Home management
Clothing care
Cleaning
Meal preparation and cleanup
Shopping
Money management
Household maintenance
Safety procedures
Care of others
Educational activities
Vocational activities
Vocational exploration
Job acquisition
Work or job performance
Retirement planning
Play or leisure activities
Play or leisure exploration
Play or leisure performance

terms may be unfamiliar to you and are defined in the Glossary at the back of the book (4).

By evaluating the client's performance components, the occupational therapist attempts to identify the root causes of the limitations in occupational performance. Once these have been identified, the therapist will be able to set appropriate goals and design treatment activities intended to improve weak or damaged performance components or to compensate for them. Treatment goals are usually discussed with the client and mutually agreed upon. It is essential that the client's needs and wishes be taken into account when planning a therapeutic program, since the client's interest and active participation are critical to the achievement of a successful outcome. In planning a therapeutic program, the occupational therapist relies on his or her knowledge of effective activities used by other occupational therapists for this type of dysfunction, on results of research, and on past experience working with this type of disorder.

CHANGING CONCEPTS OF THERAPEUTIC ACTIVITY

Activities are the tools of occupational therapy, but what kind of activities and how are they applied? In the early days of the field, arts and crafts activities were heavily used. They were considered a first step toward vocational training, and a strong work orientation was present in many of the early descriptions of therapeutic activities. Haas (5), writing in 1925, described a comprehensive occupational therapy program in the men's division of Bloomingdale Hospital, an institution for the mentally ill. Haas, an early occupational therapist, was a craftsperson and a craft instructor. He utilized activities such as industrial brush making, chair caning, basketry, metal work, jewelry making, construction of concrete garden furniture, stringing tennis rackets, making tennis and basketball nets, and furniture making. The therapeutic uses of each activity were described, with case studies showing the benefits achieved by some of the residents of the institution. High-quality work was expected and good work habits were encouraged.

As times and conditions changed, occupational therapy media changed. Fidler (6), writing in 1948, suggested a method of analyzing potential treatment activities in terms of their psychological characteristics. She recommended that the mental as well as the physical processes demanded by an activity be considered, and she urged that therapists consider the opportunities an activity provided for creative expression, expression of feelings, assumption of social roles, and adaptability.

Table 4.2. Performance Components

- Sensory motor components
  - Sensory integration
    - Sensory awareness
    - Sensory processing
      - Tactile
      - Proprioceptive
      - Vestibular
      - Visual
      - Auditory
      - Gustatory
      - Olfactory
  - Perceptual skills
    - Stereognosis
    - Kinesthesia
    - Body scheme
    - Right-left discrimination
    - Form constancy
    - Position in space
    - Visual closure
    - Figure-ground discrimination
    - Depth perception
    - Topographical orientation
- Neuromuscular components
  - Reflexes
  - Range of motion
  - Muscle tone
  - Strength
  - Endurance
  - Postural control
  - Soft tissue integrity
- Motor components
  - Activity tolerance
  - Gross motor coordination
  - Crossing the midline
  - Laterality
  - Bilateral integration
  - Praxis
  - Fine motor coordination
  - Visual-motor integration
  - Oral-motor control
- Cognitive integration and cognitive components
  - Level of arousal
  - Orientation
  - Recognition
  - Attention span
  - Memory
    - Short-term
    - Long-term
    - Remote
    - Recent
  - Sequencing
  - Categorization
  - Concept formation
  - Intellectual operations in space
  - Problem solving
  - Generalization of learning
  - Integration of learning
  - Synthesis of learning
- Psychosocial skills and components
  - Psychological
    - Roles
    - Values
    - Interests
    - Initiation of activity
    - Termination of activity
    - Self-concept
  - Social
    - Social conduct
    - Conversation
    - Self-expression
  - Self-management
    - Coping skills
    - Time management
    - Self-control

Kathlyn Reed, in her Slagle lecture of 1986, pointed out that changing values and social and economic trends have a strong influence on occupational therapy media. Changing technology also plays a role (7). Today occupational therapy staff members use computer software programs to give some clients specific practice in fine motor skills, cognitive abilities, and communication skills. Simulations of work tasks help clients to reenter the workplace and resume their previous employment. Biofeedback methods enable some clients to reduce stress and learn to relax. Cooperative group activities help clients learn to interact constructively with others and to share work or leisure activities. Therapists' knowledge of a wide range of activities allows them to be creative in their selection of appropriate treatment media with their clients. As society changes, occupational therapy media will change in order to remain relevant to the clients served.

TOOLS OF OCCUPATIONAL THERAPY

Mosey (3) in 1981 identified six "legitimate tools" of occupational therapy. We will look at these tools in detail and will describe how occupational therapists use them in programs of intervention.

Nonhuman Environment

The physical surroundings are one tool that the occupational therapist can manipulate to help the client achieve security, mastery of environmental interactions, and as a source of pleasure and relaxation. For example, the therapist or therapy assistant may suggest environmental modifications that will make an elderly client's home a safer and more convenient place to live.

Conscious Use of Self

Occupational therapists and therapy assistants learn to use their personalities as a therapeutic tool to alleviate client anxiety, provide reassurance or information, and assist the client in mobilizing and using inner resources. *Use of self* means that the therapist engages in planned interactions with clients to help them toward their therapeutic goals. Therapists must be well aware of their own feelings and reactions when engaged in such interactions and must be able to express their feelings as well as be sensitive and receptive to those of their clients. Effective use of self depends heavily on the therapist's people skills and the ability to communicate clearly and directly.

Teaching-Learning Process

Each therapist-client interaction can be viewed as a teaching-learning situation in which the therapist helps clients to experience, learn, and practice new behavior that will enable them to function more effectively in daily life. The therapist and therapy assistant are teachers, and study of learning theories and principles helps make the learning process easier and more effective for the client.

Use of Purposeful Activities

Purposeful activity involves interaction with both the human and nonhuman environments and is one of the ways in which people achieve mastery or competence. Activities may be realistic, symbolic, or a little of both. In occupational therapy, purposeful activities usually relate to the domains of work, leisure, or self-care. They may be performed in the natural environment or may be simulated. For example, handicapped homemakers may be taught adapted cooking methods in their own kitchens or in a simulated kitchen in a hospital occupational therapy clinic. To be effective, purposeful activities used as therapy must be relevant to the needs, interests, and capacities of the client. They must be sufficiently interesting that the client will be motivated to perform them, and they must lead to functions that the client wants to be able to perform in his or her daily environment. New activities are constantly being added to the occupational therapy repertoire.

In 1991 Taylor and Manguno published the results of a study of the use of various treatment activities in occupational therapy. They found that self care and social skills activities were used most frequently by occupational therapists in all practice specialties. Therapists in mental health settings tended to use crafts more often than did therapists working in programs for the physically disabled; however, noncraft activities were used more frequently than craft activities in all of the facilities surveyed (8).

Activity Groups

Activity groups are made up of individuals who share common concerns or who need to work on similar problems or deficiencies. Because we all function in many kinds of group situations, we need to know how to relate to group members effectively, how to get our own needs met within groups, and how to recognize and help meet the needs of other group members. Mosey (3) describes activity groups as laboratories for learning, because they provide opportunities for individuals to try out and practice ways of dealing with others in a relatively safe environment. Activity groups involve a "doing" process. They differ from verbal therapy groups in that the group members work on purposeful activities as well as take part in group discussion. The activity helps to focus the group's attention on problems and issues in need of resolution and provides a structure and organization that many clients need. Many people find it easier to talk about themselves when they are engaged in an activity. Cooperative interaction is fostered, since the group must complete a common task. The occupational therapist or therapy assistant serves as a facilitator for the group and guides it toward positive interactions and resolution of conflicts. Therapists using group techniques must be familiar with group dynamics, communication, and group leadership methods.

In 1985 Duncombe and Howe (9) conducted a survey of occupational therapy practice to determine how occupational therapists used group techniques. They found that 60% of the therapists surveyed in all areas of practice were using group treatment approaches. Of these, 54% reported using activity groups, while 24% were using verbal groups. Specific types of groups being used included exercise groups, cooking groups, activities of daily living groups, self-expression groups, task groups, arts and crafts groups, feeling-oriented discussion groups, reality-oriented discussion groups, sensorimotor groups, and education groups.

Activity Analysis and Synthesis

The occupational therapist and the therapy assistant must be skilled in the process of analyzing activities for their potential therapeutic value. Activity analysis is the process of examining the task or activity in terms of its smallest performance components. The task of selecting an appropriate treatment activity is essentially one of matching an activity to the specific needs of the client. If the match is a good one, the activity chosen will help the client achieve his or her therapy goals.

Activity analysis may be general in nature or may be related to a specific theoretical frame of reference. A general activity analysis looks at the factors that have traditionally been accepted as part of the domain of occupational therapy. The sample activity analysis outline shown on pp. 45–46 is an example of this general approach. Another way of analyzing an activity is in terms of a specific theoretical frame of reference. For example, Kielhofner and his colleagues have developed a form of activity analysis that is derived from the model of human occupation. They analyze a given activity by placing it in the context of the whole range of human occupation. To use this type of activity analysis one must be familiar with the model on which it is based and be able to apply the theoretical constructs of that model.

To effectively analyze any activity, one must be familiar with the activity, the materials used, the necessary tools, and the processes involved. The therapist or therapy assistant should have had direct experience with the activity. In educational programs that prepare registered occupational therapists and certified occupational therapy assistants, the study of activity analysis and the learning of a broad range of potentially therapeutic activities comprise an important part of the curriculum.

SELECTION OF THERAPEUTIC ACTIVITIES

Cynkin (2) offers some guidelines for the selection of appropriate therapeutic activities. She notes that treatment activities must be meaningful to the client and appropriate to the setting in which they are being used. They should be practical—easily administered and compatible with the amount of time available for treatment. They should be versatile and adaptable so that they can be graded and adjusted to different client needs. It should be possible to grade the activity in terms of difficulty, physical and psychological demands, cognitive requirements, and/or social characteristics. Therapeutic activities should lend themselves to a step-by-step progression and to a systematic, structured approach. One activity may build on another, so that each takes the client further toward achievement of a treatment goal. The therapist must be alert to a client's changing needs and must be able to adapt the treatment activities accordingly. In planning the sequence of treatment, the therapist must anticipate events likely to occur during the treatment process and should be prepared to vary the program as needed (2).

EXAMPLES OF THERAPEUTIC ACTIVITY USE

Work

Let us now look briefly at some recent reports of how activity has been used as treatment in the three occupational performance areas of work, use of leisure time, and self-care. In May of 1985 the *American Journal of Occupational Therapy* devoted an entire issue to work evaluation in occupational therapy. In a paper describing the historical involvement and interest of occupational therapy in work, Marshall (10) pointed out that in its earliest years occupational therapy was developing work programs for the mentally ill. By the late 1930s, prevocational evaluation was becoming part of the practice of occupational therapy, and therapists were using crafts to develop skills that would be readily transferable to industry. The emphasis on work evaluation and training continued until the 1950s, when professionals in the field of vocational rehabilitation began to assume more of the responsibility for work evaluation and training programs. Occupational therapy largely neglected these areas until the 1970s, when there was a resurgence of interest in work roles and the contributions occupational therapy could make to preparing clients for work.

Therapists working with physical limitations have frequently been involved with work evaluation and training programs. Bettencourt and his colleagues (11) have described a comprehensive program of work simulation used with clients who had back injuries. The program was sponsored by an insurance company that provided rehabilitation services for policyholders who had been injured on the job. Treatment included client education, focusing on anatomy, body mechanics, and energy conservation so that clients would fully understand their treatment program. Activities were then begun to develop the physical abilities and skills needed for specific job performance. Elaborate equipment was developed for the program, including a balance monitor to determine distribution of weight by the client and a multiwork station that simulated carpentry construction tasks, plumbing jobs, and electrical wiring jobs. A truck simulator was used to practice driving skills, and a pneumatic lift platform simulated lifting tasks. An upper extremity simulator provided graded practice with a variety of industrial tools. Much of the equipment was computerized and provided immediate feedback on the amount of muscular effort being exerted and other parameters of function. Such sophisticated programs provide close approximation of the work tasks that clients will be returning to and can directly prepare them to resume their jobs.

Leisure

The use of leisure time is another area in which occupational therapy makes use of activity to contribute to the client's health and well-being. Occupational therapy has long been interested in the role of play in the growth and development of children. Gliner (12) has suggested that purposeful activity is an essential component in the learning of coordination and motor skills. He saw the therapist's role in motor development as one of structuring client-environment interactions in a purposeful way to allow for the development or refinement of motor skills. Ayres (13) and her colleagues working with learning-disabled and autistic children have used a variety of movement experiences and games to improve perceptual and motor planning skills.

With adult clients, constructive use of leisure time is frequently a focus of occupational therapy intervention. Citizens of the United States seem to have particular problems with finding time for leisure activities and with enjoying the leisure time that they do have. A 1992 study showed that the hours of work have been increasing for many American workers while hours devoted to leisure are declining. Parents, especially single parents, are hard hit by this phenomenon and struggle to balance work, household responsibilities, and quality time with their children. When the time spent commuting to work is added in, the picture looks even worse. Many people are forced to take second jobs to make ends meet. The increase in work hours has been especially great for women, who now take less time off for childbirth, caring for young children, and for family emergencies (14).

For too many people, leisure time is filled by sitting before the television set rather than pursuing personal interests. University of Michigan researchers found that companionship was a key element of satisfying leisure activities. Their national study of 1000 subjects showed that it was activities involving social interaction that were most highly valued as recreation (15). Occupational therapists and therapy assistants know that a reasonable balance of work, leisure, and self-care activities helps to promote a healthy life-style. There seems to be a strong need for occupational therapists to call attention to the need for leisure and to help the well population develop satisfying ways of using their leisure time. Retirement planning is another area where the skills of occupational therapists can contribute by helping people make the transition from the world of work to the productive use of leisure. Broderick and Glazer (16) conducted a study of 60 retired men and found that those who had a high level of preretirement participation in leisure activities were the most likely to show a high degree of planning for their retirement. Those retired persons who were the most socially active also showed the most positive attitudes toward retirement. There is a definite role for occupational therapists and therapy assistants in helping the aging population find fulfilling leisure activities that can be carried into the retirement years.

Arnetz (17) reported the results of a study conducted in Sweden on the effects of a social activation program carried out in a senior citizen apartment building. She found that residents who participated in a six-month activity program showed a threefold increase in their activity level following the program. The people who benefitted most were those who had been the most passive and isolated prior to the study. Arnetz concluded that occupational therapy programs play an important role in preventing social isolation in elderly persons who live in institutional environments.

Self-Care

Self-care has been a traditional focus of occupational therapy services in the past and continues to be a necessary part of the treatment program of many clients. Traditionally, the phrase *activities of daily living* (frequently abbreviated ADL) has included feeding, dressing, personal hygiene, travel and transportation, and other abilities needed to function in daily life. In our society, independence in such tasks is highly valued and most of us are reluctant to accept help. Attention to the performance of daily living skills is essential to help many clients retain their sense of self-worth and competence.

With the advent of sophisticated electronic equipment, occupational therapists and therapy assistants have found new ways of making the performance of daily tasks easier for severely disabled clients. In a 1984 report, Seplowitz (18) described the case of a 39-year-old quadriplegic client who had suffered secondary neurologic complications. Seplowitz was able to adapt an inexpensive remote control unit, which enabled the client to operate his stereo, dictaphone, lights, television, telephone, CB radio, and tape recorder by himself. He was also able to operate his home computer with the use of hand splints. These adaptations allowed him to remain mentally active and productive and gave him some degree of control over his immediate environment. Seplowitz noted that advances in medical care and technology are enabling severely disabled clients to live longer. Such individuals are being discharged from medical facilities earlier than in the past and have very complex needs. Occupational therapy can play a major role in helping these people to be as productive and in control as they wish to be, even though seriously limited in their performance abilities.

Training and practice in self-care activities is also useful for clients with psychosocial disturbances or developmental disabilities. Many clients are unable to live independently in the community because they lack essential self-care skills. Learning to manage money, shop sensibly, perform household maintenance tasks, do laundry, or cook for themselves are skills that can be taught, either individually or in groups. With opportunities to learn and practice such skills, many disabled persons can live and function adequately in community settings.

SUMMARY

Additional examples of the use of activity are found in the individual case studies in Section II of this text. We have looked at some of the ways that occupational therapists and therapy assistants use activities to accomplish therapeutic goals with clients. The concepts of occupational performance and performance components are important in understanding the use of purposeful activity as a treatment medium. The occupational performance areas of activities of daily living, work, and leisure are the focal points around which occupational therapy intervention takes place. When disease or injury causes limitations in these performance areas, clients may appropriately be referred for occupational therapy services.

Discussion Questions

1. Activities can be used to maintain health and prevent problems as well as improve impaired functions. Can you think of some ways that you can utilize activities to maintain good physical and psychological health?
2. Think of a new skill that you have recently learned. What kind of cognitive abilities are required to perform this skill? What kind of movements? What kind of social or psychological abilities?
3. Occupational therapy activities are constantly changing as new media are developed and as the needs of clients change. List some recently developed activities, materials, or pieces of equipment that might have application in occupational therapy.
4. Imagine that a group of people share a common need to be able to live in their homes or apartments without requiring constant help and support from their families or friends. How could an activity group be used to help them develop independent living skills?
5. Do the meanings of activities vary from one culture to another? Give an example of how an activity might be interpreted differently by people from different cultural backgrounds.
6. Constructive and satisfying use of leisure time may be a goal in some occupational therapy intervention programs. List several activities that might be useful in helping clients develop better social interactions with others through recreational opportunities.
7. Are some activities in our society gender related? Discuss some activities that might be considered primarily male or female oriented.

GENERAL ACTIVITY ANALYSIS

1. *Basic Considerations*

What equipment is needed to perform the activity?
What materials are needed?
How much time is required to complete the activity?
What is the cost of the activity?
What safety precautions should be considered?
What age group is the activity appropriate for?
Does the activity have a gender association?
Does the activity require prior knowledge or technical skill?

2. *Sensory Qualities of the Activity*

Which sensory systems must register and process information in the activity?

__tactile __visual
__proprioceptive __auditory
__vestibular __gustatory
__olfactory

Which perceptual skills are needed to perform the activity?

__stereognosis __position in space
__kinesthesia __visual closure
__body scheme __figure-ground discrimination
__right-left discrimination __depth perception discrimination
__form constancy __topographical orientation

3. *Neuromuscular Requirements of the Activity*

Does it require integration of primitive reflex patterns?
What range of motion is required?

__ active
__ passive
__ active resistive

How much muscle tone and muscular control is needed?
What degree of coordination is required?
How much muscular strength is needed?
How much endurance must the client have?
How much postural control is needed?

4. *Motor Requirements of the Activity*

Does the activity require a prolonged tolerance of physical exertion?
What kind of gross motor coordination is needed?
Does the activity require crossing the midline?
Does the activity require awareness of left and right sides of the body?
Does the activity require integrating the two sides of the body?
Does the activity require motor planning ability?
What degree of fine motor coordination is needed to perform the activity?
What degree of visual-motor integration is needed?
Does the activity require oral-motor control? To what degree?

5. *Cognitive Integration and Cognitive Components of the Activity*

What level of arousal is needed to perform the activity?
What degree of orientation is needed?
Must the client recognize certain elements in order to perform the activity?
What kind of attention span does the activity require?
Does the activity require memory? What kind?

__short-term __remote
__long-term __recent

Does the activity require the sequencing of elements in a given order or pattern?
Does the activity require the ability to categorize elements?
Does the activity require concept formation? To what degree?
Does the activity require the mental manipulation of objects in space?
Is problem solving required to perform the activity? Does the activity depend on generalization of learning? Does the activity require the integration of learned concepts?
Does the client need to be able to synthesize previously learned concepts into new patterns?

6. *Psychosocial Skills and Components*

Is the activity related to specific life roles?
Is the activity related to certain personal values held by the client?
Does the activity fall within the client's range of interests?
Is the client required to initiate the activity? Can the client end the activity when he or she wishes? Does the activity aid in the development of self-concept?
Does the activity require social interaction with others?

Does the activity permit verbal or non-verbal communication with others?
Does the activity allow the client to express his or her thoughts, feelings, and needs?
Is the activity culturally appropriate for the client?
Does the activity help the client to identify and manage stress and related reactions?
Does the activity help the client learn to manage time?
Does the activity help the client learn to control his or her own behavior?

(Adapted from Uniform Terminology for Occupational Therapy, ed. 2. AOTA, *AJOT* 43(12):808–814, 1989.)

REFERENCES

1. AOTA: Purposeful activities. *AJOT* 37(12):805–806, 1983.
2. Cynkin S: *Occupational Therapy: Toward Health Through Activities*. Boston, Little, Brown & Co., pp. 33, 47–58, 1979.
3. Mosey A: *Occupational Therapy: Configuration of a Profession*. New York, Raven Press, pp. 74–79, 89–118, 1981.
4. AOTA: Uniform terminology for occupational therapy, ed 2. *AJOT* 43(12):808–814, 1989.
5. Haas L: *Occupational Therapy*. Milwaukee, Bruce Publishing Co., pp. 38–50, 1925.
6. Fidler GS: Psychological evaluation of occupational therapy activities. *AJOT* II(5):284–287, 1948.
7. Reed KL: Tools of practice: heritage or baggage? *AJOT* 40(9):597–605, 1986.
8. Taylor E, Manguno J: Use of treatment activities in occupational therapy *AJOT* 45(4):317–322, 1991.
9. Duncombe LW, Howe MC: Group work in occupational therapy: a survey of practice. *AJOT* 39(3):163–170, 1985.
10. Marshall E: Looking backward. *AJOT* 39(5):297–300, 1985.
11. Bettencourt et al: Using work simulation to treat adults with back injuries. *AJOT* 40(1):12–18, 1986.
12. Gliner JA: Purposeful activity in motor learning theory: an event approach to motor skill acquisition. *AJOT* 39(1):28–34, 1985.
13. Ayres A: *Sensory Integration and the Child*. Los Angeles, Western Psychological Services, pp. 135–156, 1979.
14. Mastrangelo R: Americans don't have time for fun. *Advance for Occupational Therapists* 8(14):8, 1992.
15. Creighton C: Therapeutic activities study shows free time unfulfilling for many. *OT Week* 2(16):4, 1988.
16. Broderick T, Glazer B: Leisure participation and the retirement process. *AJOT* 37(1):15–22, 1983.
17. Arnetz BB: Gerontic occupational therapy—psychological and social predictors of participation and therapeutic benefits. *AJOT* 39(7):460–465, 1985.
18. Seplowitz C: Technology and occupational therapy in the rehabilitation of the bedridden quadriplegic. *AJOT* 38(11):743–747, 1984.

SUGGESTED READINGS

Allen CK: Activity: occupational therapy's treatment method. *AJOT* 41(9):563–575, 1987.

Boyer J, Colman W, Levy L, Manoly B: Affective responses to activities: a comparative study. *AJOT* 43(2):81–87, 1989.

Creighton C: The origin and evolution of activity analysis. *AJOT* 46(1):45–48, 1992.

Cynkin S, Robinson A: *Occupational Therapy and Activities Health: Toward Health Through Activities*. Boston, Little, Brown & Co., 1989.

Engle JM: Relaxation training: a self-help approach for children with headaches. *AJOT* 46(7):591–596, 1992.

Falk-Kessler J, Momich C, Perel S: Therapeutic factors in occupational therapy groups. *AJOT* 45(1):59–66, 1991.

Heck SA: The effect of purposeful activity on pain tolerance. *AJOT* 42(9):577–581, 1988.

Lamport NK, Coffey MS, Hersch GI: *Activity Analysis Handbook*. Thorofare, NJ, Slack Inc., 1989.

Larson KB: Activity patterns and life changes in people with depression. *AJOT* 44(10):902–906, 1990.

Levine RE: The influence of the arts-and-crafts movement on the professional status of occupational therapy. *AJOT* 41(4):248–254, 1987.

MacRae A: Should music be used therapeutically in occupational therapy? *AJOT* 46(3):275–277, 1992.

Peloquin SM: Sustaining the art of practice in occupational therapy. *AJOT* 43(4):219–225, 1989.

Rosenfeld MS: Occupational disruption and adaptation: a study of house fire victims. *AJOT* 43(2):89–96, 1989.

Sladyk K: Traumatic brain injury, behavioral disorder, and group treatment. *AJOT* 46(3):267–270, 1992.

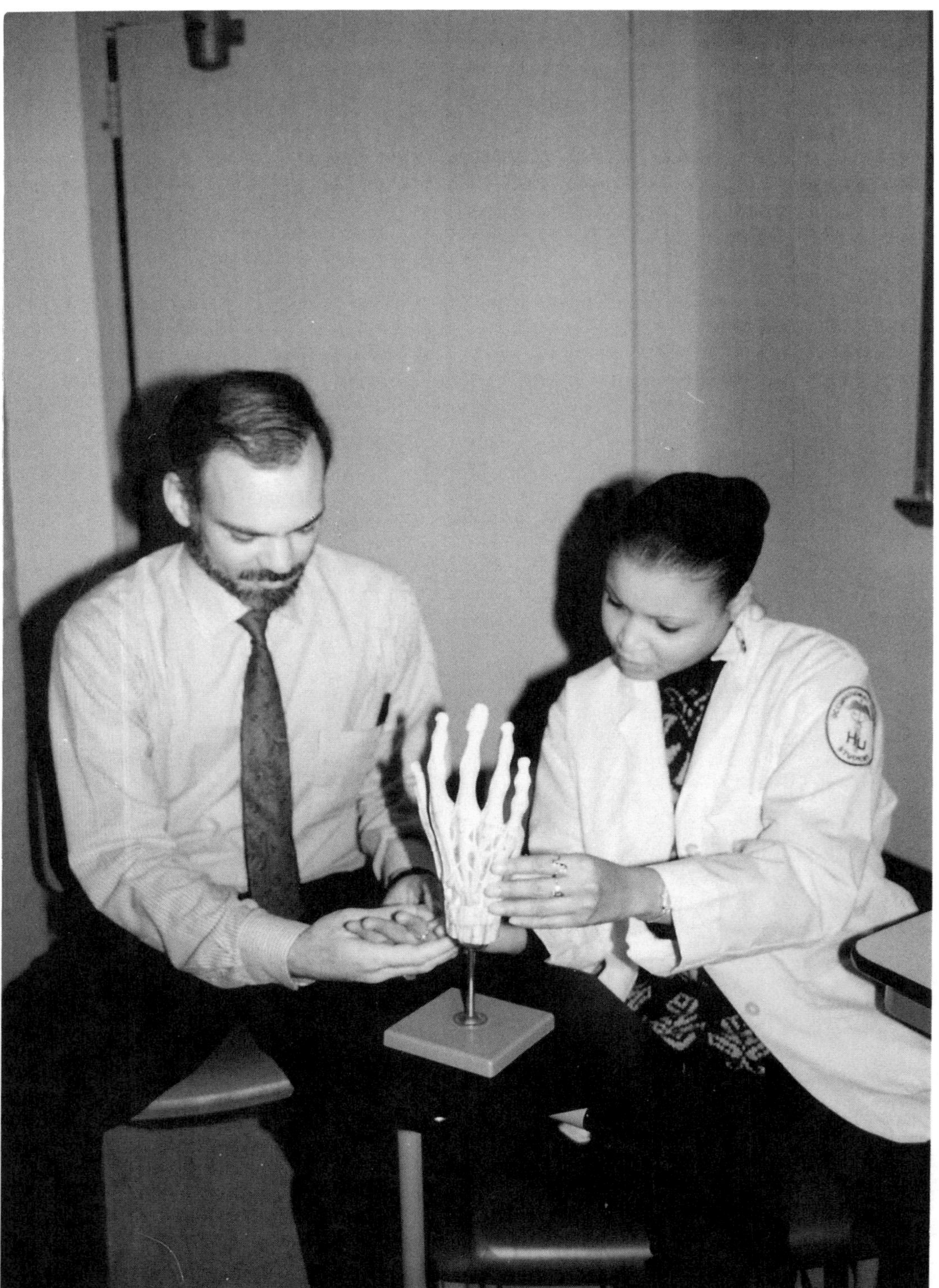

5 Education and Certification Patterns

Three different levels of personnel are involved in the delivery of occupational therapy services. The registered occupational therapist (OTR) is a graduate of a baccalaureate, certificate, or an entry-level master's degree program. This education prepares students to evaluate and treat deficiencies in occupational performance areas and their components and to manage occupational therapy service programs. The certified occupational therapy assistant (COTA) is a graduate of a certificate or associate degree program of technical education. The COTA graduate is prepared to collaborate with OTRs in providing occupational therapy services and participating in program management. The COTA may also direct activity programs (1, 2). The occupational therapy aide usually has no formal education in the field but receives on-the-job training that equips him or her to assist with routine procedures in occupational therapy programs. These three types of personnel work cooperatively to help clients achieve their treatment objectives. In addition, an occupational therapy department may include volunteer workers who provide important supplementary services to the program. In this chapter the type of educational preparation required of the OTR and the COTA is discussed and the certification process is described.

The OTR is probably the best known, having been on the scene the longest time. As early as 1906 Susan Tracy, a nurse, was teaching a short course to nursing students on invalid occupations that emphasized the value of activity for bedridden patients. Later, Julia Lathrop, Dr. William R. Dunton, Eleanor Clarke Slagle, and others conducted training programs to prepare personnel to work in "occupation therapy." By 1918 there were four schools offering an education in occupational therapy in Milwaukee, Philadelphia, Boston, and St. Louis. By 1949 all occupational therapy education programs were required to be located in colleges or universities and to be authorized degree programs. In 1932 the American Occupational Therapy Association (AOTA) began its registry of qualified occupational therapists who had completed the required program of study and were prepared to practice in the field. In 1935 the AOTA, together with the American Medical Association, began to accredit educational programs in order to maintain minimum educational standards and assure some uniformity of educational preparation. Educational programs for the OTR have continued to develop; in 1992 there were 75 such programs, with 15 more developing (1).

EDUCATION OF THE REGISTERED OCCUPATIONAL THERAPIST

To be admitted to an educational program preparing OTRs, a prospective student must meet the admission requirements of the college or university to which he or she is applying. A high school diploma or equivalent is required, and there may be specific requirements for high school preparation in mathematics, English, science, and social studies. A high school background in speech and English composition is helpful, since communication skills are highly valued in occupational therapy. Also desirable is a foundation in the biological and behavioral sciences so that the student may build on these areas in college course work. A background in liberal studies is beneficial, as these subjects will contribute to the student's overall preparation for working in a helping relationship to others.

A listing of all educational programs for OTR and COTA education in the United States is available from the American Occupational Therapy Association. Students are advised to contact the program of their choice for specific information about entrance requirements, the educational program offered, and the time and financial resources needed to complete the program.

Once accepted by a college or university, the student will embark on preprofessional course work. A common pattern in many baccalaureate degree programs is two years of preprofessional education, two years of professional education, and six to nine months of supervised fieldwork. In some curricula, students may be admitted directly into the professional program as juniors. Some colleges offer certificate or master's degree education for entry into occupational therapy. Such programs are designed for persons who hold a baccalaureate degree in another field and are usually more intensive than the standard baccalaureate program. They may also require that certain courses be completed before entry into the professional program, so students should be careful to inquire about prerequisites for admission. Although all accredited programs meet AOTA's minimum standards, they may differ in their emphasis and in their course sequencing patterns. One accredited program may stress biomedical studies, while another may emphasize the human development process or human learning theories. These differences are to be expected, since AOTA's educational standards are intentionally broad to allow for individual differences between colleges. Students are advised to inquire about the program's philosophy and emphasis when they seek information about educational programs so that they are fully informed about the nature of the education they will receive.

The most recent revisions to AOTA's *Essentials and Guidelines for Accredited Educational Programs for the Occupational Therapist* were completed in 1991 and were adopted by AOTA and the American Medical Association, who jointly accredit these programs. According to this document, the goal of entry level education for the OTR is to prepare practitioners who are able to do the following:

1. Evaluate and assess performance areas and their components;
2. Provide occupational therapy services to maintain or improve function and to prevent deficits in activities of daily living, work, and play/leisure and in the underlying performance components;
3. Manage occupational therapy service;
4. Incorporate values and attitudes congruent with the profession's standards and ethics; and
5. Demonstrate an attitude of inquiry for creative analysis and problem-solving.

The document also points out that entry-level professional education lays a foundation for other roles of the experienced therapist, such as those of administrator, consultant, educator, researcher, and health planner.

The 1991 *Essentials and Guidelines for Accredited Educational Programs for the Occupational Therapist* require that the educational program include content in the following areas:

1. Liberal arts;
2. Biological, behavioral, and health sciences;
3. Occupational therapy theory and practice;
4. Management of occupational therapy services;
5. Research;
6. Professional ethics; and
7. Fieldwork education:
   Level I: observational and participatory experiences to enrich didactic coursework.
   Level II: a minimum of 6 months su-

pervised practice providing occupational therapy services to clients.

Educational programs arrange these content areas in different ways; however, it is fairly common to find the liberal arts and science courses included in the preprofessional part of the curriculum. This content may include courses in English composition, literature, psychology, sociology, biology, speech, anatomy, physiology, kinesiology, and philosophy. The preprofessional program may also include a number of electives so that students may pursue other studies of personal interest to them. Near the end of the preprofessional program, the student may apply for admission to the professional part of the educational program. Admission requirements and methods vary considerably from one program to another; the student should seek information about the admission process directly from the program of his or her choice.

Once admitted to the professional program, the student studies subjects directly related to occupational therapy theory and practice. Aspects of human performance are studied in detail, looking at both the normal and abnormal aspects of function. Human occupation throughout the life cycle is analyzed, and the student learns activity processes that can be used to maintain existing functions or to improve deficiencies in function. Students are exposed to concepts of health and disease, health maintenance, and prevention of disability. A variety of physical and psychosocial disorders that may interfere with normal occupational performance are studied, and students learn intervention or management techniques for use with these disorders. Learning experiences are not limited to the classroom. Level I fieldwork provides observational and practice experiences in clinical settings, introducing students to the application of occupational therapy concepts and procedures. Such fieldwork is usually supervised by the course instructor or by experienced occupational therapists employed in clinical settings. Level I fieldwork is a vital part of the curriculum and gives the student a better idea of how occupational therapy is used in client care. Students gradually learn how to carry out assessment and treatment procedures with clients and become more comfortable in the therapeutic relationship.

Professional education in occupational therapy is not intended to prepare specialists. Rather it is aimed at giving the student general knowledge and skills that are the basis of all occupational therapy practice. Because of this general focus, both physical and psychosocial disorders are studied, as well as developmental disabilities and limitations related to the aging process. It is only after students have mastered the general concepts and shown the ability to apply them clinically that they may wish to limit their practice to one disability or age group. Specialization usually occurs after some years of clinical practice and requires advanced study of the specialty area through continuing education, advanced clinical experience, or graduate education.

The professional curriculum also includes content on the management of occupational therapy services, research concepts and applications, professional ethics, and values and attitudes related to work in a helping profession. The student who has completed all or a significant portion of the professional coursework then enters the level II fieldwork phase of education. Level II fieldwork is student participation (usually on a full-time basis) in a clinical program or programs that offer supervised experience in occupational therapy practice. The AOTA's *Essentials and Guidelines for an Accredited Educational Program for the Occupational Therapist* require a minimum of six months of level II fieldwork, but many educational programs exceed this minimum.

The purpose of level II fieldwork is to provide an in-depth experience in providing occupational therapy service to clients. These fieldwork placements promote the development of clinical reasoning and reflective practice, transmit the values and ethical beliefs of the profession, communicate and model professionalism, and help the student develop a repertoire of assessment and treatment methods related to deficits in human performance (1). The student's work is closely supervised by an experienced therapist who is available to consult with the student, answer questions, and assist when needed. The fieldwork student is gradually assigned more responsibility for the care of clients and is expected to complete all of the documentation related to client care that the clinical setting requires. By the end of the fieldwork period, the student is expected to be functioning at the level of an entry-level occupational therapist and should be able to assume full clinical responsibilities.

The supervising therapist carefully assesses the fieldwork student's clinical abilities and prepares a detailed report that is discussed with the student. This report is returned to the educational program that prepared the student and is scored on a pass-fail basis. Students who pass their level II fieldwork successfully are then declared eligible by their educational program to take the national OTR certification examination. Students who fail level II fieldwork may reschedule additional fieldwork (within the regulations of their specific educational program) until they are declared eligible to write the certification examination. (The examination is discussed later when we look at the certification process.)

EDUCATION OF THE CERTIFIED OCCUPATIONAL THERAPY ASSISTANT

We saw in Chapter 3 that the need for a technically educated occupational therapy staff member originated from a serious staff shortage during the 1950s. There were not enough occupational therapists to meet service needs, and the expanding scope of occupational therapy practice compounded the problem. In 1953 the AOTA House of Delegates approved a study of the feasibility of educating occupational therapy assistants. The results of the study affirmed the need for an assistant level worker and in 1958 the first occupational therapy assistants were being educated for practice in psychiatric facilities. By 1960 COTAs were being prepared for general practice as well.

The earliest educational programs were only three months long and were often located in hospitals. In 1959 the AOTA amended its bylaws to permit the certification of COTAs and began approving COTA educational programs. By 1963 COTA students were being offered a unified curriculum that included both psychiatric and general practice studies, and many of the educational programs had been transferred to community colleges and technical schools. COTA education gradually lengthened to 9 to 12 months, but today most programs are two-year associate degree programs. In 1992 there were 74 established COTA educational programs with 12 more being developed (3, 4). Until 1977, occupational therapy assistants were certified immediately after graduating from an approved program, but in 1971 a proposal was made to establish a national examination for certification purposes. The first COTA certification examination was held in 1977, and passing the examination continues to be the requirement for certification today.

Just as with educational programs for the OTR, the AOTA developed *Essentials and Guidelines* (standards) for COTA educational programs. These standards closely paralleled those for OTR education, but with some differences that reflected the differences in function of the two types of workers. One major difference was in the depth and complexity of the curriculum. Technical programs generally placed less emphasis on knowledge of occupational therapy theory and did not provide in-depth study of the biomedical and behavioral sciences. They tended to emphasize instead the "doing" aspects of the field—occupational therapy methods and procedures used in daily practice.

According to AOTA's 1991 *Essentials and Guidelines for an Accredited Program for the Occupational Therapy Assistant*, technical education in the field was intended to prepare workers who could do the following:

Collaborate in providing occupational therapy services with appropriate supervision to prevent deficits and to maintain or improve function in activities of daily living, work, and play/leisure and in the underlying components;
Participate in managing occupational therapy service;
Direct activity programs; and
Incorporate values and attitudes congruent with the profession's standards and ethics (3).

In the 1991 revision, content requirements for COTA educational programs included the following:

1. General education;
2. Biological, behavioral, and health sciences;
3. Occupational therapy principles and practice skills; and
4. Fieldwork education:
   Level I: observational and participatory experiences to enrich didactic education.
   Level II: a minimum of 12 weeks of in-depth supervised experience in providing occupational therapy services.

Just as with educational programs for the OTR, technical education programs tend to vary in their approach and emphasis, although all are expected to meet AOTA's minimum educational standards. Thus some programs stress preparation for employment in long-term care facilities, while others focus to a greater extent on home health care or employment in community agencies. The philosophy and emphasis of a program should be investigated by prospective students, since it pervades the educational program and influences the type of education provided.

In a two-year associate degree program, the first year is often spent in general studies that prepare the student for the study of occupational therapy principles and practice in the second year. Observation and practice experiences in clinical settings (level I fieldwork) are required in COTA education just as at the OTR level, and these experiences are tied in with classroom learning. Twelve weeks of level II fieldwork is required; however, some schools exceed this minimum. Level II fieldwork is usually done on a full-time basis and provides the student with direct clinical experience under the close supervision of an experienced OTR or COTA. This practice experience enables the student to apply the knowledge learned in the classroom to actual cases and is an important part of the curriculum.

Just as with the OTR student, the clinical performance of the COTA fieldwork student is observed and a written performance assessment is completed by the supervisor. This report is sent back to the student's school and is scored pass or fail. Students who pass the level II fieldwork and who have completed all other educational requirements are declared eligible to take the national certification examination for occupational therapy assistants.

FINANCIAL ASSISTANCE

Today all forms of higher education are expensive and most students will require some sort of financial assistance during their student years. More than half (69.7%) of all OTR students and 57.7% of COTA students enrolled during 1991 were receiving some form of financial aid. It is recommended that students ask about the availability of financial aid when they are visiting educational programs. Some programs offer special scholarships for occupational therapy students, and many state occupational therapy associations provide scholarship support. Some employers of occupational therapy personnel will provide financial support to students in return for employment in their facilities after graduation.

For graduate students, teaching and research assistantships may be available as well as traineeships and fellowships (1).

CERTIFICATION PROCESS

Certification is an official recognition by an authorized body that individuals have completed the necessary academic and examination requirements to qualify for practice in a given field. In occupational therapy, certification is provided by the American Occupational Therapy Certification Board (AOTCB), which operates independently from the AOTA and which administers national qualifying examinations. Membership in the AOTA is separate from certification, and one may be certified as an OTR or COTA without becoming a member of the organization.

The certification board controls the certifying examinations and is responsible for their content. Monitoring and scoring of the examinations are the responsibility of a private testing agency under contract with the AOTCB. Examinations are scheduled twice a year for OTR and COTA candidates. No two examinations are exactly alike. Each year new questions are added and out-of-date or less discriminating questions are withdrawn so that the examination reflects the current thinking and practice of the field.

When OTR and COTA candidates have been declared eligible by their educational programs to take the appropriate examination, the AOTCB sends candidates information on the location of testing centers and application forms for the examinations. A testing fee is charged to students who apply, and general information on examination content is provided. Both examinations are intended to objectively measure the knowledge and skills required by entry-level OTRs and COTAs in clinical practice and are based on role delineation studies of OTR and COTA roles and functions.

A multiple-choice format is used for both examinations. After the examinations have been scored by the testing agency, candidates are notified of whether they passed or failed, along with their total score and subscores on specific parts of the examination. Candidates who fail the examination may retake it an unlimited number of times. Upon passing the examination, the candidate is issued a certificate by AOTCB that verifies their certification. The certificate is reissued every five years.

Although AOTCB certification is voluntary, states that have regulatory laws governing occupational therapy practice use AOTCB certification for determining eligibility for state licensure or practice (5). If candidates wish to practice in a state that regulates occupational therapy practice, they *must* apply to the state regulatory board for a license or permit to practice in that state. Only after obtaining the state license are they legally qualified to practice in that state. Certified individuals are entitled to use the initials OTR or COTA after their names and may represent themselves as qualified practitioners. Graduates of foreign educational programs in occupational therapy (professional level) that are approved by the World Federation of Occupational Therapists may apply to take the national occupational therapy certification examination if they wish to qualify for practice within the United States (6).

In addition to being the certifying agency for OTRs and COTAs, the AOTCB has the additional responsibility of investigating cases of alleged unethical or incompetent occupational therapy practice. If an OTR or COTA is found to have engaged in unethical or incompetent practice or is found to be too impaired to practice occupational therapy, the AOTCB is authorized to take disciplinary action. Penalties can range from a reprimand to the withdrawal of certification (7).

STATE REGULATION

By the 1990s most states were requiring some form of state licensure for OTRs and COTAs. Licensure is a process by which an agency of the state government grants permission to persons who meet established qualifications to engage in a given occupation or to use a particular title. Licensure is intended to protect the public from unqualified practitioners who may cause harm through improper or inappropriate services. Licensure attempts to guarantee a minimum educational standard for practitioners and to provide for a minimum quality of service. In 1991, a total of 49 United States jurisdictions had some type of law regulating the qualifications of occupational therapy practitioners and their practice. Thirty eight states plus the District of Columbia and Puerto Rico had licensure laws. Three states had passed registration laws and two had trademark laws. By 1993 only Colorado had not yet regulated occupational therapy practice (8, 9).

The majority of states with licensure acts require that practitioners be graduates of an accredited or approved educational program in occupational therapy, show evidence of successful completion or fieldwork requirements, and pass a qualifying examination in the field. Candidates who seek employment in states requiring licensure may request that the AOTCB forward their examination results to the appropriate state licensing board for review. Applicants may also be asked to complete an application form and pay a state licensing fee. Currently all states with occupational therapy regulatory laws accept the results of the AOTCB certification examinations, so there is no need to pass a separate qualifying examination when moving from one state to another.

WHICH EDUCATIONAL PROGRAM IS RIGHT FOR ME?

Students are sometimes uncertain which level of occupational therapy practice may suit them best. Both OTRs and COTAs perform valued services to clients. The OTR educational programs require more time to complete and are usually more costly, since they are located in colleges and universities. The COTA programs are shorter, introduce the principles of the field, and graduate workers who are immediately employable in direct service programs. Students who choose the COTA route may later continue their education at the OTR level. This laddering process is encouraged, and more COTAs are entering OTR programs each year.

For several years the AOTA sponsored a career mobility project, whereby COTAs could undertake an intensive program of individual study and supervised fieldwork to become eligible to take the OTR certification examination. A number of persons earned their OTR certification through this process, but it was recognized that this was a very difficult way to qualify. Relatively few who undertook it completed the process. The program was abandoned in favor of encouraging COTAs to qualify for the next practice level through completion of an OTR educational program. College programs were simultaneously urged to eliminate barriers to COTA graduates who wished to enter an OTR educational program. Most colleges have made genuine efforts to achieve this and try to make the transition from COTA graduate to OTR student as smooth as possible. Although many COTAs are very happy with their work and are satisfied to remain at the COTA level, others may wish to continue their professional education and should be given every opportunity to do so. Students are advised to discuss their career goals with faculty members of both educational levels if they are in doubt about which type of program to enter. Visiting occupational therapy clinical programs and observing the roles of the OTR and COTA can also be helpful in deciding which level of practice will be the most satisfying.

HIGHER EDUCATION IN OCCUPATIONAL THERAPY

There are two other educational levels in occupational therapy that should briefly be mentioned. Graduate education is becoming ever more important in the field, and most occupational therapy personnel agree that there are some types of jobs where specialized knowledge and skills are needed. Many areas of practice are becoming highly technical, and practitioners find that they need more knowledge in these areas than their entry-level education has given them. To meet such needs, occupational therapists may seek continuing education on an informal basis or may enter a master's or doctoral degree program.

In 1992, 28 colleges and universities in the United States offered postprofessional master's degree programs in occupational therapy (1). These programs are open to persons with a baccalaureate degree or equivalent in the field and offer advanced study of specific aspects of occupational therapy. Three universities offered doctoral programs in occupational therapy in 1992; many others offered doctoral programs in related fields (1). In 1991 a total of 608 students were enrolled in postprofessional master's degree programs, with 1/4 being full-time students and 3/4 part-time. A total of 83 students were enrolled in doctoral programs in that year (1, 4).

There has been a great deal of concern in recent years over the lack of occupational therapists who hold doctoral degrees. Such people are needed urgently to teach at the college level and to conduct research and generate and test theory in the field. These functions require knowledge gained at the doctoral level, and the AOTA is encouraging more students to enter doctoral programs. When embarking on an education in occupational therapy, it is wise to think ahead. Not all occupational therapists remain clinicians. Many become teachers, administrators, researchers, writers or editors, health planners, or consultants. It is important that beginning students consider all of these roles when planning their professional education. Shortages exist in occupational therapy at all levels, but the need for people with advanced knowledge and skills is particularly urgent.

TRENDS IN OCCUPATIONAL THERAPY EDUCATION

Enrollment in occupational therapy educational programs was up 11.5% in 1992 over the previous year, with increases seen in every type of educational program. A slow rise is also being seen in the number of minorities, males, disabled, and older students. Table 5.1 shows the demographic characteristics of occupational therapy students in 1991. The number of COTAs who were enrolled in OTR educational programs was holding steady in 1991 at 5.7% of the total number of OTR students (1).

The rapidly changing practice environment is demanding higher level skills and more specialized knowledge. It is likely that more practitioners will be entering graduate programs in the future to retool for new specialty areas and to develop management and research skills. It has become increasingly important for entry-level educational programs to remain current with practice developments to insure that their graduates are prepared for occupational therapy practice of the 1990s.

CONTINUING EDUCATION

Students are sometimes surprised to learn that graduation from an OTR or COTA program is not the end of their professional education. The truth is that at this point the real education is just beginning. In any profession that is growing and changing, it is vital that practitioners keep up with new developments and new knowledge in the field. This can be achieved in many ways: through professional reading, through participation in professional meetings and conferences, through discussion and communication with colleagues, and through attendance at continuing education programs and workshops. However one chooses to do it, all colleagues in a professional field must accept the responsibility to keep their skills sharpened and their knowledge up-to-date so that they can provide optimal services to their clients. This means a lifelong commitment to professional education. There is always more to be learned; this process of continued learning makes for a competent professional who is able to make significant contributions to health care and to the advancement of the profession.

Table 5.1. Demographic Characteristics of Occupational Therapy Students, 1991

Characteristic	OTR Students (%)	COTA Students (%)
Ethnic minority	10.6	17.5
Male	8.6	9.8
Disabled	1.4	3.7
Older than 25 years	23.7	50.3

Discussion Questions

1. If you are enrolled in an OTR curriculum, is there a COTA curriculum in your area? Obtain a copy of each curriculum and discuss the similarities and differences between the two. If you are a COTA student, compare your curriculum with that of an OTR program.
2. Are there some personal characteristics that might be desirable in one who wishes to pursue a career in occupational therapy? Discuss some of the personal traits that might be desirable in an OTR and a COTA.
3. Discuss the areas of advanced study that interest you. What are some areas of academic study that would be related or complementary to occupational therapy?

References

1. AOTA: *1992 Educational Data Survey, Final Report*. Rockville, MD, AOTA, 1992.
2. AOTA: Essentials and guidelines for an accredited educational program for the occupational therapist. *AJOT* 45(12):1077–1084, 1991.
3. AOTA: Essentials and guidelines for an accredited educational program for the occupational therapy assistant. *AJOT* 45(12):1085–1092, 1991.
4. AOTA: Listing of educational programs in occupational therapy. *AJOT* 45(12):1093–1111, 1991.
5. AOTCB: *Questions Asked Most Frequently by Students about Certification*. Rockville, MD, AOTCB, 1992.
6. AOTCB: *1992 Candidate Handbook, Certification Examination for OTR and COTA Candidates*. Rockville, MD, AOTCB, 1992.
7. AOTCB: *Disciplinary Action: A Process to Protect the Public*. Rockville, MD, AOTCB, 1991.
8. AOTA: *Occupational Therapy State Regulatory Update*. Rockville, MD, AOTA, 1991.
9. Joe BE: New Jersey wins licensure effort. *OT Week* 7(13):9, 1993.

Suggested Readings

Donohue MV: Progressive career patterns versus mandated entry-level education. *AJOT* 44(8):759–762, 1990.

Dunn W, Rask S: Entry level and specialized practice: a professional encounter. *AJOT* 43(1):7–9, 1989.

Ezersky S, Havazelet L, Scott A, Zettler CL: Specialty choice in occupational therapy. *AJOT* 43(4):227–233, 1989.

Marshall E: A survey of occupational therapy curricula. *AJOT* 45(10):932–935, 1991.

Rider BA, Brashear RM: Men in occupational therapy. *AJOT* 42(4):231–237, 1988.

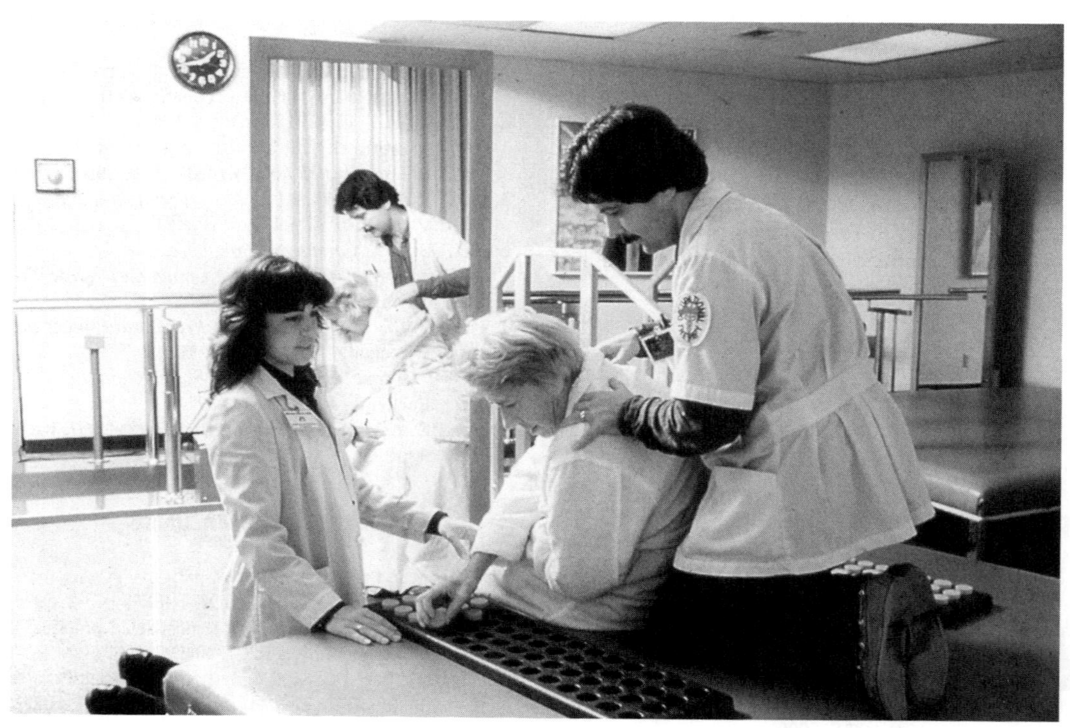

6 Clinical Roles and Functions of the OTR and COTA

In Chapter 5 the similarities and differences in the education of registered occupational therapists and certified occupational therapy assistants were discussed. In this chapter we examine how these two levels of personnel function in the work setting. When training programs for COTAs were first developed in the 1950s, the curriculum was designed to prepare people for work in psychiatric hospitals, since these hospitals had the greatest shortage in personnel at the time. Later, nursing homes were also found to be in need of personnel to direct activity programs for their residents. Another curriculum was developed to meet this need, and COTAs were trained in one of these two programs. By 1963, the two educational programs had been merged into a single curriculum that combined study of psychiatry and general practice. The first group of graduates from the combined curriculum worked in general hospitals and provided diversionary activities, ordered equipment and supplies, and made adapted equipment designed by the OTR (1). From this time on, COTAs were given general preparation for occupational therapy practice.

By the early 1970s, a number of OTRs were expressing concern over the roles and functions of COTAs. Some OTRs felt that COTAs were assuming roles that properly belonged to the OTR and were performing functions for which they were not adequately trained. Many more COTAs were practicing without direct OTR supervision than had been anticipated when the assistant level was established. Some highly competent COTAs were indeed performing at levels equal to that of some OTRs, and administrators who were facing increasing operational costs were likely to hire the least costly person to fill the position. In 1973 the AOTA identified six levels of occupational therapy positions: aide; entry-level COTA; experienced COTA; entry-level OTR; experienced OTR; and specialized practitioner, administrator, researcher, or instructor. In 1976, data were collected for a role delineation study of COTAs and OTRs. This study, which attempted to clarify the functions of the two groups, was published in 1981. It provided some guidelines for how the two levels of personnel could be utilized in delivery of occupational therapy services, but was criticized for its methods and its small sample size. An additional weakness of the study was that it focused only on entry-level workers (workers with less than one year of clinical experience). Critics pointed out that experienced COTAs and OTRs could legitimately assume higher levels of responsibility and that this was not addressed by the 1981 document (2). In 1985 this problem was corrected by the publication of another occupational therapy personnel classification that described the roles of both entry-level and experienced personnel. The 1985 personnel classification looked at entry, intermediate, and advanced levels of function for both the OTR and the COTA. It also included the roles of occupational therapy supervisors and department managers or directors. Because of these additional levels of function, it more clearly showed the differences between levels of experience and job functions.

Another role delineation study was published by the AOTA in 1990 and looked only at entry-level practice competencies. This report replaced the 1981 study and included greater emphasis on values, attitudes, research, and ethics as components of practice. It was also more specific about the tasks of the OTR and the COTA. The role delineation was used to develop job descriptions for each level of personnel and to provide regulatory boards, employers, and educators with a standard set of competencies that could be expected of entry-level OTRs and COTAs (3).

COTA ROLES AND FUNCTIONS

According to the 1985 document (4), the primary function of the entry level COTA is "to *implement* occupational therapy services for patients and clients under the supervision of an occupational therapist." *Entry level* is defined as less than one year of practice experience as a COTA. The entry-level COTA is expected to have competency skills in the delivery of occupational therapy treatment, and the document describes a number of critical performance areas for the entry-level COTA (Table 6.1). Close supervision is required for the entry-level COTA in clinical performance, and general supervision by an OTR or an experienced COTA is recommended for administrative functions.

In the 1990 role delineation, the assessment of client needs is clearly seen as the responsibility of the OTR, with the COTA contributing to the process under the OTR's supervision. Program planning is also viewed primarily as a function of the OTR. The COTA plays a larger role in implementing the intervention plan, with the degree of supervision determined by the COTA's level of competence in the specific treatment methods to be used. Documentation and discontinuation of service are perceived as OTR responsibilities. The 1990 study seems to give the COTA a greater role in service management than previous studies have done. Research has been and continues to be an OTR function.

This most recent document makes it clear that when an OTR delegates a task to a COTA there must be assurance that the same result will be obtained as if the OTR carried out the task. Thus verifying the service competency of an entry-level employee becomes critical to good service delivery. The document recommends that the supervising OTR observe correct performance of the procedure on at least three separate occasions in order to document service competency of the inexperienced COTA (3).

An intermediate-level COTA has one or more years of clinical practice as a COTA. This more experienced worker is expected to possess all of the entry-level competencies as well as the ability to implement programs to improve independent living skills and the ability to use a variety of treatment activities. The intermediate-level COTA may also be developing advanced skills in areas of special interest. This staff member is expected to perform all of the entry-level COTA functions and additional functions that are consistent with the additional experience and training. General supervision by an experienced OTR or an advanced level COTA is recommended for administrative functions.

The advanced-level COTA has three or more years of experience in a specialized area of practice. At this level, COTAs function in staff positions but demonstrate a higher level of performance than that of intermediate-level COTAs. Assigned job responsibilities vary from one facility to another, but these highly skilled staff members have advanced competencies in their specialty area and are capable of sharing their knowledge through education, publication, or participation in clinical studies. The advanced-level COTA is a skilled practitioner who requires only general supervision in clinical service and in administrative functions. The advanced-level COTA may function more independently in some types of clinical practice, but when the client's condition is unstable, supervision by an OTR is recommended (4, 5).

Table 6.1. COTA

	Entry	Intermediate	Advanced
Experience	Less than 1 year of practice experience as COTA	One or more years of practice as a COTA	More than 3 years experience
Competencies	Compentence in delivery of OT services under the direction of an OTR	Entry-level competence plus skill in implementing a variety of independent living skills and treatment activities	Demonstrates advanced clinical, educational, or administrative skills; shares knowledge through education, publication or clinical studies.
Examples of performance areas	Transmits requests for service to OTR; contributes to client assessment; assists OTR in planning and implementing treatment; reports client observations to OTR; maintains necessary documentation as directed by supervising OTR	Entry-level competencies plus greater independence in performing selected assessments, reports observations to OTR and other team members; assists in the documentation of treatment protocols, department records and procedures; provides in-service and community education; supervises entry-level COTAs, OT aides, volunteers, and COTA students	Performs assigned tasks at a higher level than an intermediate COTA and demonstrates greater knowledge of areas of practice; may contribute to a variety of department functions
Supervisory support	Close supervision of clinical performance by an intermediate or advanced OTR and general supervision of management functions by an experienced OTR or COTA	General clinical supervision from intermediate or advanced-level OTR and general management supervision by experienced OTR or advanced-level COTA	General clinical supervision from intermediate or advanced-level OTR; general management supervision by experienced OTR

Frequently COTAs are employed by nursing homes, group homes, and residential settings as directors of resident activities. In this type of position the COTA is able to function fairly independently in providing an ongoing program of meaningful activities to promote the overall health and well-being of residents. As an activity director, the COTA is directly responsible to the administrator of the facility and administers as well as implements the activity program. Keeping records of programming and resident participation are part of the COTA's role in this setting, as are ordering supplies and equipment, supervising volunteers, aides, and students, and managing the program budget. Activity programs of this kind are not considered occupational therapy, because they meet general rather than specific needs. If a COTA activity director finds a resident with specific functional problems who could benefit from occupational therapy intervention, an OTR should be consulted to evaluate the resident and develop a treatment plan (6).

ROLES AND FUNCTIONS OF THE OTR

The entry-level OTR has less than one year's practice experience as an OTR. According to the 1985 personnel classification (4), the primary function of this worker is "to provide occupational therapy services to patients/clients, including assessment, treatment planning and implementation, related documentation, and communication." Competencies as a general practitioner of occupational therapy are required. The personnel classification lists a number of critical performance areas for the entry-level OTR. This staff member is viewed as having greater responsibility for assessment and documentation of client problems than the entry-level COTA (Table 6.2). There are also greater responsibilities for administrative functions, and the entry-level OTR may be given some supervisory duties. Close supervision of the entry-level OTR's clinical performance and direct supervision of administrative functions should be given by an intermediate or advanced-level OTR.

The 1990 entry level role delineation generally affirmed these expectations and clarified the concept that the entry-level OTR must also establish his or her service competency in specific clinical procedures. Consultation is included as a form of intervention and the entry-level OTR is viewed as capable of case and colleague consultation. System consultation, in which the OTR addresses the needs of a larger system or agency, is seen as appropriate only for an experienced practitioner. Service management is described as a shared responsibility with the COTA, as are the maintenance of professional competencies, promotion of the profession, and ethical behavior (3).

An intermediate-level OTR has had one or more years of practice experience as an OTR. This staff member must demonstrate all of the established entry-level OTR skills and should be able to use a variety of treatment approaches independently. This practitioner may be developing advanced skills in one or more areas of occupational therapy and may be assigned higher level departmental functions. General supervision by an experienced OTR is recommended for clinical performance, and administrative supervision by an OTR with administrative experience is suggested.

The advanced-level OTR holds a graduate degree in occupational therapy or a related area and/or certification by an organization or group that offers continuing education, examination, or advanced practice requirements in a specialty area of practice. These practitioners must have three or more years of practice experience in a specialty area of occupational therapy practice. Their skills should reflect a broad range of experience and a greater depth of knowledge than the two previous OTR levels. At the advanced level, OTRs should show ability to integrate clinical theory and practice at a high level, resulting in evaluation and treatment services that are innovative, complex, and efficient. Advanced practitioners are expected to share their knowledge through staff and student education, publications, clinical studies, or research. The duties are likely to be diverse, and advanced practitioners should serve as a resource to their occupational therapy colleagues and to members of related professions in their areas of expertise. No supervision is required for these staff members when they are working in their specialty area of practice and only occasional supervision when working in nonspecialty areas. General supervision for administrative functions is recommended.

Two additional positions that require specialized skills were described for the OTR in the 1985 personnel classification: occupational therapy supervisor and department manager/director. The primary duties of a supervisor are to "supervise OTRs, COTAs, students, volunteers, and aides." Supervisors may also provide direct client service, but this may be omitted if they are responsible for super-

Table 6.2. OTR

	Entry	Intermediate	Advanced	Supervisor	Manager/Director
Experience	Less than 1 year experience	More than 1 year experience	More than 3 years	More than 3 years	More than 3 years
Competency	Competencies as general OT practioner	Demonstrated independence in use of varied treatment approaches	Broad range of experience and depth of knowledge; innovative, complex, and efficient clinical practice; shares knowledge with others	Thorough understanding of department policies and procedures; leadership potential; intermediate or advanced clinical skills	Thorough knowledge of OT and management principles and practices; understands department's objectives and functions and can communicate them to others
Examples of performance areas	Receives referrals for service; performs screening and assessments, plans and implements treatment procedures; documents services; complies with agency standards; supervises COTAs, aides, volunteers, and students	All entry-level tasks, plus greater development and provision of record keeping systems, continuing education; review of service program; of documentation of treatment protocols and procedures	Integrates clinical theory and practice at an advanced level; participates in providing student and staff education; publication, clinical research	Participation in staff selection, evaluates job performance, coordinates education and work schedule; implements departmental policies; assists with documentation of department goals and objectives; assists department manager	Hires and evaluates staff; develops and implements department policies and procedures; participates in organizational planning; represents department to other units of organization, ensures compliance with government and professional standards
Supervisory support	Close supervision of clinical performance; general administrative supervision by experienced OTR	General supervision of clinical performance; and general administrative supervision by experienced OTR	General clinical supervision as required; general administrative supervision by experienced OTR	General supervision of clinical performance by department manager and also of administrative responsibilities	General supervision by administration personnel of the organization

vising a large group of people. Coordination of occupational therapy fieldwork may be another role for the OTR supervisor. Additional education related to supervision is recommended for this job classification, and at least three years of clinical experience is considered necessary before assuming a supervisory role. This position requires an understanding of personnel and department policies, demonstrated leadership skills, good communication skills, and the ability to organize time, material, and personnel effectively. An occupational therapy supervisor should possess intermediate or advanced clinical skills. General supervision in clinical and administrative functions is recommended.

The final OTR position described in the 1985 document is that of occupational therapy department manager or director. This function includes "planning, organizing, directing, controlling, and coordinating all aspects of the department or service." Continuing education relevant to management and administration is a prerequisite for this position, and some practitioners may hold graduate degrees in administration and management. The amount of experience required to assume such responsibilities will vary with the size and scope of the department, but three years of clinical experience is suggested as a minimum requirement, with at least one of those years being spent in a supervisory role. Individuals who assume management positions must have "a thorough knowledge of occupational therapy and of management principles and practices; demonstrate understanding of department objectives and functions; and conceptualize, interpret, and integrate occupational therapy services into the relevant organizational context." The occupational therapy department manager works under the general supervision of the administrative personnel of the organization.

Tables 6.1 and 6.2 identify some of the key differences between the different levels of occupational therapy personnel. Generally the COTA is viewed as an implementer of occupational therapy services—the front-line worker who carries out vital client interventions. The COTA is viewed as having less responsibility for specialized assessment of client deficits, treatment planning, and independent delivery of services. Supervision is required for all three levels of COTA personnel, although the advanced-level COTA may need only minimal supervision. This document suggests that the OTR is expected to carry greater responsibility for assessment, treatment planning, supervision of treatment services, documentation, and administrative functions. At higher levels, responsibilities steadily increase, with additional education being needed to help the practitioner master more complex clinical and administrative skills. An entry-level OTR, however, might rely heavily on the experience and skills of an intermediate- or advanced-level COTA and might consult with that individual on many clinical and administrative matters.

SUPERVISION

Issues of supervision for both entry-level OTRs and COTAs are addressed in the 1990 document. Entry-level OTRs are urged to practice under the supervision of an experienced OTR initially. If this is not possible, it is recommended that an OTR be available for consultation or in a mentor relationship with the entry-level therapist (3).

COTA supervision is more stringent. The AOTA issued a new set of supervision guidelines for COTAs in 1990 for application in clinical settings. They state that, while the OTR has legal and ethical responsibility to provide supervision to the COTA, the COTA also has a legal and ethical responsibility to obtain adequate supervision. The degree of supervision will vary with the setting, the client population, and the service competence of the COTA.

Supervision may be either close or general. Close supervision usually means direct, on-site, daily contact. General supervision may be provided through frequent meetings and regular communication between supervisor and employee. In states that regulate occupational therapy practice, the state practice law supercedes any AOTA guidelines (7).

The 1990 role delineation recommends that the following things be considered when deciding on the appropriate level of supervision:

1. Current occupational therapy practice standards and guidelines;
2. Therapy needs within the life environment;
3. Complexity of evaluation and intervention methods used;
4. Proficiencies of the supervisee;
5. Regulations, policies, and procedures of the department or agency;
6. State laws and regulations; and
7. Reimbursement requirements (3).

ETHICAL CONSIDERATIONS

The 1990 role delineation recognized that all occupational therapy staff members have a responsibility to demonstrate ethical and professional attitudes. The following statements embody professional beliefs and attitudes that are expected of all occupational therapy practitioners.

1. All individuals have equal rights, privileges, and status.
2. All individuals have the right to expect the freedom to exercise choice in their lives.
3. Professionals adhere to moral and legal principles, including standards of accuracy, objectivity, honesty, and integrity.
4. Professionals are self-disciplined and are able to use sound judgment in their daily work.
5. Professionals are dedicated and concerned with the welfare of others and are advocates for those options that benefit their clients (8).

Appendix 2 of this text shows the Occupational Therapy Code of Ethics (1988) to which practitioners are expected to adhere in their daily practice.

OTR-COTA TEAMS

In recent years OTR-COTA teams have become recognized as an effective way to deliver occupational therapy services. In 1987 Blechert, Christiansen, and Kari identified some ways that OTRs and COTAs could function more effectively as a team and stressed the importance of respecting one another's knowledge and contributions to client care (9).

Egan has quoted members of OTR-COTA teams as saying that good communication, understanding of one another's roles, and a partnership concept helped them to develop close professional relationships. They emphasized that team members need to develop a cooperative rather than an adversarial relationship and must be able to depend on each other (10).

In 1991 the AOTA began to recognize exemplary OTR-COTA teams by giving an annual COTA/OTR Partnership Award. This award reflected the growing importance of OTR-COTA teams in clinical practice. In 1992 the AOTA announced a self-study program that will help to identify appropriate OTR and COTA roles in public school occupational therapy practice. It is clear that occupational therapy service is enhanced by the use of effective intraprofessional teams, and we can expect to see more of them as health care delivery becomes more complex.

EMERGING ROLES FOR COTAs AND OTRs

In the AOTA's 1990 Member Data Survey, members of the organization were asked to list their primary and secondary job functions. The results are shown in Tables 6.3 and 6.4. As one would expect, the majority of both OTRs and COTAs listed direct client service as their primary function. It is interesting to note that small percentages of COTAs listed administration, consultation, supervision, and teaching as primary functions. Even greater percentages of COTAs listed these areas as secondary functions (11). The COTA role is rapidly changing along with changing health

Table 6.3. Primary and Secondary Functions of OTRs

Function	Primary (%)	Secondary (%)
Administration	12.5	14.1
Consultation	6.5	33.1
Direct client service	72.3	16.6
Public relations/information	0.5	4.9
Research	0.5	1.8
Supervision	4.3	16.1
Classroom teaching	2.5	2.3
Fieldwork teaching	0.3	8.9
Other	0.5	2.2

Table 6.4. Primary and Secondary Functions of COTAs

Function	Primary (%)	Secondary (%)
Administration	3.5	11.4
Consultation	1.5	24.8
Direct client service	88.5	12.3
Public relations/information	0.7	10.3
Research	0.2	1.1
Supervision	2.3	14.6
Classroom teaching	2.3	5.9
Fieldwork teaching	0.3	13.3
Other	1.0	6.1

care priorities, and new roles are emerging for both levels of personnel.

One of the most important new roles to develop for the OTR is that of case manager. In the complex and confusing health care environment of the 1990s, it was becoming necessary for some health professional to take on the task of coordinating and organizing the many services that a given client might be receiving from multiple agencies. OTRs found that they had many of the skills needed for this task. A case manager may work for a health insurance company, a hospital, or an employer. The case manager tries to insure that the client receives the right services at the right time and at a reasonable cost. This is a demanding job that requires good knowledge of local resources and health care delivery patterns. It is certainly not an entry-level competency, but for the experienced therapist, case management offers the opportunity to use acquired experience and skills to benefit groups of clients. The AOTA has developed a position paper on the role of occupational therapists in case management, and we are likely to see greater numbers of therapists assuming this role (12).

COTAs are also seeing their roles expand as new practice areas develop. In 1991 some COTAs were working as environmental consultants who advised on environmental adaptations for persons with functional limitations. Others were serving as patient advocates and were entering private practice in specialty areas such as ergonomics, job evaluation, and work hardening (13). At least one COTA was employed in a medical equipment company where she functioned as a sales representative and a medical equipment specialist (14).

As OTRs and COTAs enter new practice roles, there are bound to be some frustrations. COTAs have often felt that they had to fight to achieve higher levels of responsibility.

Some OTRs have been and still are reluctant to permit COTAs to function more independently in their areas of expertise. COTAs have sometimes been left out when new programs were being planned or when standards were being written. Many experienced COTAs have felt that their skills were not being fully utilized (15). As it heads into an unsettled period for health care, occupational therapy cannot afford to overlook any of its resources. It is likely that COTAs will become even more indispensable to occupational therapy programs as health care resources are stretched to their limits.

Discussion Questions

1. Invite an OTR-COTA team to visit your class and discuss their roles. How did they work out complementary roles?
2. What promotional opportunities are there for OTRs and COTAs in your area?
3. What innovative roles are OTRs or COTAs assuming in your local area?
4. Read some job descriptions of OTR/COTA positions in your area. What roles and functions are described, and what level of experience is required for the positions?
5. Many students enter occupational therapy because of its direct service opportunities. For the experienced practitioner, however, there are likely to be supervisory or administrative responsibilities as well. How do you feel about assuming these roles later in your career?

References

1. Hirama H: A chronological review. In Ryan S, ed. *The Certified Occupational Therapy Assistant: Roles and Responsibilities*. Thorofare, NJ, Slack, 1986, pp. 23–24.
2. Shapiro D, Brown D: The delineation of the role of entry-level occupational therapy personnel. *AJOT* 35:306–311, 1986.
3. AOTA: Entry-level role delineation for registered occupational therapists (OTRs) and certified occupational therapy assistants (COTAs). *AJOT* 44(12):1091–1102, 1990.
4. Schell BA: Guide to occupational therapy personnel. *AJOT* 49:803–810, 1985. (Approved by the Representative Assembly, April, 1985).
5. Ryan S: Therapeutic intervention: an overview. In Ryan S, ed. *The Certified Occupational Therapy Assistant: Roles and Responsibilities*. Thorofare, NJ, Slack, 1986, pp. 149–152.
6. Ryan S: The Role of the COTA as an activities director. In Ryan S, ed. *The Certified Occupational Therapy Assistant: Roles and Responsibilities*. Thorofare, NJ, Slack, 1986, pp. 295–304.
7. AOTA: Supervision guidelines for certified occupational therapy assistants. *AJOT* 44(12):1089–1090, 1990.
8. AOTA: *PATRA: The Professional and Technical Role Analysis Project, Final Report*. Rockville, MD, AOTA, 1988.
9. Blechert T, Christiansen M, Kari N: Intraprofessional team building. *AJOT* 41(9):576–582, 1987.
10. Egan M: COTAs and OTRs in conversation. *OT Week* March 19, 1992, pp. 14.
11. AOTA: 1990 member data survey. *OT Week* 5(22):6, 1991.
12. Special issue on case management. *OT Week* 5(12):4–9, 1991.
13. Tapper BE: Expanding their roles. *OT Week* 5(24):14–15, 1991.
14. Copley J: The role of the COTA in a medical equipment company. *Occupational Therapy Forum* Aug 26, 1987, pp. 12–13.
15. Fox S: COTAs talk about their frustrations and their future. *Adv Occup Ther* 7(22):6–7, 1991.

SECTION II

PRACTICE ARENA OF OCCUPATIONAL THERAPY

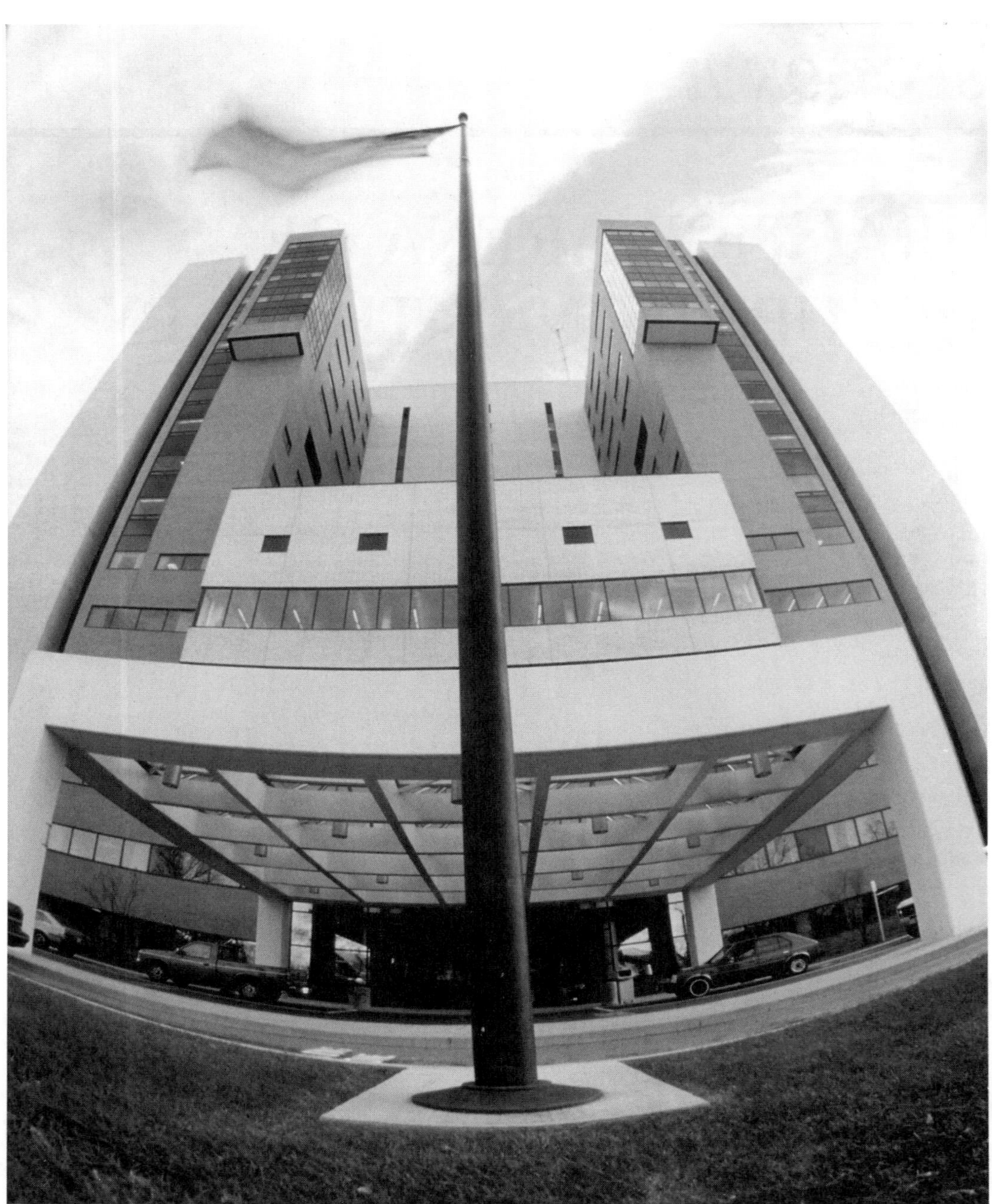

7 Health Care Funding and Services in the United States

Joseph P. is a small farmer who has had a hard time financially for the past ten years. He cannot afford health insurance and is not poor enough to qualify for Medicaid in his state or old enough to qualify for Medicare. A few months ago his health began to rapidly deteriorate. He had difficulty breathing and finally went to see a local doctor. The doctor ordered a lung biopsy at a local nonprofit hospital. The hospital demanded $300 as an advance payment before they would admit Mr. P., but he did not have the money. His doctor was forced to admit him as an emergency patient in order to get around the advance payment. The biopsy showed an advanced stage of lung cancer. Mr. P's doctor knew that Joseph needed radiation treatment, which was available only at a for-profit hospital in a nearby community, but that hospital refused to admit Mr. P since he was uninsured. After several weeks of effort, a legal aid society forced the hospital to admit him but it was far too late. Joseph P. died three months later, the victim of a fragmented and profit-oriented health care system.

Why is health care in such a crisis today in the United States? How did it get this way? In order to answer these questions we must review the current health care environment in the United States and look at how health services and the funding of health services evolved.

CURRENT HEALTH CARE SCENE

Health care in the United States today is the nation's second largest industry, surpassed in size only by the defense industry. In 1992 the United States was spending over 12% of its gross national product (GNP) on health care—the highest rate in the developed world. By contrast, the British were spending only 6% of their GNP on health care. Swedish citizens were spending 5%, and Canadian nationals were spending 9.5%.

Although the United States ranked first in health care costs during the 1990s, its citizens were not necessarily receiving the world's best health care services. One index of the adequacy of health care services is the infant mortality rate. Only a few years ago the United States ranked 14th among the countries of the world in infant mortality. In 1990, according to UNICEF, it ranked 21st, behind such areas as East Germany, Singapore, and Hong Kong. The mortality rate for black babies in the United States was double that of the rate for white babies (1).

In 1986 the average American visited a doctor 5.4 times a year. During 1987 the American Hospital Association reported a total of 34.4 million hospital admissions, with an average length of stay of 6.4 days (2). In 1990 the average American family was spending at least 10% of its income on health care. Fifteen per cent of the population had no health care insurance at all.

Hospitals continue to be the largest segment of the health care industry, and hospital costs account for 2/3 of the average medical bill. The number of community hospitals has declined steadily since 1985 due to their difficulty competing with larger, better-funded hospitals. Since 1980, 558 community hospitals have closed, mostly in rural areas.

Other components of the industry are nursing homes and long-term care facilities, clinics for ambulatory care, mental health services, outpatient surgical centers, clinical laboratories, pharmacies, pharmaceutical companies, medical equipment suppliers, and a variety of specialized care services.

Unlike most other industrialized countries, the United States does not have a single, unified system of health care. American health care most closely resembles a large shopping mall where a variety of health services are available from public or private vendors for a variety of prices. It includes a bewildering variety of institutions, clinics, laboratories, government agencies, business organizations, and independent practitioners. In the United States, health care has developed along the lines of private business, with fee-for-service being the traditional pattern of payment. To understand the status of health care in the United States, it is necessary to review how services developed and how they reached their present form.

PREINDUSTRIAL PHASE

In discussing the evolution of health care in America, Ehrenreich (3) describes two phases of development: the preindustrial phase that went up to the 1930s and the industrial period from the 1930s to the present. This is a useful distinction, since health care services in the 19th and early 20th century resembled a cottage industry and functioned quite differently from those of today. In the early years of the nation, health care was largely the responsibility of each individual or family. Doctors were rare, so people had to care for most illnesses or injuries on their own. Books on home medical care provided some guidance, and in many communities persons with a special talent for healing developed reputations as lay practitioners. The few physicians who were available had a minimal education. Their real training occurred primarily during an apprenticeship to an experienced doctor. What medical services there were rested in the hands of these independent practitioners, and the few hospitals that existed were custodial institutions (hospices) for the destitute or the mentally ill. In 1910 the Flexner report brought to light the poor quality of many medical schools that were then in operation. The report helped to establish higher educational standards for medical education, and many substandard medical schools were forced to close as a result of this tightening of educational requirements. Those that survived were substantially modernized and improved.

By 1910, hospitals had begun to play a more important role in health care. In Europe, hospitals had evolved from charity institutions to public facilities staffed by physicians who were employed by the hospital. In the United States, however, a mixed economy of hospitals developed. Some hospitals were public, tax-supported institutions; others were nonprofit institutions run by religious or charitable organizations (voluntary hospitals); still others were private, for-profit institutions (proprietary hospitals). Hospitals were financed through patient fees; they charged the individual on a fee-for-service basis. With the development of nursing as a trained profession, the division of labor in health care began. By the end of the 19th century, hospitals had developed into a sizable industry that was organized along business lines. As standards of cleanliness and personal care improved, hospitals overcame their previous reputation as "pest houses" and became an important adjunct to medical care. Gradually hospitals began to limit their care to the acute phases of illness rather than to its full course. Other institutions began to develop to serve the needs of patients who required long-term nursing care. These included nursing and convalescent homes as well as sanitariums for the treatment of specific diseases such as tuberculosis.

As hospital budgets increased, new patterns of financing hospital care were inevitable. The number of charity cases treated declined as hospitals became more business oriented. Although state and local governments operated their own hospitals and accepted patients who were unable to pay for their care, these institutions were unable to keep up with the health care needs of the poor, the chronically ill and disabled, and the unemployed. Gradually a two-tiered system of health care evolved: a highly developed private sector for those who could afford to pay for care and an underdeveloped public sector that provided care for the poor and those with chronic medical problems. Public institutions were filled with patients who had tuberculosis, alcoholism, and mental disorders—diseases of social disorganization (4). Public health in America was relegated to a secondary status and lagged far behind private medicine in prestige and financial resources. The underfinanced public health establishment was never able to assume a leadership or coordinating role in health care.

In the early years of the 20th century, hospitals functioned fairly independently, with local trustees, physicians, and administrators deciding on the policies and procedures for their particular institution. There was little attempt to integrate services in hospital care, ambulatory care, or public health. Group practice (the organization of a group of physicians into a clinic), which could offer a broader array of medical services than the individual practitioner, began to develop in the 1880s. The Mayo Clinic in Rochester, Minnesota, was the prototype for this type of practice. Typically, doctors financed such clinics and became their owners while other doctors became their employees. Thus a new type of profit-making organization entered American medical practice. Group practices gradually spread throughout the country, although many physicians continued to practice independently. By the 1920s, other health-related industries were developing, such as the pharmaceutical industry and hospital equipment industries.

As the demand for medical services grew, doctors were forced to delegate some of their responsibilities as health care providers. They did this in three ways: (*a*) by using young doctors in training to help provide hospital care; (*b*) by encouraging responsible professionalism in a number of related health care fields; and (*c*) by employing women in auxiliary health care service roles. Professionalism was encouraged to free the physician from the need to directly supervise every aspect of care. Doctors, however, maintained their position of authority over other health care workers and never relinquished their role as direct intermediary between the patient and the health care system. The subordinate health care professions eventually became rigidly stratified, with a large gap between their status and that of the physician.

Throughout the preindustrial period of development, physicians had been able to maintain control of the health care market and services. Even in the 19th century, however, a small number of Americans had begun to carry some insurance against sickness through an employer, a fraternal order, a trade union, or a commercial insurance company. The need for health insurance centered around four basic types of costs:

Individual loss of income;
Individual medical costs;
Indirect costs of illness to society; and
Social costs of medical care.

By the end of World War I, all of the European countries had developed some form of coverage of health care costs for their citizens. Most of these plans were part of a general program of social insurance against the risks that interrupted the income of workers: industrial accidents, sickness and disability, old age, and unemployment. Such plans were worker-oriented and were intended to stabilize incomes and offer some degree of protection against catastrophic events. In the United States, however, government was highly decentralized and there was much less government involvement in programs of social welfare. There was no national sponsor for the types of programs developed in the European countries and no structure on which to build such programs.

From the beginning of the 20th century, various types of national health insurance plans had been proposed, but each time they were defeated. Labor organizations did not favor the concept. Employers saw compulsory health insurance as contrary to their interests. The private insurance industry, which was beginning to do a flourishing business in private sickness insurance, was strongly opposed to a national health insurance plan. The most vehement opposition came from the physicians themselves and their national organization, the American Medical Association (AMA). Doctors feared that they would lose their autonomy under such a system, and they also believed that national health insurance would place limits on their income.

By the 1920s and 1930s a concern was developing over the cost of medical care. As the middle class began to feel the effect of higher costs for health care services, they began turning in larger numbers to private insurers who offered at least partial coverage of costs. With the impact of the Great Depression of the late 1920s, there was renewed interest in a program of national health insurance. Unemployment insurance, however, was considered to be an even higher priority and took precedence. Old age benefits were also a major concern, and in 1935 Congress passed the Social Security Act, which provided a minimum income for retired persons and some additional welfare health care costs, although that had not originally been part of the package.

EARLY INDUSTRIAL PHASE: 1930–1950

The severe economic depression resulted in a sharp drop in spending for medical care. Doctors and hospitals, whose incomes had fallen abruptly, no longer felt that they could provide free services to the poor and began to ask state and local welfare departments to pay for the cost of health services for this population. Welfare departments began to do so on a temporary basis, and this set the precedent for government financing of health care for low-income groups. In the mid-1930s the AMA softened its opposition to private health insurance, as more and more people began to take advantage of such plans. Physicians were now seeing that private insurance coverage could increase rather than decrease their incomes and need not substantially interfere with the doctor-patient relationship. In 1946 the AMA created the Associated Medical Care Plans, the precursor of Blue Shield, and entered into their own version of private health insurance (5). Another type of insurance plan, Blue Cross, was developed by the hospital industry.

After World War II, President Truman included a program of national health insurance in his election platform, but the AMA and other health care interests opposed the plan and it was abandoned, except for some funding to expand hospitals and allow new hospital construction. The strong fear of "socialized medicine" prevented compulsory health insurance from developing, and the groups that had formed an alliance to support it eventually drifted apart. By 1952 over half of all Americans had purchased some health insurance. Labor unions had now entered the scene and had successfully bargained for health care benefits for their members (6). The extent of coverage was highly variable, however, and the persons most likely to be insured through employer plans were workers living in urban industrial areas. The unemployed, those living in rural areas, the elderly, and the chronically ill—those who needed it most—remained uninsured.

Private health insurance plans offered three different types of benefits:

1. Indemnity benefits (in which the insurer reimbursed the consumer for partial costs of medical care);
2. Service benefits (in which the insurer paid the physician or hospital for services rendered, often in full); and
3. Direct services (in which the insurer directly provided health care services to

the consumer in return for prepayment).

Each type of insurance plan contained some mechanism for cost control and limitation of services.

In the 1930s and 1940s, indemnity and service-benefit plans predominated. Slowly, however, a few direct service plans began to appear. These early health cooperatives enrolled members for a set monthly or annual fee and provided a full range of health services. They built their own clinics and hospitals and employed their own staff to provide ambulatory care. Popularly known as health maintenance organizations (HMOs), they emphasized prevention and health maintenance in addition to offering sickness care. Their coverage was usually more comprehensive than indemnity or service-benefit plans; however, start-up costs were high and, since no government aid was available to them in the 1950s, they were largely local ventures. They attracted widespread interest, however, since they seemed to be effective in controlling health care costs by stressing prevention, providing maximum ambulatory care services, using physician extenders, and minimizing hospitalization (4, 7).

INCREASING INDUSTRIALIZATION: 1950–1970

With the increased use of health insurance, the industrial phase of health care delivery had begun. By the early 1950s, commercial insurance plans were gaining ground over the service-benefit plans of Blue Cross and Blue Shield. As commercial health insurance expanded, the nature of the health care industry changed. Individual policies were still being sold, but the bulk of health insurance was now being marketed for groups as employee health benefit plans became one of the standard fringe benefits of employment. Starr, in his book *The Social Transformation of American Medicine* (4), sums it up by saying:

> *America had taken a different road to health insurance than the one taken by European societies, and it arrived at a different destination. The original European model began with the industrial working class and emphasized income maintenance. From that base, it expanded in both its coverage of the population and the range of benefits. . . . But in America, there was no institutional structure for health insurance when the middle class encountered problems in paying for hospital costs during the 1920's and when the hospitals encountered problems in meeting their expenses during the depression. . . . America developed an insurance system . . . to improve access of middle-class patients to hospitals; an insurance system developed under the control of the hospitals and doctors that sought to buttress the existing forms of organization.*

The evolution of health insurance was a direct outcome of the private enterprise system that had developed in the United States.

In the years that followed World War II, an immense medical research establishment developed in the United States. From the early part of the 20th century, the chief sources of mortality had been shifting from infectious to chronic disease. Research into the causes of cancer, heart disease, and other life-threatening diseases had become a high priority. The public was also concerned about some of the behavioral problems that were being seen with greater frequency: alcoholism, drug use, and delinquency. The federal government generously supported medical research in many areas, and private foundations supplemented this effort by providing private funding for health research and projects. Hospitals had benefitted from increased governmental support as well. The Hill-Burton Act of 1946 had provided construction funds for community hospitals in underserved areas, and many small hospitals were able to expand under this program. Medicine was becoming highly specialized and more and more young doctors were choosing to enter lucrative specialty practices rather than general practice. The higher levels of education required for specialization helped to raise health care costs even further.

By the early 1960s it was recognized that large segments of the population did not have access to adequate medical care. Congress had provided funding to educate greater numbers of health care workers and had encouraged the development of community-based mental health services and ambulatory care clinics; despite this, health care resources were unevenly distributed and not readily available to the underprivileged. The antipoverty and civil rights programs, begun during the Kennedy administration and continued by President Johnson, helped to focus awareness on the health needs of the poor, the elderly, and minority groups. By 1965 there was adequate Congressional support for passage of the Medicare and Medicaid programs. Medicare provided both compulsory hospital insurance (part A) for persons over the age of 65 under the umbrella of the Social Security Act and a government-subsidized voluntary insurance program to cover physicians' bills (part B). Medicaid provided for federal grants to the states for programs of medical assistance for the poor. States were given considerable discretion in how Medicaid funds would be applied, and eligibility requirements varied widely. The objective of both programs was to enable the poor and the elderly to "buy into" the private health care system. Despite these measures, the gap between health care services available to the middle-class and low-income groups actually widened. By the 1970s a large group of people still lacked financial protection for periods of illness or disability. Part-time workers, the recently unemployed, and the working poor who earned too little to afford private insurance but too much to qualify for public assistance were still left out of the picture.

COST-CONTAINMENT MEASURES: 1970–1985

The 1970s brought a wave of disillusionment with the health care system in general and physicians in particular. Health care costs had soared out of control, and the government was forced to intervene in a direct way. In 1970 a federal program was authorized that provided funding to establish HMOs. State governments began to enact tougher laws regulating the health care industry and requiring state approval (certificates of need) for the construction of new hospitals and nursing homes. In 1973 a federal law was passed requiring businesses with more than 25 employees to offer at least one qualified HMO as an option in employee health insurance coverage. In 1974 a new health planning law established 200 Health Systems Agencies (HSAs) that were given responsibility for drawing up three-year plans, reviewing proposed new health projects, and recommending action to the states and the federal government on certificates of need and the use of federal funds. Health care planning was now seen as an urgent need and as the responsibility of the public sector. A proposal for national health insurance came very close to being introduced by the Nixon administration, but, as in the past, other needs took priority and it did not reach Congress.

By 1979 there were 217 HMOs operating throughout the country, and they were providing health care at significantly lower costs than traditional medical practices. With the election of Ronald Reagan to the presidency, a wave of political conservatism swept the country, which affected health care as well as other segments of the economy. The Reagan administration believed that America's health care problems could best be resolved by reducing government involvement to a minimum and relying instead on competition and the incentives of the marketplace to contain health care costs and restructure services. Consumers, doctors, hospitals, and even the insurance companies were reluctant to lose the benefits of federally funded programs and the public programs of medical assistance and voiced their opposition strongly. The Reagan administration was forced to modify its position and left the Medicare and Medicaid programs in place; however, substantial cuts in funding were made in public health services and medical assistance for the poor. There was also much less inclination for the government to continue its efforts to regulate the health care industry.

RISE OF FOR-PROFIT HEALTH CARE CHAINS

During the 1980s a new type of health care organization appeared. This was the large health-care corporation that bought up hospitals and other health service organizations and proceeded to operate them along corporate lines. These large corporate enterprises in health care became highly visible and were extremely attractive to private investors. Relman (8) wrote that we were seeing the rise of a "medical-industrial complex" in the United States, with the large health care chains becoming a central element in the delivery of health services. By 1991 25% of all nonfederal acute care hospitals were investor-owned and this percentage was expected to increase (1). Humana was the largest of the hospital chains with 82 hospitals, and in 1991 was expected to earn revenues of over $6 billion. Second in size was the Hospital Corporation of America (HCA) with 75 acute care hospitals and 53 psychiatric hospitals. National Medical Enterprises was third with 38 hospitals (1).

Proprietary nursing homes were an even bigger business, with many owned by small investors or physicians. About a third of the diagnostic laboratories were owned by profit-making companies. Other health services were also being taken over by business interests. Home care services, formerly provided by public health programs or community agencies, were growing rapidly and included such services as nursing care, homemaking assistance, physical and occupational therapy, respiratory therapy, and pacemaker monitoring. Additional related services such as mobile computerized tomography (CT) scanning, cardiopulmonary testing, industrial health screening, rehabilitation counseling, dental care, weight-control clinics, alcohol- and drug-abuse programs, and fitness centers were being aggressively marketed by private entrepreneurs. Two areas of special interest are hospital emergency room services and long-term hemodialysis programs for patients with end-stage renal disease. Large corporations have taken over these services in some areas and provide them to hospitals on a contract basis.

The move toward corporate control and management of health services may have both positive and negative effects. On the one hand, it may result in slowing down health care cost increases through strong central management of the corporate structures and increase the efficiency of health care delivery. On the other hand, health care may not respond to the classic laws of supply and demand, since the consumer of health care is often not really free or knowledgeable enough to shop around for the best bargain in health care services. Also, private enterprises exist to sell their services. The more they sell, the more profit they make. This sales emphasis has the potential for consumer exploitation in health services and will require some type of regulation. Lindorf (1) points out that for-profit hospitals do not locate in low-income or minority neighborhoods and they tend to provide very little charity care. Also, most of the for-profit hospitals have deliberately chosen not to provide emergency room services since this type of care tends to lose money for the hospital. Some health care corporations have made attempts to buy or lease teaching hospitals for their prestige value and their key role in health care research and advanced medical practice (1). Apparently health care corporations are here to stay, but their overall impact on the health care environment remains to be seen. Nonprofit hospitals have tended to follow the lead of the for-profit chains in order to compete for patients, and so the influence of the for-profits is greater than their numbers would indicate.

MULTIPLE HEALTH CARE SYSTEMS

American health care evolved in a free-enterprise system as a network of private business enterprises. Government has played a role when necessary to guarantee health services for the underprivileged in society, to promote research, and to regulate the health care industry. According to Torrens (9), there are at least four health care systems operating in the United States today. First, there is the system of health care used by middle and upper income groups (frequently referred to as *the* American health care system). Each individual or family puts together a set of services to meet their needs and pays for them out of their own resources or through private insurance. This service system revolves around the physician, who coordinates services to some degree and calls on specialized services as needed. Local community hospitals are used most frequently by this group of consumers. The individual services used have little formal connection with one another, and the only thread of continuity in care is provided by the physician or by the consumer.

A second system of health care is used by the poor, the inner-city dwellers, and minority groups. Again there is no formal system but rather a loose network of services that the individual or family uses to meet immediate needs. These groups tend to have no continuity of care through a single provider. Some routine prevention services such as immunizations are available through local health departments, and the hospital emergency room is often used as a source of treatment for acute illness or injury. City or county hospitals are most frequently used when hospitalization is required, and outpatient clinics of public hospitals may provide some ambulatory care. To some extent these patients are now beginning to enter private hospitals and nursing homes because of reimbursement through Medicare and Medicaid funds. Health care is generally unplanned and unmonitored for these groups.

A third system of health care is that provided by the military services. Extensive health care services are available to all active military personnel and their families. This is a highly organized system and is available everywhere military personnel are found. This system emphasizes total care, with a particular emphasis on preventing illness and injury.

A fourth health care system is that of the Veterans Administration, which was designed to provide medical care for retired, disabled veterans. It is a hospital-based system, with 171 hospitals located within the continental United States, and now provides some outpatient care as well. Torrens notes that the two civilian systems are informal and haphazard in their organization. There are many health situations that fall between the cracks, and entry into each system requires a certain amount of know-how. These multiple systems of health care make for areas of overlap and areas of scarcity of services. No one authority plays a coordinating role.

Mechanic (10) says that physicians in the United States have concentrated on developing private, entrepreneurial medicine rather than on building a rational system of health care. Because demands for care have always exceeded the resources available, various forms of rationing have existed. The most basic form is fee-for-service medicine. Care has been available only to those who could purchase it, and this was in effect a method of rationing resources. A second method is by implicit rationing. In countries that have a government-sponsored health insurance system, health care is rationed through centralized budgeting for health expenditures or by limiting the resources available to insured consumers. Today most societies are moving toward the explicit rationing of health care, in which limits are set on total expenditures for health services but rational decisions are made as to which services will be supported. Mechanic contends that under the latter system the physician's role shifts from that of expert to that of bureaucrat:

> *The locus of control for medical decision-making is a key variable in examining the implications of medical care for social life more generally. . . . In a bureaucratic structure, physicians are rewarded more for being good*

managers and researchers . . . than for providing interested and humane care. (10)

According to Mechanic, the bureaucratization of medicine is inevitable, and he warns that the humane aspects of health care may be neglected in the effort to make the technology of health care work.

HEALTH CARE TRENDS IN THE UNITED STATES

Two significant pieces of legislation were passed in the late 1980s and early 1990s that had an impact on health care and public welfare. In 1987 Congress passed the Omnibus Budget Reconciliation Act of Nursing Home Reform (OBRA). This act set new criteria for staffing patterns, required prompt assessment of residents' needs, paid greater attention to residents' rights, and raised the standards for quality of care in nursing homes. It was applied to nearly 15,000 long-term care facilities across the country and did much to improve the level of care in those facilities. Nursing homes have more and more become the location for convalescent and rehabilitative care as hospital costs have risen and hospital stays have become shorter.

In 1990 President Bush signed the Americans with Disabilities Act (ADA). This far-reaching legislation protected millions of disabled United States citizens from discrimination and provided them with greater access to employment, transportation, and communications systems. The ADA has been called a civil rights act for the disabled and will benefit around 36 million Americans with disabilities.

President Reagan had signed the Medicare Catastrophic Coverage Act of 1988 but the resulting outcry from older citizens forced its repeal. Intended to cover the costs of catastrophic illness for Medicare recipients, it imposed a substantial premium on Medicare subscribers to cover costs. Many of the elderly population found that the new government-sponsored insurance duplicated coverage that they already had in existing Medigap health insurance policies. They objected strenuously to paying for extra coverage that they didn't need. Another objection centered around the fact that the bill failed to provide coverage for long-term care, and with more of the population living to advanced ages, this was viewed as a serious deficiency.

Other attempts to expand Medicare and Medicaid were more successful. OBRA improved the way providers were reimbursed for Medicare-covered services, and a new fee schedule was prepared and was to be phased in by 1996. In 1990 an Early and Periodic Screening, Diagnosis, and Treatment Program (EPSDT) was established by the federal government to provide services to the 0- to 21-year-old population as an expansion of Medicaid. This program was intended to provide early diagnosis and intervention for childhood disorders of children from low-income households.

The United States was facing a serious crisis in health care during the 1990s as cost of services continued to escalate despite private and public attempts at cost controls. Access to health services was another major issue. Due to a sluggish national economy, many people were losing their jobs and also losing their health insurance. The middle class was beginning to face the same lack of access to health care that the poor had faced for decades. Quality of care also seemed to be declining as hospitals and other health care facilities struggled to contain costs and compete for the consumers' health care dollar. By 1992 a number of health care reform bills had been introduced to Congress and were making their way through legislative committees.

REFORM PROPOSALS

The proposed health care reforms tended to fall into three general categories. The most limited approach attempted to make health care more affordable for the average person. Tax breaks and limited regulation of health insurance premiums were proposed to help small businesses and the self-employed buy affordable health insurance. A second approach was to try to expand the employer-based health insurance system. Often referred to as "the pay or play plan," this type of approach would expect employers either to provide their employees with a minimum health insurance package or to pay the government to enroll them in a public health insurance program. This program would maintain employer-based health insurance but would offer businesses an option on how to provide health benefits. The third option, and the most extreme of the three approaches, would create a universal public health insurance plan that would cover all United States citizens and be funded through a combination of premiums and taxation. Each approach had its advocates, and in the 1992 presidential election, health care reform became a major issue that the candidates were forced to address (11, 12).

Since action on the federal level was moving so slowly, a number of states decided to enact their own health care reforms. Minnesota passed a comprehensive HealthRight program that was to take effect in 1996. Vermont established a common benefit plan for all health insurers that went into effect in 1992, and its legislature was studying the possible adoption of either a single-payer plan or a universal access health care plan. In 1974 Hawaii had passed a Prepaid Health Act that gave basic health insurance coverage to all employees who worked 19.5 or more hours a week. This was followed in 1989 by the State Health Insurance Program that covered the unemployed and those who worked less than 19.5 hours a week. Oregon in 1989 established a high-risk pool to provide health insurance to those who were uninsurable because of preexisting medical conditions. Later the Oregon Health Plan was enacted and it included Medicaid, the high-risk pool, and employer health plans. Massachusetts passed a "pay or play" type of program and a number of other states were considering single-payer legislation in 1992. It may be more realistic to look for health care reforms at the state level, since national representatives seem fearful of making any substantial change at the federal level (13, 14).

Kemper and Novak pointed out in 1992 that large amounts of money were being poured into lobbying efforts to defeat or limit health care reform proposals on the federal level. These funds were coming from political action committees (PACs) that represented organizations ranging from the AMA to pharmaceutical and insurance companies who had a vested interest in maintaining the current health care scene. The multibillion dollar health care industry would have a lot to lose if real health care reforms were enacted, and they appeared determined to protect their interests (11).

PREDICTIONS FOR THE 1990s

In 1990 Anthony Kovner, editor of *Health Care Delivery in the United States* (15), reviewed the forecasts of future trends in health care made by a number of distinguished observers. Based on these and on his assessment of current trends, Kovner predicted the following developments for United States health care in the next five years.

1. Failure of the effort to establish a national health insurance system in the United States;
2. Fewer but larger groups of health care providers competing for the consumers' health care dollars in local markets;
3. Less use of medical care by consumers on an age-adjusted basis;
4. Increased state regulation of cost, quality, and access to health care; and
5. Declining decision-making power of physicians on health care issues.

ISSUES FOR FUTURE RESOLUTION

As we progress through the 1990s, Lindorf suggests that American consumers of health care should seriously consider the following questions:

Where is United States health care headed? Government policies are presently encouraging the growth of for-profit health facilities. Is this the way we want to go?

At what point does the doctor's loyalty belong to the for-profit hospital rather than to the patient? Can the doctor remain the patient's advocate in a profit-oriented system of care?

Does the free market approach make for better health care?

Does the free market approach reduce health care costs? So far, it has not appeared to do so.

Will the gap between health care for the affluent and that for the poor become even greater as a result of business-oriented health care?

What can be done to guide the health care industry's development so that it becomes an affordable and a democratically controlled system of care? (1)

Discussion Questions

1. Is health care a right or a privilege? Do you believe that every person has an inherent right to health services?
2. Should local communities have the right to control their local health care resources as they do their public schools?
3. How do minorities and low-income groups obtain health care in your community?
4. Is there a for-profit hospital in your area? How do its services and costs compare with local nonprofit hospitals?
5. Whose problem is it to control health care costs? The government? The hospitals? The doctors? The insurance companies? Consumers?
6. Should health care policies and decisions be made by the federal government to ensure the public good, or should they be left to private provider organizations?
7. What type of health insurance do you and your family have? Do you know what it covers? Are there any services that are specifically excluded?
8. Does your state have a health plan that lists the state's priorities for allocation of funds to health services? If so, what are the top priorities?
9. Should hospital and health insurance managers be licensed by the state so that they can be legally held accountable to the public when abuses or negligence occurs?
10. How can consumers influence public policies on health care?

References

1. Lindorf D: *Marketplace Medicine*. New York, Bantam Books, 1992.
2. Jonas S: Population data for health and health care. In Kovner AR, ed. *Health Care Delivery in the United States*, ed. 4. New York, Springer, 1990, pp. 31–49.
3. Ehrenreich B: The health care industry: a theory of industrial medicine. In Lee PR, Estes CL, Ramsay NB, eds. *The Nation's Health*. ed 2. San Francisco, Boyd & Fraser, 1984, pp. 187–195.
4. Starr P: *The Social Transformation of American Medicine*. New York, Basic Books, 1982, pp. 30–198, 235–449.
5. Numbers RL: The third party: health insurance in America. In *The Nation's Health*, ed 2. San Francisco, Boyd & Fraser, 1984, pp. 196–204.
6. Munts R: *Bargaining for Health: Labor Unions, Health Insurance, and Medical Care*. Madison, University of Wisconsin Press, 1967, pp. 81–100.
7. Luft HS: Definition and scope of the HMO concept. In Lee PR, Estes CL, Ramsay NB, eds. *The Nation's Health*, ed 2. San Francisco, Boyd & Fraser, 1984, pp. 243–250.
8. Relman AS: The new medical-industrial complex. In Lee PR, Estes CL, Ramsay NB, eds. *The Nation's Health*, ed 2. San Francisco, Boyd & Fraser, 1984, pp. 233–242.
9. Torrens PR: Overview of the health services in the United States. In Lee PR, Estes CL, Ramsay NB, eds. *The Nation's Health*, ed 2. San Francisco, Boyd & Fraser, 1984, pp. 223–232.
10. Mechanic D: The growth of medical technology and bureaucracy: implications for medical care. In Lee PR, Estes CL, Ramsay NB, eds. *The Nation's Health*, ed 2. San Francisco, Boyd & Fraser, 1984, pp. 205–215.
11. Kemper V, Novak V: What's blocking health care reform? *Common Cause Magazine*, Jan/Feb/Mar 1992, pp. 8–13, 25.
12. Fein R: Prescription for change. *Modern Maturity* Aug/Sept 1992, pp. 22–30, 34–35.
13. Joe B: Health care reform: a high priority for states. *OT Week* 6(29):16–17, 1992.
14. Joe B: States take lead in health care reform. *OT Week* 6(30):12–13, 1992.
15. Kovner AR (ed): Futures. In *Health Care Delivery in the United States*, ed. 4. New York, Springer, pp. 510–532, 1990.

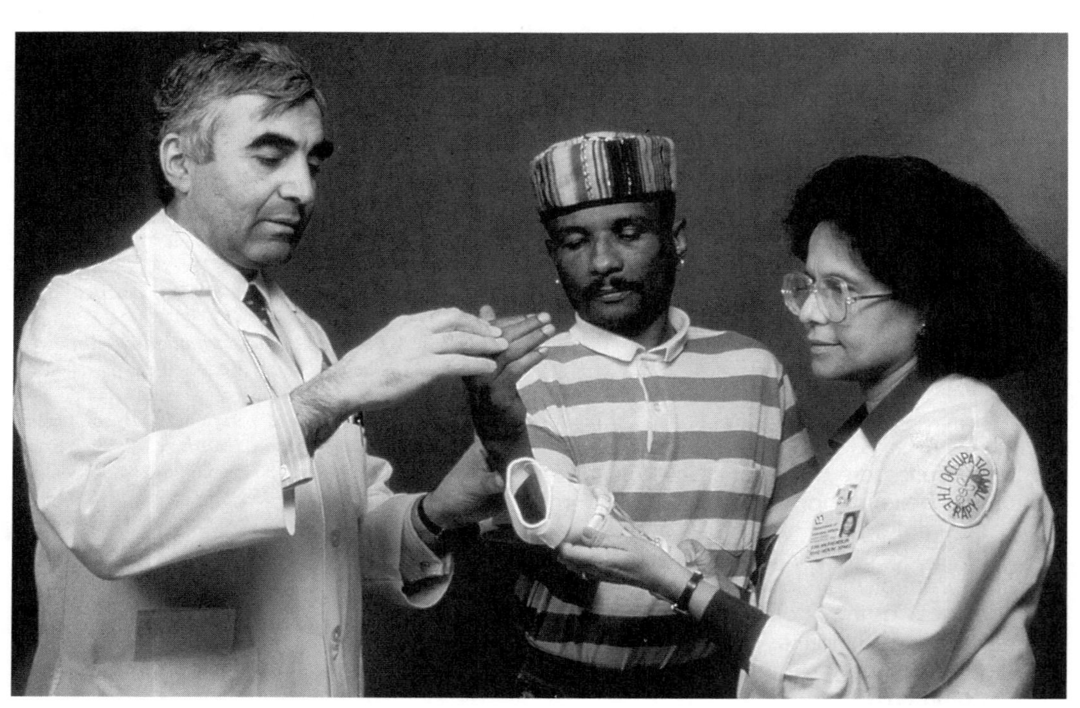
THERAPY

8 Working Together: The Health Care Team

Martha K. Stavros, ACSW, BCD, and Daraleen C. Sitka, OTR

Graduate occupational therapists have the opportunity to practice in a variety of professional settings but most will function as part of a team effort. The volume, complexity, and cost of effective service delivery today requires the collaborative efforts of many disciplines. The shift away from the narrow medical model that viewed the client as a machine with a faulty part has yielded to the larger conceptualization of the patient as a whole person. The recognition that the person treated is not only a physical body but a social, psychological, cultural, and spiritual being has increased both the number of treatment specialists and has also underscored the importance of teamwork (1).

The words used to describe team practice in recent history reflect the changes in the way teamwork is viewed. Early in the first half of this century, the medical model gave way to interdisciplinary health care. "Inter," according to the Random House College Dictionary (revised edition, 1988) is a prefix that suggests action "among, between, or done mutually." Even more recently, however, the literature of team practice has introduced the term "transdisciplinary team" and the word change may well reveal what is new about teams. "Trans" suggests a focus "beyond, through, or changing thoroughly" (Random House College Dictionary, revised edition, 1988). It indicates that not only is there a universal awareness of the complex nature of the individual patient and his/her family, but also that the client and the team exist in an ecosystem that must be taken into consideration if effective long-term care is to take place.

To understand team practice, therefore, occupational therapists need to appreciate their unique contribution to a body of professionals and clients that not only serve the needs of individuals but also affect the whole treatment system in which treatment takes place (2). This chapter describes some of the team members that might be assembled to meet the needs of clients in various settings, discusses the mechanics of team function, and suggests skills that promote successful team participation. It also takes a look at two of the biggest identified challenges to the health care team: ethics and cost containment.

TEAM MEMBERS

The membership of a health care team is determined by the setting, requirements of the patient, and family. In a hospital, the occupational therapist is routinely joined by the following and an effective health care team is formed:

Physicians: In the hospital, physicians usually lead the health care team. An attending physician is ultimately responsible for medical outcome; physician residents, under the direction of the attending physician, provide much of the day-to-day care.

Nurse: Many interdisciplinary teams now use a nursing system, in which one nurse accepts primary responsibility for the development of a treatment plan that carries out team decisions and reinforces therapies on the patient unit.

Physical therapists: These professionals work closely with occupational therapists but focus primarily on gross motor functions, such as strength, range of motion, ambulation, transfers, balance skills, and mobility.

Speech and language pathologists: These team members outline the nature of communication problems and work to improve auditory-reading comprehension, verbal expression, writing skills, nonverbal communication skills, memory, and cognition (3).

Social workers: The patient and family are assessed by the social workers and treated for their emotional reaction to disability. Social workers facilitate family function and investigate concrete issues related to health care, such as finances and resource needs. The social worker is also concerned with mobilizing the human as well as durable resources needed to develop carryover in the discharge plan.

Psychologists: These team members work with social workers to enable families and patients to adjust to disability. Psychologists administer and interpret appropriate psychometric tests when indicated and treat psychological issues that influence service delivery.

Specialized vocational counselors: Vocational counselors interact with health care teams, the community, and government funding sources to assist clients to return to work.

Also present on many in-hospital health care teams are dietitians, who monitor nutritional needs, and biomedical engineers, who assist with the assessment and acquisition of equipment, especially when it is highly specialized. Respiratory therapists assess respiratory needs and prescribe respiratory support mechanisms. Pastoral care personnel offer spiritual support and counseling.

In school health care teams, the occupational therapist will normally interface with classroom teachers and special educators through both consultative and direct care services. These educators and teachers are the individuals who carry over treatment recommendations from clinic to classroom experience. School social workers and school psychologists interface with team, family, and community mental health resources. School administrators and principals are also regular members of the team, as are student counselors (5). Also found in the school setting are speech and language pathologists, educational prescriptionists (who assess children's auditory and visual processing abilities), physical therapists, and teacher aides. Physicians do not take a direct role in school programs but provide medical information as needed and allow linkages between educational systems and medical care.

Many other professionals expand or change the makeup of the health care team, depending on the setting and team goals: the psychiatrist in a psychiatric setting; lawyers, judges, and police, when legal matters are involved; funding personnel, such as insurance representatives, social security and department of social services personnel; visiting nurses, community mental health workers, and private industry staff, when community reentry or work-hardening programs are underway; residential placement staff and personal care attendants (who are trained with the clients).

One more professional who has recently been added to treatment teams in many settings is the ethicist or, in some cases, a single representative of an entire ethics committee that was established to protect and affirm the rights of the individual. The reason for this addition is directly attributable to the growing complexity of care and a greater sensitivity to human rights. Deciding who will be allowed to access the resources of the treatment team under what circumstance is a recurring issue. The awareness of the highly technological services available and the limitations of time and money are two reasons that it is necessary to keep ethics as a focus of team practice.

All of the health care professionals on the transdisciplinary team need to know the group goal as well as the goal of each of the other disciplines on the team. "This requires a high level of group interaction and knowledge of the sum of many parts" (5). The occupational therapist, like the other professionals involved, uses the team as a source of information and support for therapy (4). Successful health care teams are models of interdisciplinary or transdisciplinary practice.

TEAM MEETINGS

Although ethical considerations have affected team process, it is the cost-containment factor more than any other that is influencing the team's work. Cost containment mandates an ever-increasing need to speed up service delivery and to move the bulk of intervention to services outside of the expensive hospital environment. The overall effect of making cost management a primary focus is complex and far reaching, but from the perspective of teamwork, it can be said that the team now includes at least two new dimensions of activity for the occupational therapist: consultation services before a patient is admitted and a heavy emphasis on outpatient treatment. It is also predictable that patients on all levels of service will be moved out of the hospital "sicker and quicker" (6). This means that the referring services are moving the clients to outside rehabilitation settings with physical and emotional conditions that we would have thought unstable in years past.

Effective, cost-efficient, and ethical performance depends greatly on communication among team members. Today, therefore, the occupational therapists may be required to meet with other team members at as many as five different stages of care. Each serves three goals:

1. Collaborative assessment (consult rounds and initial staffings;
2. A follow-up evaluation of the treatment plan (paper rounds or gym rounds); and
3. The involvement of patient and family (family meetings).

In decades past, these were spaced to allow ease of transition to various stages of care. Today they are compressed into much shorter lengths of stay that force team members to be ready at every stage to offer information that affects change as soon as possible.

Especially in a hospital setting, the inclusion of occupational therapists in the selection of patients (consult rounds) is happening in response to the need to identify as early as possible the clients who can best make use of the services of the transdisciplinary team. The immediate goal is to move the patients along the continuum of care as efficiently as possible to reduce unnecessary days in the treatment facility. A 1992 study about the efforts of one acute care hospital to reduce the average length of stay and ensure the best use of the inpatient environment suggests that this is best accomplished if a representative from each treating discipline goes on consult rounds with the physicians (7). In this way a concensus can be arrived at about what can or cannot be done for the person evaluated. This suggests that the occupational therapist on consult rounds should be prepared to offer recommendations about what services occupational therapy could provide and how occupational therapy services would affect the long-term rehabilitation of the client.

After the patient is selected, the challenge is to get ready for the initial staffing. This team meeting is scheduled as early as possible after a client has been identified. Before the team comes together formally for the first time, it is generally assumed that each professional involved has made an initial assessment and is prepared to contribute to joint problem identification, data collection, problem evaluation, goal setting, outcome prediction, and determination of activities to achieve this outcome (3). Each setting outlines the exact parameters of the individual team member's participation in assessment and development of a treatment plan. Ordinarily the team will expect the occupational therapist to have information regarding the following:

Performance of daily living activities;
Possible equipment needs;
Preliminary cognitive/perceptual evaluation;
Information on accessibility of home, school, work setting;
Vocational information;
Preliminary suggestions concerning use of resources, such as onsite work evaluators and personal care attendants; and
Some estimation of time required for intervention.

Rounds, or some other type of follow-up evaluation of the health care team's treatment plan, is the tool that best shows the dynamic characteristics of team practice. Having established initial goals and a treatment plan, team members reconvene regularly to evaluate these and adjust them according to new information. Because each member shares in the responsibility and accountability for outcome, the meetings involve collaborating, communicating, and consolidating knowledge that changes the treatment plan as appropriate (1). The occupational therapist, like all other team members, must be prepared to cite specific examples of change and recommend continuation or alteration of goals or the treatment initially established.

Some health care teams expand the concept of rounds to include on-site clinic or classroom visits. In such cases, the team members go to the treatment area to watch therapy procedures to better understand the treatment recommendations. In the occupational therapy clinic, the therapist uses such occasions to increase team members' awareness of actual client performance. In the clinic of another discipline, occupational therapists increase their understanding of that professional's goals and interventions to modify or to improve their own goals and interventions.

Family meetings are common to almost all health care team efforts, since the family's involvement is generally indispensable to the carryover and maintenance of achievements made by the intervention of the team with the client. The value of team-family meetings depends largely on the clarity of reporting done by each therapist and the projection of a unified set of goals and expectations by the team. The team that is well practiced at active listening attends closely to the questions and suggestions of family members to enhance the treatment plan or to improve communication regarding its goals. Very often the therapeutic area that is the responsibility of the occupational therapist is of great practical value to the patient and family. The following are typical questions: "Will my son need someone with him all the time?" "Can my wife maintain her job?" "Will my mother be able to manage personal care?" The occupational therapist provides the information in the presence of the other discipline specialists, who support or modify it with their own reports. For example, an occupational therapist, physical therapist, and physician might report good functional skills, while the neuropsychologist reports cognitive deficits that increase care needs beyond what a family may have expected.

Family involvement is so critical to most treatment plans that family and patient can be considered members of the health care team. The family and patients' understanding of professional jargon and the quality of their emotional involvement in the issues being discussed is, however, different. Family-team meetings should be stripped of medical terminology and conducted with a simplicity and clarity that does not reduce the quality of information shared with other team members. Anxiety in family members who are in the presence of many professionals reporting huge quantities of information may interfere with comprehension. Every effort must be made to reduce the formality of the occasion and to ensure the participants that the team values their involvement. Because the client is very often present, the occupational therapist can build on his or her rapport with that individual to increase the comfort level of the family. This can be done most effectively by referring questions regarding certain interventions to the client and requesting the client's acknowledgment or opinion.

Team meetings are based on client needs as well as the on mandates of individual settings. In a school situation, the occupational therapist will participate in team meetings that fulfill the state laws requiring the assignment of special education labels and resources. Legal procedures may involve preliminary meetings with attorneys to prepare for court hearings. Community services ideally require interdisciplinary meetings with referring health care teams to develop carryover plans consistent with treatment already performed inside hospitals or institutions.

In each setting, the team meetings bring together professionals with individual expertise to apply to a common goal or purpose. Although there is an organized division of labor, each person must accept the responsibility for making and implementing decisions in his or her own area of expertise. The team sessions support each person's formal and informal involvement for an integrated delivery of service (1).

Just as the occupational therapist is now often involved in the selection of clients before service, he or she is integral to the discussion of discharge planning at the end of treatment as well. Although much study and effort is going on to determine who should ultimately be responsible for the discharge planning, it is important that each person on the team cooperate in that process. Leonard J. Marcus has noted that the health care system in the United States is characterized by many separate organizations that each manage a piece of the total care plan for an individual patient (8). The person treated encounters many disparate services and different personnel during an episode of illness, especially if treatment lasts for a protracted period of time. The occupational therapist can help by keeping in mind that there are goals for each level of service. Good team effort requires seeing each movement to another level on the continuum of care as another discharge, and every therapist in or outside the milieu in which he or she is presently functioning as another member of the whole team.

SKILLS NEEDED FOR GOOD TEAMWORK

The old adage, "a chain is as strong as its weakest link," fits the challenge of interdisciplinary health care team practice very well. Not only must the occupational therapist and each other member of a successful team bring a high level of personal competence to the group, but he or she must develop communication skills that facilitate group process. Furthermore, as a team member, the individual therapist is challenged to develop special characteristics that support the group's ability to set team goals and develop team programs that are superior to individual interventions.

Because the complexity of modern health care has given rise to a vast network of professions, each of which specializes in a segment of the person's total care needs, the totality of the health delivery system depends on the quality of each professional's individual contribution to the whole. Because no one discipline can master all parts of the care plan, each professional is expected to have particular expertise in his or her own area. This is not only true because the client needs each unique intervention but because all members of a health care team tailor their involvement according to information they have gathered from the work of every other member. Thus, the whole depends largely on the parts. The quality of each person's contribution greatly affects the quality of the total service delivery.

The complexity of the health care system establishes the need for excellence among the members of the team who serve the client in hospitals, schools, and community services. That same complexity mandates a commitment on the part of each professional to continue to learn and grow after formal education requirements have been met. Not only must occupational therapists develop their skills in occupational therapy by means of continuing education programs, in-service education, and regular reading of professional journals and literature, but they must pursue and improve their skills in team participation as well. Duconis and Golin (9) suggest that this is done in three ways: (*a*) preprofessional training done in school before certification, involving curriculum-integrated courses of specific training in team skills; (*b*) continuing education programs after college, such as workshops, seminars, and formal postgraduate courses offered to individuals or groups; and (*c*) team development with the help of hired consultants trained to facilitate team practice.

The team skills that need to be added to the occupational therapy expertise are many, but the most essential is communication. If an interdisciplinary team is going to do good work, the members must develop their ability to speak, listen, write, and read effectively. To express occupational therapy issues and to learn about the evaluation of client needs by other disciplines, the therapist's communication must be as clear as possible.

The spoken word in formal and informal settings is the heart of the team process. Because most teams function with limited time, the expression of findings, recommendations, and questions needs to be brief, precise, and objective. The responsibility to listen to what is shared is equally important. Because not all members will be effective speakers, the good listener is active, asking questions that clarify information or requesting repetition or examples to ensure that the facts are understood. There is an important distinction between passive and active listening. Passive listening is the noninvolved relaxed listening one might use at a concert or in a light social exchange. Active listening, which is required on a health care team, involves an active effort not only to hear what is being said but to analyze it in relation to other information one has on a case. This other information could be the occupational therapist's own assessment or a treatment goal previously established by the team.

Not only must team members speak and listen well, they must also read and write accurately. No matter what the setting, the occupational therapist, like every other staff member, will be required to document assessments, interventions, and recommendations in some written form. Documentation responsibility has always been a serious charge for the professional, but it is especially so today when the written word has powerful legal significance. Beyond that, however, the information charted by members of a health care team provides ongoing guidelines for other team members who are providing complementing interventions or piggybacking their own plans for the client with those of another therapist. The written documentation must be up to date, precise, and brief. Lengthy or unnecessarily anecdotal charting is often distracting and overlooked because of the time it takes to read it.

The responsibility to read the documentation of other team members parallels the responsibility to listen actively. Because interdisciplinary practice is an integration of multiple efforts, the charge to know what each team member is doing is very serious. Because there is a professional as well as a legal mandate on each team member to write down assessments and care plans, there is an equally serious responsibility for other team members to read what is written.

Given and Simmons (10) cite eight other personal and team characteristics that support effective health care team function:

1. Open-mindedness, or the willingness to accept differences and the perspective of others;
2. Independence, because the ability to function independently is required to achieve team goals;

3. Negotiation skills, because team members need to assert their perspective but remain willing to achieve a consensus by practicing give and take;
4. The willingness to accept new values, attitudes, and perceptions as appropriate;
5. Tolerance of constant review and the challenges of other team members;
6. The ability to risk;
7. Personal identity and integrity;
8. The ability to accept and assume a team's philosophy of care after it has been established by consensus.

Given and Simmons also suggest that good team players can tolerate frustration, because team process is often arduous and always more time-consuming than individual effort. The professional on a team not only has to be flexible so as to adjust to new situations but must also operate from a basic personal security that allows open-mindedness without experiencing a sense of threat (10).

Team function depends on each member's ability to state his or her opinions positively to assert recommendations with assurance. Furthermore, each member needs to participate in the group process that is identified in each setting to resolve inevitable conflict and then proceed with a spirit of cooperation and flexibility to carry out the plan that is the result of consensus.

According to Etzioni (2) and Thompson (4), the movement away from multidisciplinary to interdisciplinary and now transdisciplinary practice for health care teams has allowed a departure from traditional hierarchal patterns that is stimulating new insights, perspectives, and innovative therapy. Nevertheless, the change requires not only the development of a new set of skills for the participants but new and important group skills as well.

The team members must know each other's roles to avoid making unreasonable demands. They need to recognize that, at times, there will be a blurring of traditional roles and therefore a need to accept shared responsibility. The development of expertise in one area does not rule out an opinion or skill in another. In good team process, the occupational therapist may be the most appropriate person to assist with some psychosocial intervention that might ordinarily be seen as the social worker's task. The social worker may be able to help a client with adjustment while he or she participates in activities of daily living (ADLs) that are usually the province of the occupational therapist. Such sharing requires a high level of trust among team members, not only to allow participation in one another's area of expertise but to accept the appropriate guidance of the more expert member when doing so. Teams, therefore, have to accept shifting leadership. There has to be a spirit of cooperation instead of competition, and resolution of issues should follow consensus, not coercion or compromise (3).

Health care team practice is still more of an ideal than a reality in many places where occupational therapists practice. Nevertheless, paralleling the growing recognition that occupational therapy, like many other areas of professional expertise has mastered an important segment of the whole health care system, there is a movement toward group intervention. Duconis and Golin (9) polled 175 professional schools in the late 1970s. Of the 124 schools that responded, only 34% offered specific course work in team process. However, 90% responded that they recognized the growing need and most said that the concepts of team practice were an integrated part of the existing curriculum.

CASE STUDY WITH TEAM INTERVENTION

In today's fast-paced, budget-minded service centers, it is seldom or never that an individual therapist gets to follow a case to its conclusion. Rather, a client may pass through many stages and meet several occupational therapists along the way. An example is DB, a 63-year-old male psychology professor who came to the emergency room with severe bilateral strokes. Stabilized there only briefly, the patient was moved to the Intensive Care Unit where the occupational therapist on the consult service evaluated him along with the physiatrists, nurse, physical therapist, and social worker. It was decided that DB had sufficient potential to be transferred to the inpatient unit. He was moved to the rehabilitation floor to begin an intensive program that included care by the doctors, a primary care nurse, a physical therapist, an occupational therapist, a speech and language therapist, social worker, dietician, psychologist, and a continuing care nurse. In this particular case, occupational therapy focused on the areas of swallowing, compensatory strategies for DB's paralysis on one side of the body, and the evaluation and treatment of visual spatial deficits. However, because the client had sustained massive insults to his brain and had been started on rehabilitation very early in his recovery period, he proved to be too lethargic to participate. Therefore the transdisciplinary team could not keep him in the acute care hospital more than 3 weeks.

During staffing and rounds, it was determined that the long-term goal of getting him back home where his wife could take care of him might be achievable if DB were transferred to the less costly skilled nursing facility (nursing home) until he was up to the rigors of a full rehabilitation program. Although there was no serious ethical dilemma in this case, it was decided that it would be an inappropriate use of resources to keep DB in an environment that was too demanding for his stage of recovery. The task of the occupational therapist became one of preparing good guidelines for the treatment personnel in the nursing home to assure the progress necessary to get DB back into the hospital at a later date. Notes, phone calls, and fax messages were sent to the occupational therapist at the nursing home.

Later, when the social worker indicated that the insurance coverage for DB's skilled nursing home care was coming to an end, the occupational therapist and several other members of the hospital rehabilitation team went to the hospital's outpatient clinic where DB had come in for a routine appointment to determine his eligibility for inpatient admission. The occupational therapist re-evaluated DB's swallowing ability as well as the important activities of daily living that could reduce costly care after being discharged to his home. It was determined by all members of the team that DB was now ready for an aggressive inpatient program. He was admitted for a 6-week stay. During this time the occupational therapist assisted DB to master many of the skills he needed to have a limited level of autonomy in his home environment. He learned how to dress using the functional side of his body, was able to swallow pudding-like consistencies of food, improved his upper body strength sufficiently to assist with transfers, became able to use a urinal independently, and developed some reading strategies to overcome visual neglect. He did not become independent by any means, but the carefully orchestrated teamwork made it possible for DB to go home at last. The services of the inpatient team were transferred to a team of community-based therapists who continued to work with him at home. The hospital occupational therapist paved the way for the community-based therapist by supplying good notes of his hospital progress and made additional recommendations by phone. The outpatient occupational therapist is presently using DB's home environment to determine further goals for greater independence.

The importance of team effort to maximize outcomes for clients in today's treatment centers can hardly be overemphasized. Team practice, which simultaneously targets multiple levels of need while keeping an eye on cost control and ethical issues, is clearly a better model for successful care management. It is expensive, however, and for that reason new therapists may feel great pressure to do excellent work without adequate time. The fear is that mistakes will be made or some part of the treatment plan will be unfinished. That is always a concern, but the advantage of teamwork is that it supports the interventions of individual team players. Under the stress of short hospital stays and low budgets it is far more likely that a client will get most of what he or she needs if treated by a whole team than by one individual acting under the same pressures. In the case of DB, it was clear that his successful transition to his home environment was possible because many professionals with varied expertise worked together to make it happen.

Discussion Questions

1. Why have ethical issues become such an important concern in today's health care environments?
2. Communication skills are critical to effective team functioning. How can students improve their personal communication skills to prepare for future work settings?
3. How could the interpersonal skills required for transdisciplinary team practice be developed?
4. How many levels of care were represented by the case of DB? How did the treatment goals vary with each level of care?
5. Cost considerations played a role in DB's treatment program. Discuss how the treatment program might have been different if DB had been a Medicaid patient.
6. How much do you know about the other health disciplines that you might someday be working with? How can you learn more about what they know and what they do?

REFERENCES

1. Melvin JL: Interdisciplinary and multidisciplinary activities and the A.C.R.M. *Arch Phys Med Rehabil* 8:379–380, 1980.
2. Etzioni A: *A Comparative Analysis of Complex Organizations*. New York, Free Press, 1961, pp. 1–22.
3. *Roles: Policies and Procedures Manual*. Ann Arbor, University of Michigan Hospitals, 1985, pp. 1–15.
4. Thompson JO: *Organization in Action*. New York, McGraw-Hill, 1967, pp. 51–65, 132–143.
5. Hopkins H, Smith HD (eds): *Willard and Spackman's Occupational Therapy*. Philadelphia, JB Lippincott, 1983, pp. 380, 686–688.
6. Kosecoff J, Kahn KL, Rodgers, WH, Reinisch EJ, Sherwood MJ, Rubenstein CV, Draper D, Roth CP, Chew I, Brook RH: Prospective payment system and impairment at discharge; the" quicker and sicker" story revisited. *JAMA* 264(15):1980–1983, 1990.
7. LaBan MM, Muzljakovich D, Perrin JC: Improving the efficiency of patient selection for continuing rehabilitation in a general hospital; the Stroke Option Rehabilitation Team—a commentary. *Am J Phys Med Rehabil* 71(1):55–56, 1992.
8. Marcus LJ: Discharge planning: an organizational perspective. *Health & Social Work* 12:1, 1987.
9. Duconis A, Golin A: *Educating for Team Work: The Interdisciplinary Health Care Team*. Germantown, MD, Aspen Systems, 1979, pp. 153–166.
10. Given B, Simmons S: Interdisciplinary health care team: fact or fiction? *Nurse Forum* 2:165–184, 1977.

SUGGESTED READINGS

Bailey DB Jr: A triaxial model of the interdisciplinary team and group process. *Exceptional Children* 51:17–25, 1984.

Bailey D, et al.: Measuring individual participation on the interdisciplinary team. *Am J Ment Defic* 88:247–254, 1983.

Bailey DB, et al.: Participation of professionals, paraprofessionals, and direct care staff members in the interdisciplinary team meeting. *Am J Ment Defic* 89:437–440, 1985.

Bryand J: The health team. In *Health and the Developing World*. Ithaca, NY, Cornell University Press, 1969, pp. 139–199.

Duncombe LW, et al.: Group work in occupational therapy: a survey of practice. *Am J Occup Ther* 39:163–170, 1985.

Feiger SM, Schmitt MH: Collegiality in interdisciplinary health teams: its measurement and its effect. *Soc Sci Med* 13A:217–229, 1979.

Johnston A, Cummings V, Pooler L: Teammates are equal partners. *Canadian Nurse* 64:36–41, 1968.

Wagner RJ: Rehabilitation team practice. *Rehabil Couns Bull* 20:206–217, 1977.

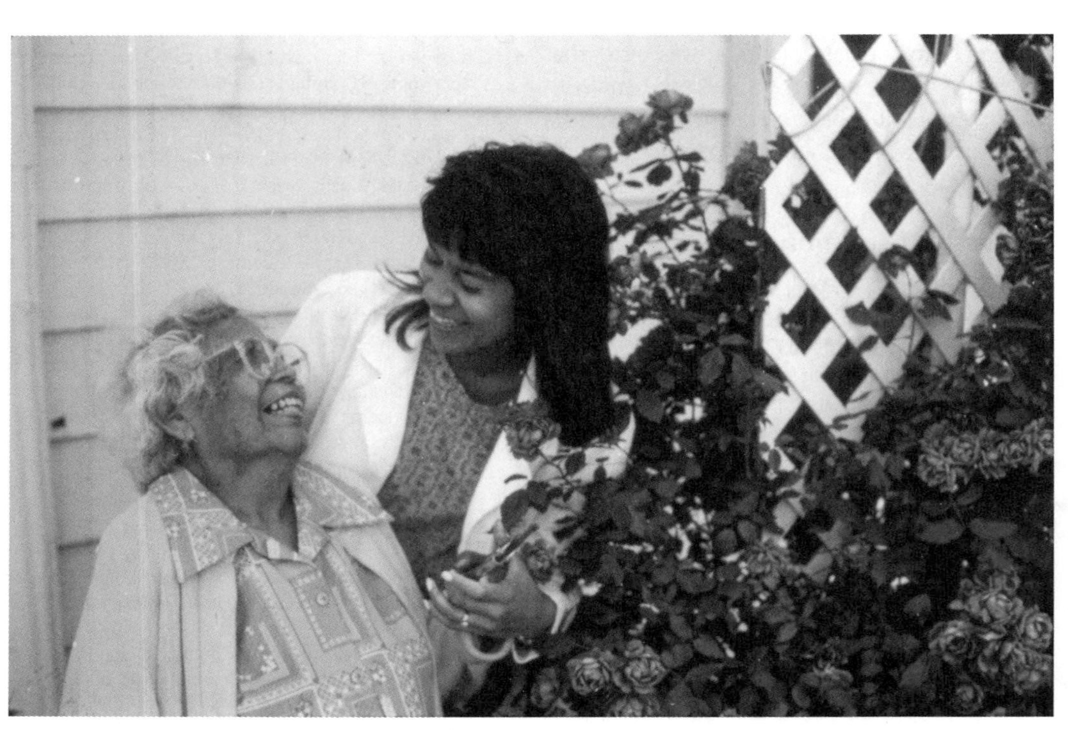

9 Concepts of Occupational Therapy Practice

Occupational therapists and therapy assistants work with a diverse population and practice in a variety of settings. This chapter introduces some of the specialized areas of occupational therapy practice. Some typical settings in which occupational therapists practice and some trends in occupational therapy service delivery today are discussed.

GENERAL PRACTICE OR SPECIALIZATION

In the early years of occupational therapy, practice tended to fall into only two specializations. One type of practice was focused on mental disturbances and was located in an institution for the mentally ill. The other type focused on physical illnesses and disabilities and was located in a general hospital. In developing countries, this broadly based type of practice is still typical, and therapists must be prepared to work with a variety of diseases or disabilities. In the United States, however, and in other countries with highly developed medical resources, occupational therapists have begun to limit their practices to specific types of disabilities or to specific age groups. This is partly an attempt to cope with an ever-increasing knowledge explosion in science and medicine. It is also an effort on the part of occupational therapists to offer their clients the benefits of advanced study and training in complex procedures and theoretical aspects of practice. By the early 1990s, AOTA had recognized nine separate specialty areas within the field: developmental disabilities, gerontology, mental health, physical disabilities, sensory integration, administration, work programs, technology, and education. More than half of the OTRs who responded to the AOTA's 1990 Member Data Survey considered themselves specialists rather than generalists. To facilitate communication among members who practice in a given specialty area, AOTA has created special interest sections in these nine areas. Members of these groups meet at state and national conferences, sponsor continuing education in their area of interest, promote research, publish materials related to their interest area, and serve as an information resource on practice within the area of specialization. In 1992, therapists who were working in the areas of school practice, home health, and wellness and health promotion were petitioning AOTA for recognition as special interest sections of the national organization.

The OTRs and COTAs have the choice of remaining as general practitioners or of specializing in a more limited area of practice. Specialization is usually achieved through graduate education, work experience in the specialty area, or continuing education. In 1987, the AOTA's Representative Assembly passed a policy on specialty certification, which approved the recognition of members who had achieved advanced competence in a specialized area of practice (1). The method whereby members would earn specialty certification was not specified, but by 1991, an advanced competency examination had been developed for pediatric practitioners. Those who successfully passed the examination were board certified as having advanced knowledge and skills in this practice specialty. Other specialty certifications may be added in the future.

Ezersky and her colleagues surveyed over 400 occupational therapists to determine whether they were practicing in specialty areas and what influenced their choice of specialty. They found that the largest group in their sample (43.4%) was working with physical disabilities. This was followed by 25.5%, who were working in pediatrics; 13.2% in mental health; 10.5% in geriatrics; and 7.4% in developmental disabilities or other areas. Variables influencing their choice of specialty included field work experiences, feelings of greater competence in one specialty area, availability of employment in a given specialty, consistency with personal interests and values, and an empathy for a certain type of patient (2).

In a comparable study, Wittman and her colleagues found that 16% of their sample had already made a specialty choice while in the preprofessional phase of their education. Another 13% made their choice during their occupational therapy professional education, and 62% said that their choice had been made during level II field work. Selection of practice specialties remained relatively consistent over time (3).

WORK SITES

The employment sites where occupational therapists and therapy assistants work are as varied as the client populations. In 1985, the AOTA published a report on the occupational therapy workforce that documented changes that were taking place in service delivery sites. It found that hospitals were still the most common work setting, but both levels of personnel were beginning to move into school systems, home health agencies, outpatient clinics, private practices, residential care facilities, and skilled nursing homes (4). The 1990 Member Data Survey conducted by the AOTA found that general hospitals continued to be the most common work site for OTRs, followed by school systems, rehabilitation hospitals, and private practices. For COTAs, skilled nursing homes were the most common work site, with general hospitals, rehabilitation hospitals, and school systems coming next in order (5). Table 9.1 shows the primary employment sites reported by OTRs and COTAs who were AOTA members in 1990.

GROWING AND DECLINING PRACTICE SITES

According to the AOTA 1990 Member Data Survey growth was occurring in outpatient clinics, private industry, rehabilitation hospitals, skilled nursing homes, and private practices. COTA employment continued to rise in school systems but OTR employment in schools had fallen back to its 1980 level. Residential care facilities were another growth area for COTA employment. The number of practitioners working in mental health settings continued to decline. In general, employment of occupational therapy personnel has grown in private, profit-making institutions. COTAs are twice as likely as OTRs to be working in fields other than occupational therapy (5).

AGE GROUPS SERVED

Table 9.2 shows the age groups that AOTA members were working with in 1990. There has been a general decline in the number of practitioners working with mixed age groups as practice became more specialized and as specific services were established for certain age groups. OTR practitioners were more often working with children or adult clients, while COTAs were working more frequently with adults and the elderly. The increased numbers of personnel employed in programs for older citizens reflect the increasing numbers of this segment of the population and also mirror an increased level of funding to support geriatric programs (5).

HEALTH PROBLEMS SEEN

Table 9.3 lists the health problems most frequently seen by OTRs and COTAs in 1990. During that year, the largest proportion of OTRs was working with patients who had strokes (cerebrovascular accident, CVA), developmental delays, hand injuries, and learning disabilities. Conditions seen most fre-

Table 9.1. Primary Clinical Employment Settings of OTRs and COTAs in 1990

Setting	OTRs (%)	COTAs (%)
Community mental health center	1.1	1.7
Correctional institution		
Day care program	0.9	1.7
HMO (including PPO, IPA)	0.4	0.1
Home health agency	3.6	1.5
Hospice program	0.0	0.0
General hospital (all units)	25.4	19.0
Pediatric hospital	1.7	0.7
Psychiatric hospital	4.6	6.6
Outpatient clinic (free standing)	3.7	2.2
Physician's office	1.2	0.3
Private industry	0.8	
Private practice	7.7	2.7
Public health agency	0.9	0.6
Rehabilitation hospital center	11.4	10.9
Research facility	0.2	0.2
Residential care facility, including group home, independent living center	2.7	5.9
Retirement or senior center	0.2	0.8
Schools (including private)	18.6	17.0
Sheltered workshop	0.4	1.6
Skilled nursing home/intermediate care facility	6.4	20.1
Vocational or Prevocational program		0.8
Voluntary agency (Easter Seal, U.C.P.)	1.0	1.1
Other	2.5	2.3
Total	99.9%	99.8%

Table 9.2. Primary Age Range of Clients, 1990

Age Range	OTRs (%)	COTAs (%)
Less than 3 years	7.6	2.1
3–5 years	10.1	8.1
6–12 years	14.3	11.7
13–18 years	2.7	3.7
19–64 years	37.2	37.2
65–74 years	16.9	16.6
75–84 years	9.8	16.0
85+ years	1.3	4.6
Total	100.0	100.0
Total pediatrics	34.7	25.5
Total adult	37.2	37.2
Total geriatrics	28.2	37.2
Total	99.9	99.9

Table 9.3. Most Frequent Health Problems of Clients, 1990

Health Problems	OTRs (%)	COTAs (%)
Alzheimer's disease	0.6	2.2
Amputations	0.1	0.3
Arteriosclerosis	0.1	0.3
Arthritis/collagen disorder	0.9	1.0
Back injuries	3.4	3.0
Burns	0.4	0.1
Cancer (neoplasms)	0.2	0.3
Cardiopulmonary diseases	0.7	0.4
Cerebral palsy	9.7	6.0
Congenital anomalies	0.3	0.1
CVA/hemiplegia	27.1	30.3
Developmental delay	12.9	8.9
Diabetes	0.1	0.1
Feeding disorders	0.3	0.0
Fractures	2.3	3.0
Hand injuries	9.5	3.2
Hearing disabilities	0.1	0.3
HIV infections, including AIDS	0.1	0.0
Kidney disorders	0.0	0.0
Learning disabilities	7.0	5.1
Neuromuscular disorders (MD, MS)	0.6	0.6
Respiratory diseases	0.1	0.2
Spinal cord injuries	1.2	1.2
Traumatic brain injuries	4.2	3.9
Visual disabilities	0.3	0.0
Well population	0.2	0.5
Adjustment disorders	0.8	1.2
Affective disorders	3.7	2.5
Alcohol/substance use disorders	0.8	1.5
Anxiety disorders	0.1	0.4
Eating disorders	0.2	0.1
Mental retardation	4.9	11.4
Organic mental disorders	0.8	2.1
Personality disorders	0.6	0.8
Schizophrenic disorders	4.1	6.6
Other psychotic disorders	0.1	0.2
Other mental health disorders	0.6	1.1
Other	0.8	1.1
Total	100.0	100.0
Physical disabilities, combined	83.4	72.0
Mental health disorders, combined	16.6	28.0

quently by COTAs included strokes, mental retardation, developmental delays, and personality disorders.

We can expect to see more occupational therapy personnel working with conditions like Alzheimer's Disease, HIV (human immune deficiency virus), and AIDS (acquired immune deficiency syndrome) as these disorders are more frequently recognized and treated. As Table 9.3 shows, only 16.6% of OTRs and 28% of COTAs were working with mental health disorders in 1990.

GEOGRAPHIC DISTRIBUTION OF PERSONNEL

The geographic distribution of OTRs and COTAs varies widely among the 50 states and U.S. territories. Figure 9.1 shows the ratio of OTRs to the U.S. population by state in 1991. While the upper tier of midwestern and eastern states was well supplied with occupational therapists, states like Mississippi and West Virginia had a very low ratio. This may well reflect overall economic conditions in those areas rather than a lack of health resources. It should be noted that the supply of OTRs in the southern and western states has improved since 1986. Only six states showed a proportion of 20 or more OTRs per 100,000 population in 1990.

Figure 9.2 shows the ratio of COTAs to the population of each state in 1991. This gives a similar picture, with midwestern and eastern states having a greater proportion of COTAs than southern, mid-Atlantic, and some western states. Only seven states showed a proportion of 4 or more COTAs per 100,000 population (5).

The maldistribution of occupational therapy personnel parallels that seen in other health care professions and presents serious problems in service delivery. The AOTA is actively working to improve the situation by encouraging the development of new OTR and COTA educational programs in underserved states.

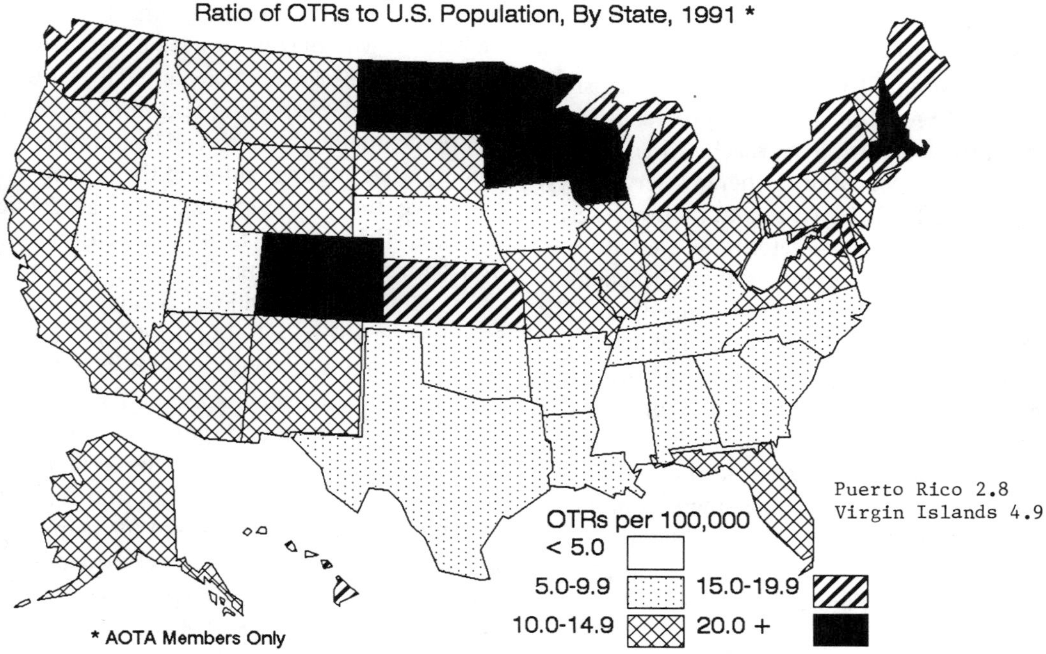

Figure 9.1. Ratio of OTRs to United States population by state 1991. Overall ratio = 11.7.

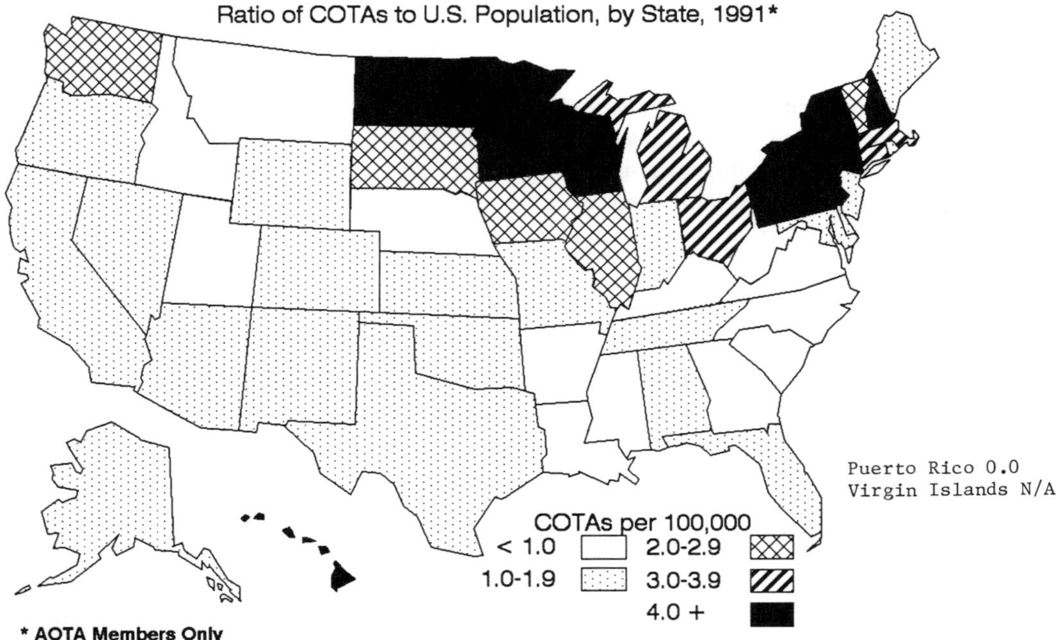

Figure 9.2. Ratio of COTAs to United States population by state, 1991. Overall ratio = 2.8.

OCCUPATIONAL THERAPY PROCESS

No matter what type of setting the OTR or COTA works in, the process for the delivery of occupational therapy services is very similar. The occupational therapy process is based on a problem-solving approach. When a client enters the occupational therapy service system, the OTR or COTA sets in motion a series of events intended to determine the nature of the performance problems that the client is experiencing. Once they are identified, the OTR and COTA design a therapeutic program aimed at helping the client regain lost abilities, develop needed skills, retain those abilities that he or she has at the desired levels, or prevent further disability. The steps in the process are screening, referral, assessment, program planning, intervention, reassessment, termination, and documentation. The process is diagrammed in Figure 9.3.

SCREENING

A client may enter the occupational therapy service system in a number of ways. Increasingly, occupational therapists are participating in screening programs to identify individuals who may be in need of services. In a school setting, for example, an OTR or COTA might administer screening tests of motor skills and perceptual abilities to determine whether kindergarten children entering the school system have the necessary skills for academic learning. Those found to have deficiencies or developmental delays may be referred for special programs of occupational therapy or other school services. In a hospital setting, certain types of diagnoses may be regularly referred to occupational therapy, inasmuch as patients with these disorders have been found to benefit from the services offered. An OTR might accompany physicians on rounds and suggest that certain patients be referred for help with specific areas of occupational performance. It is part of the OTR's and COTA's role to educate those professionals who are part of the health care team so that they recognize patients who are likely to benefit from occupational therapy. Whatever the method, some type

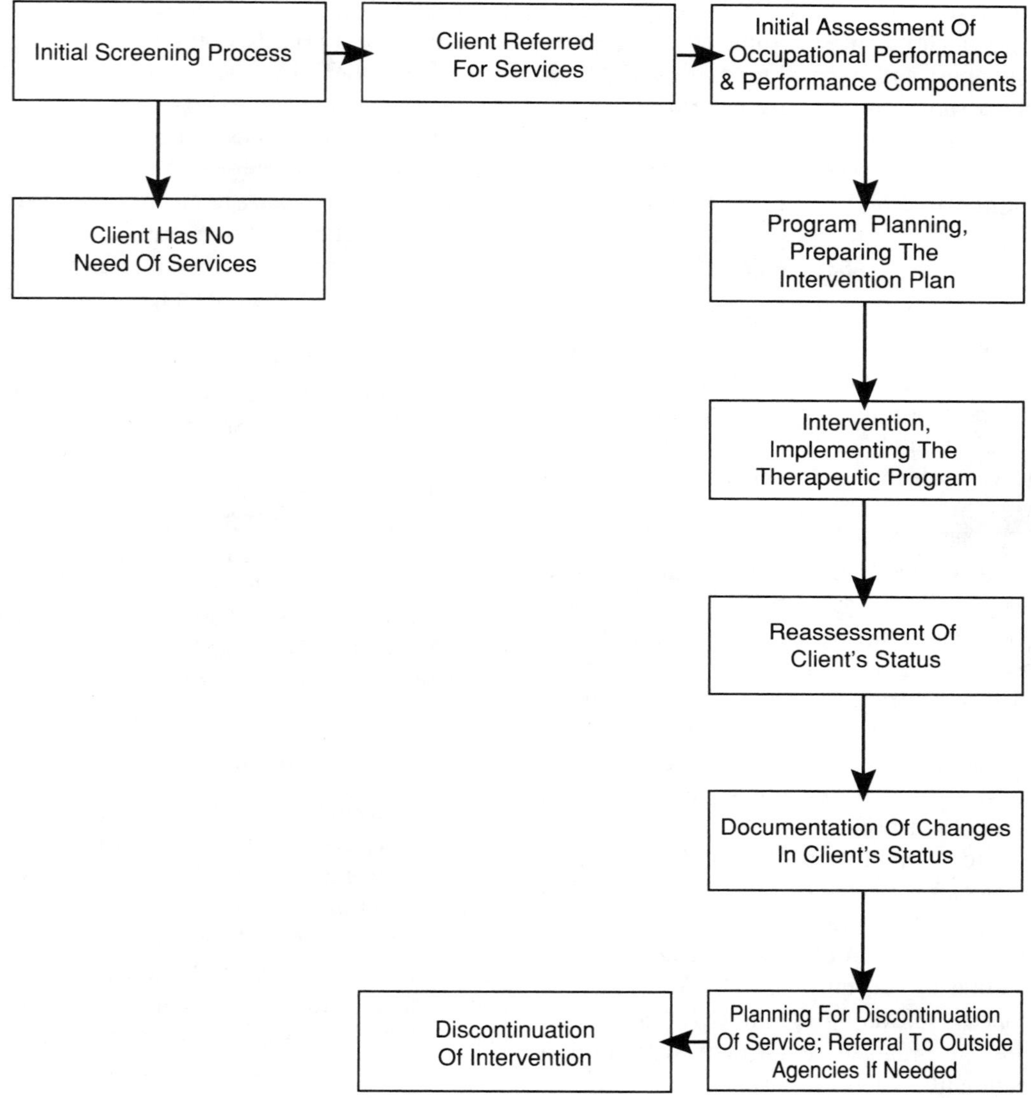

Figure 9.3. Occupational therapy process.

of screening takes place that sorts out individuals in need of occupational therapy services.

REFERRAL

Those persons who have needs that occupational therapy can help resolve should be referred, either by their physician or by another professional. Some clients may refer themselves, which is acceptable in many settings. The AOTA has taken the position that a physician's referral is not necessary for all occupational therapy services; however, a facility may require a medical referral if its accrediting agencies, state or federal laws, or third-party reimbursers require it. (Both the Joint Commission on Accreditation of Hospitals and the Commission on Accreditation of Rehabilitation Facilities require a physician's referral for occupational therapy services. Medicare regulations also require a physician's referral as do Medicaid rules in some states.) If there is no physician's referral for service, the therapist assumes full responsibility for determining the appropriate type, nature, and mode of service. COTAs become involved with clients as authorized by the supervising OTR.

ASSESSMENT

With the referral, the client enters the occupational therapy service system. The first task of the occupational therapist is to gather, analyze, and interpret any available data that can shed light on the occupational performance problems of the client. The therapist carefully evaluates the overall occupational performance of the client, considering his or her current work, family, and social roles. This area may be delegated to the COTA for evaluation. Data may include material gained from observation, from the client's medical or social history, from reports of prior treatment, and from direct interview of the client. The OTR or COTA may administer specific tests to determine the client's functional abilities and will try to identify areas of strength and areas in need of improvement. The *Uniform Terminology for Occupational Therapy,* 2nd Edition, provides a standard format of items to be evaluated (6). A copy of the document may be found in the Appendix. The AOTA has developed a software program, *O.T. Fact,* which helps to organize assessment data into a meaningful system. It enables the user to develop a functional performance profile for an individual client and can also be used to generate reports, charts, and graphs related to the client's occupational performance.

PROGRAM PLANNING

Once the data have been collected, the therapist analyzes the available information and begins to formulate priorities for the treatment process. If the result of a developmental test of motor abilities shows that a child is delayed in acquiring motor skills, the therapist will conclude that motor skill development must be a priority in the treatment program. The therapist plans a program that begins at the child's current functional level and gradually progresses until the child approaches a level of motor development compatible with his or her age or physical status.

An important part of treatment planning is the prioritizing of specific areas as a focus for treatment. Often, both long-term and short-term objectives are identified. Long-term objectives describe the desired outcome of treatment and may be quite broad. They depend on the achievement of short-term objectives. The short-term objectives describe the immediate goals—the ministeps that will lead to the desired end result. They are highly specific and are written in measurable terms so that changes can easily be documented. The client may have needs that are outside the scope of occupational therapy, and in this situation, it is appropriate for the OTR to refer the client to other professionals for the needed services.

CLINICAL REASONING

In working with their clients, occupational therapists and therapy assistants use clinical reasoning to guide their program planning and day-to-day interventions. Clinical reasoning refers to the process of thinking about and interpreting the treatment process and being able to make judgments based on observation, knowledge, and experience. By drawing on his or her accumulated experience, a therapist is often able to know which goals may be most important to the client and which therapeutic activities may have the most meaning. Occupational therapists try to consider clients' perceptions of their illnesses or disabilities and what the resulting limitations mean to them. By tuning into a client's emotional world, a therapist can better understand where a client is coming from and where he or she may wish to go. The therapist must create a situation in which the client can confront personal doubts and fears, communicate real feelings, and begin to look at what he or she can do to overcome the limitations imposed by disease or injury or to live within them.

Treatment must be individualized since no two clients are the same even though they may have the same diagnosis. Differences in attitude, culture, personal philosophy, and life situation will directly influence the nature and outcome of the intervention. The therapist constantly challenges clients to reach for more advanced goals and achievements and offers the hope of being able to resume their lives again. Clients are asked to make a commitment to their therapeutic programs. Without a real commitment on the part of the client, therapy is likely to be ineffective and frustrating.

Throughout the occupational therapy process, the therapist applies clinical reasoning to help plan, carry out, monitor, and reassess the therapeutic program. Experienced therapists do this so automatically that it looks easy, but complex clinical judgments are involved that take years of professional practice to develop.

INTERVENTION PLAN

The therapist then begins to plan an organized program of treatment to deal with the identified client needs. A written intervention plan is usually prepared, listing the short-term objectives and the methods to be used to help achieve them. Today, this is often done on the computer. Both the OTR and COTA may contribute ideas to the intervention plan. When the client is an adolescent or an adult, the therapist is likely to involve him or her in the planning process so that personal priorities can be considered. When the client is a child, the family may be consulted. When the client's and family's needs and wishes are taken into account in the planning process, they are much more likely to be active participants in treatment. Motivation and cooperation are usually better when the client and family are fully involved in the program from the beginning and when they know that their personal needs and priorities are respected.

The format of the intervention plan varies from one setting to another, as does the documentation of treatment results. Most plans are brief and succinct, including only critical pieces of information. Some plans must also include a projection of how long the treatment process is expected to take. The initial plan and subsequent documentation of changes seen may be shared with the referring physician or the treatment team. Everyone who works with the patient must understand the total treatment program and coordinate their efforts. Nothing is more disruptive to client care than conflicts among members of the care team.

INTERVENTION

After development of the intervention plan, the OTR and COTA prepare to implement the plan. Decisions are made as to which person will be responsible for the different phases of treatment. A schedule is established for regular client visits, and the actual treatment activities begin. It is important that the person who is to carry out treatment activities preplan each client visit, preparing the necessary materials and setting up any needed equipment so that the client can begin work immediately and no treatment time is wasted. The OTR or COTA may need to orient the client to each stage of the treatment program, teach procedures that are unfamiliar, and closely monitor the client's physical and emotional reactions during treatment sessions. Activities used should be compatible with the amount of time available for the treatment session and with the physical and mental capabilities of the client. Activities may be done individually or within a group environment. Many clients enjoy and benefit from group interaction during therapy sessions, and the pleasant, cheerful ambience of the occupational therapy clinic can be a powerful motivator to a client who is depressed or discouraged. The OTR and COTA offer emotional support and encouragement to clients throughout the treatment program and try to lead them to higher and higher levels of achievement until treatment objectives are accomplished. As discussed in Chapter 8, a client today may receive services from several agencies during the recovery and rehabilitation process. It is crucial that OTRs and COTAs maintain continuity of treatment by communicating with their counterparts in other facilities where the client will receive continuing services.

REASSESSMENT

Periodically during the treatment process, the OTR or COTA will reassess the problem areas and compare the data with the initial test results and with the stated treatment objectives. If adequate progress is not occurring, the therapist may need to consider changes in the treatment program or adjustments in the objectives. Sometimes the objectives are set too high for the client to achieve in a limited period of time. If the initial objectives are unrealistic, the therapist may modify them to a more reasonable level. In some situations, only limited gains may be made. When the client's ability reaches a plateau and no further progress is seen, it may be appropriate to terminate treatment. On other occasions the objective is to maintain existing abilities at their present level, preventing further deterioration of the client's performance skills. This is a valid goal, and in such cases, the therapist helps the client make use of his or her current abilities so that these abilities continue to be functional.

DOCUMENTATION

As treatment continues, the OTR and COTA regularly document changes occurring in the client's abilities or behavior. Formats for reporting progress differ from one facility to another. Usually, documentation consists of brief, factual notes on the client's progress, comparing present abilities with the initial status. Documentation of services takes up a great deal of the health professional's time, but accurate written records of the service provided and the client's progress toward objectives are absolutely essential for the service to be reimbursed. In many settings, client records have been computerized; this has greatly facilitated the entry of new data and retrieval of client information.

DISCONTINUATION OF INTERVENTION

When treatment objectives have been achieved or when maximum benefit is believed to have occurred, treatment is terminated. At this point, the OTR or COTA prepares a written summary of the occupational therapy treatment process and the results that were achieved. The report may also include recommendations for follow-up services once the client leaves the facility. When the site is a hospital or a skilled nursing facility, the physician or a treatment team may set a date for the client's discharge and make plans for any further services that are needed. Referrals may be made for continued nursing or therapy services to a local community agency. Elderly or handicapped clients may need Meals on Wheels, transportation services, or telephone follow-up. A home assessment may be needed to determine whether clients can safely manage living in their own homes. This planning is often critical to the successful independent living of clients after an illness or injury and is an important responsibility of the staff. Because many people today have no family members living nearby to assist them during periods of illness or incapacity, community services are absolutely essential to fill these needs. The OTR and COTA should be familiar with local community resources so that they can recommend appropriate services for clients when needed.

STANDARDS OF PRACTICE

This, then, is the occupational therapy process. It occurs, with minor variations, in each setting where occupational therapy is available. To encourage quality occupational therapy service, AOTA has developed standards of practice that describe the minimum acceptable standards of service for occupational therapy programs. They may be applied to all types of facilities and all client populations. The most recent standards of practice were approved by the AOTA Representative Assembly in 1991 and address the professional standing of personnel, the referral process, client screening, assessment, the intervention plan, the intervention process, discontinuation of service, quality assurance, and management responsibilities. Although the AOTA standards of practice provide guidelines for the provision of occupational therapy services, it should be noted that in states that regulate occupational therapy practice, the state practice law determines practice requirements in that jurisdiction. A copy of the current AOTA standards of practice may be found in the Appendix (7).

ETHICAL CONSIDERATIONS

As we have seen in other chapters, ethical issues are often discussed in the health care environment of the 1990s. Advances in medical practice and new technologies have made it possible to sustain life artificially for prolonged periods of time, have enabled physicians to transplant organs and reattach severed limbs, and have allowed medical scientists to create new life through in vitro fertilization. Society has had to face difficult questions. When does life really begin? When does it end, and how is death determined? Who has the authority to make life and death decisions?

Like all health care professionals, OTRs and COTAs face ethical dilemmas in their daily practice. The issues are not usually as dramatic as those faced by physicians, but they often involve decisions that are crucial to the clients being served. Occupational therapy personnel must decide which clients have the best potential to benefit from their services, whether clients can afford the optimum level of services that they need, how the client is going to cope at home after a too-short hospital stay, and what to do for a client who requests help in terminating his or her life.

As health care practitioners, OTRs and COTAs agree to practice in accordance with the *Occupational Therapy Code of Ethics* published by the AOTA in 1988 (8). This document contains both general and specific ethical guidelines and may be found in the Appendix. It is important that occupational therapy students and practitioners cultivate a strong commitment to ethical practice to warrant the trust that their clients place in them. As noted in Chapter 5, the American Occupational Therapy Certification Board (AOTCB) is authorized to take disciplinary action in cases of alleged unethical or incompetent practice. The state that licenses or regulates occupational therapy practice may also take disciplinary action in cases where the practice law has been violated. The AOTCB's grounds for discipline may be found in the Appendix.

PATIENT RIGHTS

In 1972, the American Hospital Association adopted a *Patient Bill of Rights* that listed the rights of patients while under the care of health professionals. Most hospitals and all nursing homes now routinely inform patients of their rights during admission to the facility. The patient's bill of rights includes the following points. The patient has the right to:

1. Considerate and respectful care;
2. Current and complete information concerning his or her condition, treatment, and prognosis;
3. Receive information necessary to give informed consent prior to the start of any procedure or treatment;
4. Refuse treatment;
5. Every consideration of his or her privacy concerning the medical care program;
6. Expect that all communications and records should be treated as confidential;

7. Expect the hospital to make a reasonable response to the patient's request for services;
8. Obtain information on the relationship of the hospital to other health care facilities;
9. Be advised of any human experimentation affecting his or her care or treatment;
10. Expect reasonable continuity of care;
11. Examine and receive an explanation of his or her bill regardless of the source of payment;
12. Know what hospital rules and regulations apply to his or her conduct while a patient (9).

REIMBURSEMENT SYSTEMS

Before we begin our in-depth review of occupational therapy practice, we should briefly discuss the reimbursement of occupational therapy services. Services are paid for by a variety of sources: the client's personal funds, commercial health insurers, or state and federal funds. Insurance programs (Medicare, Medicaid, worker's compensation, and private plans) pay service providers after the service has been delivered. Grant programs (the Education for all Handicapped Children Act, Community Mental Health Centers Act, the Older Americans Act, Social Security Title XX) provide ongoing funding for an overall program of which occupational therapy may be a part. There are great differences between these two types of reimbursement systems: insurance programs are highly specific as to what services will be paid for and to what extent; grant programs are more flexible as long as the broad goals of the program are met. All payment systems regulate, to some extent, the way in which services are delivered. Providers must be familiar with the regulations of reimbursement systems that pay for their services so that they know in advance the coverage allowed for the services they provide (10).

The AOTA has developed an occupational therapy product output reporting system to aid practitioners in billing and reporting their services uniformly. This system lists each service provided by occupational therapy and assigns a relative value for each 15-minute interval of service. Costs are calculated based on the service activity, the amount of time spent in the activity, and the therapist-client ratio (11). Occupational therapy services may be billed specifically as occupational therapy or they may be included in a larger service category. Table 9.4 shows the reimbursement sources reported by AOTA members in 1990 that were paying for occupational therapy services. State and local programs were important sources of funding, along with Medicare and private insurance (5).

The OTR and COTA need to be knowledgeable about the reimbursement systems in effect at their facility, since they directly participate in the billing process. Grant funds administered by a facility are subject to close scrutiny by federal or state auditors, while insurance reimbursement systems are closely monitored by the insurer. The health care provider needs some knowledge of cost accounting and fiscal management for the service department to run smoothly.

SUMMARY

Occupational therapy practice has changed as the health care system moved from its traditional fee-for-service reimbursement system to a prospective payment system with managed care. The sites of service delivery are changing, but the need for occupational therapy service continues to be strong and the profession anticipates a period of steady growth and development of occupational therapy clinical programs. A clinical reasoning process underlies clinical decision-making in occupational therapy and ethical considerations are becoming more important as health care resources are limited for many people. The occupational therapy process has been described and will be referred to again in the next chapters that look at specific practice areas of occupational therapy.

Table 9.4. Reimbursement Sources

Sources	OTRs (%)	COTAs (%)
Blue Cross/Blue Shield	6.3	6.4
Other private insurance	11.7	8.3
Medicare	23.6	26.9
Medicaid	9.6	13.5
Vocational rehabilitation agency (DVR/OVR)	0.8	1.1
Workers' compensation	8.9	5.5
Other federal programs (Champus, OVR)	3.4	3.6
State/local programs	26.3	26.6
Client direct payment	4.3	4.3
Other	5.1	3.7
Total	100.0	100.0

Discussion Questions

1. What areas of occupational therapy practice are particularly interesting to you? Have you already decided on a practice specialty?
2. What are some of the most common work settings for OTRs and COTAs in your area? Are they similar to or different from those shown in national statistics?
3. You are an occupational therapy student doing a level I field work experience at a nursing home. Another student in your class is at the same facility and one day you hear this student describing a patient she is working with to a classmate. She discusses material that she has read in the nursing notes in great detail. You believe that she is violating patient confidentiality. What should you do?
4. The geographic maldistribution of occupational therapy personnel is a serious problem that has slowed the development of services in some areas. What might some of the reasons be for this, and how could it be corrected?
5. If your state has an occupational therapy practice act, get a copy of the standards of practice. How do they compare to the AOTA standards?
6. Paperwork is a necessary part of every health professional's job. Why is it so important?
7. You are employed in an acute care hospital and have good working relationships with your colleagues. You have become friendly with a surgical nurse and sometimes have lunch with her when your work hours coincide. One day she confides in you that she has just learned that she is HIV positive. She is very upset but does not want to tell her supervisor because she is a single parent and can't take a chance on losing her job. What should you do?
8. A patient that you have been working with has no insurance coverage for the extended treatment that you think she needs. How could you help the patient get the needed treatment?

References

1. AOTA: Representative Assembly Motion on Specialty Certification. Rockville, MD: AOTA, 1987.
2. Ezersky S, Havazelet L, Scott A, Zettler C: Specialty Choice in Occupational Therapy. *Am J Occup Ther* 43:227–233, 1989.
3. Wittman P, Swinehart S, Cahill R, St. Michel G: Variables affecting specialty choice in occupational therapy. *Am J Occup Ther* 43:602–606, 1989.
4. Ad Hoc Commission on Occupational Therapy Manpower: *Occupational Therapy Manpower: A Plan for Progress*. Rockville, MD: AOTA, 1985, pp. 32–39, 55–56.
5. AOTA: 1990 Member Data Survey. *OT Week* 5:1–8, 1991.
6. Uniform occupational therapy evaluation checklist. *Am J Occup Ther* 35:817–818, 1981.
7. AOTA: Standards of practice for occupational therapy. *OT Week* 6:9–12, 1992.
8. AOTA: Occupational therapy code of ethics. *Am J Occup Ther* 42:795–796, 1988.

9. Finneran J: Patient's rights. *Occup Ther Forum* III:10–13, 1988.
10. Scott SG: Payment for occupational therapy services. In Bair J, Gray M, eds. *The Occupational Therapy Manager*. Rockville, MD: AOTA, 1985, pp. 325–340.
11. Task Force, Commission on Practice: *Occupational Therapy Product Output Reporting System and Uniform Terminology for Reporting Occupational Therapy Services*. Rockville, MD: AOTA, 1980.

SUGGESTED READINGS

Benham PK: Attitudes of occupational therapy personnel toward persons with disabilities. *Am J Occup Ther* 42:305–311, 1988.

Hansen RA: The ethics of caring for patients with HIV or AIDs. *Am J Occup Ther* 44:239–242, 1990.

Parham D: Toward professionalism: the reflective therapist. *Am J Occup Ther* 41:555–561, 1987.

Peloquin SM: The patient-therapist relationship in occupational therapy: understanding visions and images. *Am J Occup Ther* 44:13–21, 1990.

Special Issue on Clinical Reasoning. *Am J Occup Ther* 45:11, 1991.

Special Issue on Ethics. *Am J Occup Ther* 42:5, 1988.

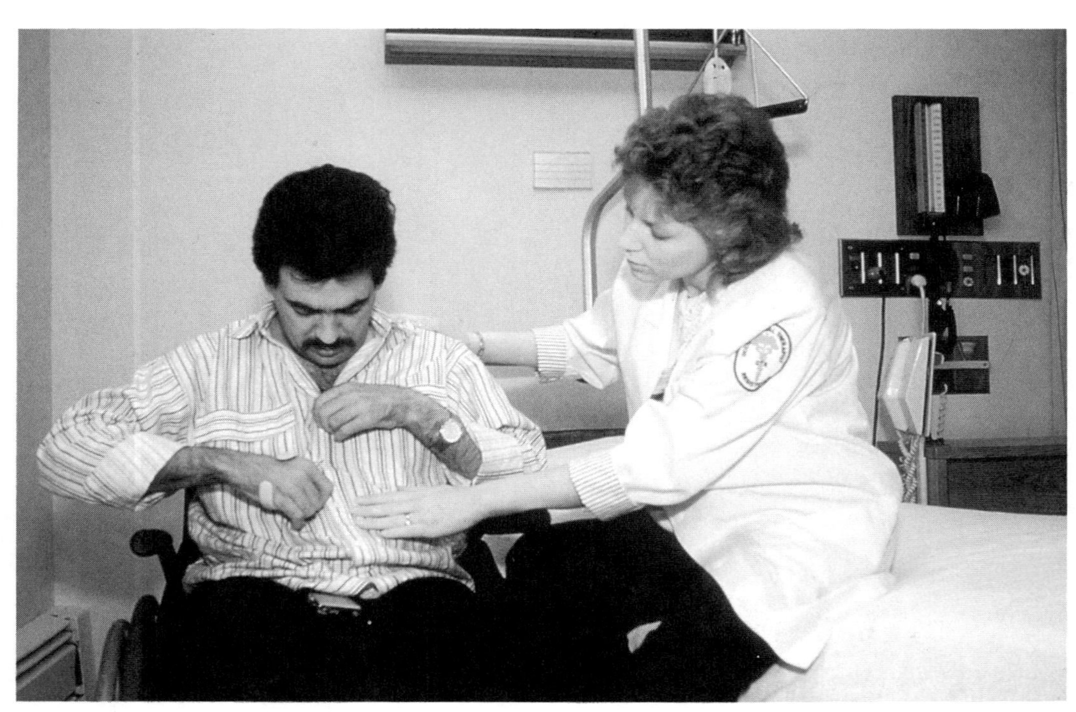

10 Practice in the Acute Care Hospital

Hospitals have always been the largest employer of occupational therapy personnel, and they continue to be. A survey of occupational therapists showed that, in 1990, 25.4% of all OTRs and 19% of all COTAs were working in general hospitals. Not all hospitals offered occupational therapy services, however. According to the American Hospital Association, only 52.5% of all hospitals provided occupational therapy in 1990. Table 10.1 shows the different types of hospitals and the percentage of each offering occupational therapy services (1).

PRACTICE SITE

The acute care hospital treats patients with immediate medical needs (a serious illness, severe injuries, or a need for a surgical procedure) and provides short-term hospital care (less than 30 days). It has always been a challenging place to work. Occupational therapy personnel must be prepared to deal with a variety of diagnostic categories and must be able to plan and implement a treatment program quickly once a patient has been referred for service. The pace tends to be rapid and maximum flexibility is needed, since the caseload changes frequently. Therapists or therapy assistants working in this setting must be particularly good at managing their time, since patient stays are short.

Table 10.1. Hospitals Offering Occupational Therapy Services in the U.S. in 1990

Hospital Type	% Offering O.T.
Federal	61.1
Psychiatric	94.1
General and other	59.2
Nonfederal	52.1
Psychiatric	66.7
Tuberculosis and respiratory disease	33.3
Long-Term general and other	84.9
Short-Term general and other	49.6
Hospital units of an institution	23.5
Community hospitals	49.6

TREATMENT TEAM

In the acute care hospital, close team relationships help make treatment of patients much more effective. Often, treatment teams are organized to deal with specific diagnostic groups. Table 10.2 shows some of the related services that are typically found in acute care hospitals.

In this setting, the team will consist of medical personnel involved in the immediate care of the patient: physicians, nurses, staff of the intensive care unit, respiratory therapists, social workers, physical therapists, speech and

Table 10.2. Therapy Services in U.S. Hospitals in 1990 (6105 Hospitals Reporting)

Service	% of Hospitals Offering Service
Occupational therapy	52.5
Physical therapy	79.0
Recreation	40.5
Respiratory therapy	81.0
Speech therapy	45.0

language therapists, nursing assistants, and technicians. Family members are important members of the treatment team and need to be fully informed about the care the patient is receiving and the family's role in the recovery process. Because hospital stays are growing shorter, the patient may be transferred to another facility for continued care and rehabilitation. More than one team may become involved in the patient's therapeutic program.

KEY CONCEPTS IN ACUTE CARE

As health care delivery has changed, the role of the acute care hospital has changed dramatically. In 1983 a prospective payment system was implemented for inpatient care of Medicare recipients. The system was based on the concept of diagnostic-related groups (DRGs). Categories were developed for 471 medical, surgical, psychiatric, and rehabilitation diagnoses. Each DRG was assigned a weighting system that determines the payment that the hospital receives for the care of Medicare patients. Among the factors considered are principal diagnosis, operating room procedures, additional diagnoses and procedures, the age and sex of the patient, and the patient's status at discharge. Under this reimbursement system, the hospital receives a fixed rate of payment for each Medicare patient treated, regardless of the number of services provided or the length of stay (2).

The prospective payment system caused major changes in health care delivery. Hospital stays grew shorter, and patients were being discharged not yet able to resume their normal patterns of living. There was an increased need for extended care facilities, home health services, and outpatient programs that could continue the treatment regimes begun in acute care hospitals. There was a comparable need for hospice programs to provide services and support to the terminally ill. More and more active treatment is taking place in these alternative care facilities and less in the acute care hospital.

CHANGING PATTERNS OF CARE

In 1990 the national economy experienced a slowdown; one result was a threat to the financial stability of many acute care hospitals. Administrators reacted by trying to cut costs even further and third-party payers tried to reduce their spending. The result was even less revenue for hospitals and increased financial pressure. Because of the economic recession there were greater numbers of unemployed people who lacked health insurance. More of the burden was shifted to Medicaid (the federal medical assistance program for the poor) and hospitals also treated some patients for no compensation. As a result of these stresses inpatient care began to decline while outpatient care increased. The federal government began to enforce reforms in Medicare reimbursement and to develop a prospective payment system for outpatient services.

Changes in medical reimbursement were long overdue. In 1990, 34.4 million Americans lacked any form of health insurance. Many of the uninsured were the working poor—employed, but not covered by an employer health plan and unable to afford private health insurance. Medicaid was inadequate to meet the increasing needs of this group and 50% of the uninsured did not qualify for its coverage in 1990. The numbers of elderly people in the population continued to increase and Medicare (the federal health insurance for the elderly) was now contributing 40.4% of the income of acute care hospitals. Even so, because of tight spending restrictions, 60% of all acute care hospitals lost money on Medicare patients in 1990 (1).

Community hospitals continued to decline as many closed and others merged with other health care groups. Since 1980, 558 community hospitals have closed and this was especially frequent in rural areas.

Acute care hospital admissions declined 13.7% from 1980–1990. The average length of a patient stay in 1990 was 7.2 days. The need for emergency and trauma services was rising.

Although 90% of all community hospitals had emergency departments that were staffed 24 hours a day, the number of certified trauma centers had declined since 1985.

In an effort to meet patient needs and to increase their revenues many community hospitals developed new services. These included long-term care units; adult day care facilities; respite care; day care for sick children of employed parents; diagnostic services for Alzheimer's disease and other dementias; comprehensive geriatric assessment services; special geriatric clinics and acute care units; senior membership programs that provided information, social activities, health and wellness programs, and emergency response systems for those who lived alone; and outpatient services for AIDs patients (1). In some states rural hospital cooperatives were established to develop rural health services and to allow small hospitals to share specialized services such as occupational and physical therapy.

There seems to have been no loss of occupational therapy positions in acute care hospitals. Frequently seen diagnoses include strokes (cerebrovascular accident—CVA), hand injuries, back injuries, traumatic brain injury, fractures, and burns. On pediatric units developmental delays are frequently seen, along with cases of cerebral palsy. Occupational therapists are now seeing patients earlier in their hospital stay (often while patients are still in the intensive care unit) and are working with more patients who are medically unstable. Many rehabilitation units have waiting lists, sometimes necessitating an extended wait before a bed becomes available. Significant growth has occurred in outpatient occupational therapy services. Because of shorter hospital stays discharge planning often begins as soon as the patient is admitted. Good communication needs to be established with community agencies and long-term care facilities to effect a smooth transition for the patient from hospital to aftercare services. In some acute care hospitals, OTRs must perform a sort of triage, making decisions about a patient's potential for recovery and identifying services to assist with his or her rehabilitation outside of the hospital. Quality assurance programs have been established in most occupational therapy departments in order to be fully accountable to hospital administration and to reimbursers.

CURRENT PRACTICE ISSUES AND TRENDS

Occupational therapy departments in acute care hospitals have responded to these changes in a variety of ways. In some departments, personnel have been reassigned from inpatient care to the growing outpatient services. Alternative work schedules have been introduced, so that maximum use can be made of facilities, staff, and equipment. Some departments now provide service 7 days a week and may be open during the evening as well as the day. Highly specialized personnel may be on call for emergency situations where their expertise is needed. Documentation of services continues to take large amounts of time for all health professionals although computerized record-keeping has speeded up the process. Occupational therapy departments are being urged to adopt productivity measures and to practice cost containment in the ordering of supplies and equipment (3).

The workload has increased for occupational therapy personnel in acute care hospitals, and OTRs and COTAs are often required to work overtime hours when severe cases are admitted and require immediate attention. Because trauma cases are increasing, advanced knowledge is needed to deal with the severe injuries and complex conditions that are being seen. Team effort is essential in the acute care hospital.

Emotional stress can run high in the intense life and death environment of acute care. Therapists need to recognize when they are experiencing job stress and actively search for ways to deal with it. Not everyone feels comfortable in the unpredictable acute care setting and it is important to recognize personal limitations and tolerances. Working in acute care presents everyday challenges to OTRs and COTAs.

SUMMARY

As hospitals engage in intense competition for the health care dollar, some loss of occupational therapy positions may occur. It is likely, however, that such losses will be offset by the development of new positions in alternative care services. Acute care services are not declining. They are only shifting to new locations. Occupational therapy will continue to be a needed service in many of these new programs. In addition, some hospitals are expanding the range of occupational therapy services to meet changing needs. Larger outpatient programs, involvement in home health care, work-hardening programs to prepare the injured worker to resume employment, and health promotion and education are only a few of these expanding service areas.

The acute care hospital is in the vanguard of major changes now occurring in health care. The nature of these changes will challenge the OTRs and COTAs who work in acute care settings for years to come. Creativity and flexibility will be needed to respond to the changing health care economy and the changing patient population. It is expected that occupational therapy personnel will adapt to these changing needs and continue to play an active role in acute care.

What is it like to work in an acute care hospital? Let's look at a typical hospital and follow the case of an occupational therapy client who was seen in an acute care setting.

Case Study: Head Injury

St. Joseph's Hospital is a 517-bed community hospital in a medium-sized midwestern city. Late one evening Laurie, an 18-year-old college student, was admitted to the emergency room of St. Joseph's. She and a group of friends had been out together and on the way home their vehicle was struck head-on by another car. Two of Laurie's friends were killed in the accident and Laurie was rushed by ambulance to the emergency room. There she was found to have sustained a severe closed head injury and facial trauma.

After being stabilized by the emergency room staff Laurie was transferred to the Intensive Care Unit (ICU) where she spent the next 9 days in a deep coma. Complications developed, including respiratory problems that required a tracheostomy and use of a respirator, and a cranial blood clot that required surgery to remove. During Laurie's second day in the ICU, she was evaluated by an OTR who found that she had abnormal posturing, no right-sided movement, flailing movements of the left extremities, and a fixed gaze with left pupil dilation and deviation to the left. Laurie could not move when asked to do so and was unresponsive to most forms of stimuli.

Initially, all communication was absent, but after 9 days in the ICU Laurie was able to respond to yes-or-no questions with eyeblinks. Laurie was then transferred to the neurology unit of the hospital. She was being tube-fed since she had no swallowing reflex and was still unable to move her right side. Increased muscle tone in her right arm made moving that arm especially difficult. Based on her evaluation results the OTR established an intervention plan with short-term and long-term goals. The immediate need was to prevent sensory deprivation and encourage Laurie's awareness of sensory stimuli. Family members were encouraged to talk to Laurie, play tapes of familiar voices, and to turn on the radio and television periodically. The OTR used tactile, visual, olfactory, and gustatory stimuli to increase Laurie's responses to sensory stimuli. Another early goal of occupational therapy was to prevent contractures and deformities that can result from lying in one position and not using the muscles and joints. Passive range-of-motion exercises were done to both arms twice a day, and the OTR advised the nursing staff on appropriate bed positioning for Laurie. A third goal was to educate the family about Laurie's condition and provide them with emotional support during this difficult period.

Laurie continued to be seen by the OTR twice a day for 30-minute sessions during the acute phase of her hospitalization. After 2 weeks Laurie was showing great improvement in her awareness of her surroundings and her medical condition was considered stable enough to transfer her to the rehabilitation floor of the hospital.

The therapeutic programs that had been begun on the neurology unit were continued on the rehabilitation unit. Laurie was beginning to be able to move her right arm, and the physical therapist was trying to elicit some movement in her legs. She was beginning to recognize visual forms and shapes but had an attention span of only 15 seconds. A splint was made by the OTR to help decrease tightness of the biceps muscle and Laurie was encouraged to use her right arm.

Within the next month, Laurie's progress was dramatic. She began to talk, to eat, and was able to breathe without the tracheostomy. She seemed ready to relearn some self-care activities, so a COTA was assigned to work with her on self-care tasks for 45 minutes each day. She gradually learned to wash her face, brush her teeth, bathe, and dress herself. She was now able to move her right arm through its full range of motion but continued to have problems with strength and coordination. Severe cognitive limitations continued to be present. Laurie had trouble with problem-solving, judgment, sequencing tasks, following directions, and memory. Rehabilitation was now focusing on improving Laurie's active and passive range of motion, improv ing the strength and coordination of her right arm, self-care training, and cognitive retraining.

Plans for Laurie's discharge were now under way. It was decided to continue her rehabilitation program on an outpatient basis, and Laurie was scheduled to visit the outpatient clinic three times a week to continue occupational and physical therapy and to be followed by her physician. While in the hospital Laurie had been taught to use a computer as part of her cognitive retraining program. Her family purchased a home computer to allow her to continue with these retraining activities at home. The OTR recommended appropriate software, gave her homework assignments, and checked her work during outpatient visits.

Although Laurie will probably never completely regain her former abilities, she made significant improvement through her therapeutic program. Her cognitive limitations continue, but she should be able to work and enjoy a full range of social and recreational activities. Laurie's multiple problems required a strong team approach and a unified intervention plan. Each discipline that worked with her contributed its special skills to Laurie's recovery and the outcome was considered a successful one.

Discussion Questions

1. Do some volunteer work in your local community hospital. Do you feel comfortable working in an acute care setting?
2. The stressful environment of the acute care hospital can lead to burnout of health care workers. How can OTRs and COTAs deal with job stress and pressure in this fast-paced setting?
3. Therapists in acute care hospitals are seeing sicker and more severely injured patients. What bodies of knowledge might be especially important to working in this health care environment?
4. In some acute care hospitals, occupational therapy departments must be staffed evenings and weekends as well as weekday hours. How do you feel about working weekend shifts, overtime, or being on call?
5. How did the OTR and the COTA work together on this case?
6. If St. Joseph's Hospital had not had a rehabilitation unit, where might Laurie have received such services?
7. How do health care workers maintain their objectivity and professionalism while working in such an emotionally charged environment?

References

1. American Hospital Association: *AHA Hospital Statistics, 1991–1992*. Chicago, IL, 1992.
2. Questions and answers about medicare prospective payment. *Occup Ther News* 38(10):4, 1984.

3. Prospective payment survey shows occupational therapy a healthy profession. *Occup Ther News* 39(10):8, 1985.
4. Jones A: Acute care intensified the challenge of therapy. *OT Week* 4:4–5, 14, 1990.
5. Evans ML: Therapists can take positive career steps. *OT Week* 2:4–6, 1988.

Suggested Readings

Daniel MS, Puccetti DD: Responding to the changing world of acute care. *OT Week* 5:4–5, 30, 1991.

Durham DP: Guidelines for working with the brain-injured patient in the acute care or rehabilitative setting. *Occup Ther Forum* III:10–12, 1988.

Ross FL: The use of computers in occupational therapy for visual-scanning training. *Am J Occup Ther* 46:314–322, 1992.

Staff: Stimulation provided to comatose patients. *Adv Occup Ther* 7:20–21,1991.

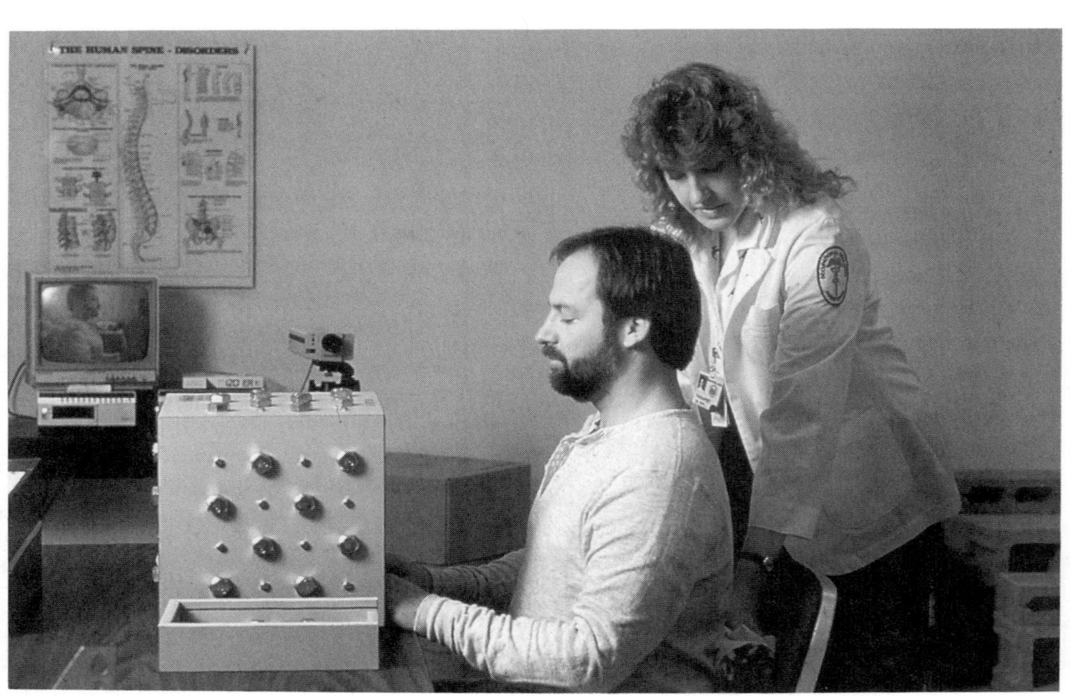
THE HUMAN SPINE - DISORDERS

11 Adult Rehabilitation Practice

Long-term care and rehabilitation of physical dysfunctions has been a traditional area of occupational therapy practice and represents one of the most common specialty areas within the field. Although practice with physical dysfunctions has undergone many changes in theoretical approach and technique, it continues to be an integral part of the medical management for many diseases and physical disabilities. Table 9.3 lists the major disorders that were being seen by OTRs and COTAs in 1990. The majority of these were physical disorders (1).

The types of physical disorders that OTRs and COTAs are working with have not changed substantially in the last 10 years, although there is an increase in the number of COTAs who are working with hemiplegic patients and a decrease in the number of OTRs and COTAs who are working with patients who have arteriosclerosis. The overall number of COTAs working with physical dysfunctions appears to have increased steadily over the last few years. According to AOTA projections, more occupational therapists will be working with cancer patients in the future, as more patients survive the disease and become candidates for rehabilitation services. The number of head trauma patients seen by occupational therapy personnel has increased and the incidence of cerebrovascular accident (CVA/hemiplegia) has declined.

One additional trend seen in practitioners who work with physical dysfunctions is that more therapists appear to be specializing. Hand therapy, specialized work in spinal cord injury, the treatment of burns, and work-related programs are all areas demanding advanced knowledge and skills and are attracting greater numbers of therapists.

PRACTICE SITES

Practice locations for the treatment of physical dysfunctions include acute care hospitals, rehabilitation centers, nursing homes and extended care facilities, outpatient services and community-based programs, public and private schools, and private practices. Each contributes a somewhat different type of care for the client with a physical dysfunction. The first place where a patient with a physical disorder is seen by occupational therapy personnel is usually the acute care hospital. Here the patient's condition is stabilized and immediate medical needs are attended to. If long-term rehabilitation services are needed, the patient may be transferred to the rehabilitation unit of the hospital if such a service is provided. If not, he or she may be transferred to a separate rehabilitation hospital or to a nursing home where long-term residential care and rehabilitative services can be offered. If the client is ambulatory, outpatient service or therapy programs offered by community agencies might be used. For children with physical disabilities, private and public schools provide therapy services as part of the overall educational program. In addition, OTRs and COTAs working in private or group practices may offer therapy on a fee-for-service basis. The occupational therapy services provided will vary with each practice location. Frequently, the physically disabled client needs a continuum of rehabilitation services, ranging from acute care of the injury or illness to long-term restorative care and follow-up as his or her condition improves. It is not unusual for a client to be seen by three or four different agencies in the course of treatment, with each providing care at a different stage of recovery.

TREATMENT TEAM

The team approach is often used in rehabilitation settings. The treatment team may be headed by a physiatrist (a physician specializing in physical medicine and rehabilitation), who refers the client for specific therapy services and supervises the medical management of the case. Other members of the team might be rehabilitation nurses, who provide daily nursing care and follow-through on therapy procedures; physical therapists, who work to restore movement and ambulation skills; speech therapists, who deal with speech and language deficiencies; social workers, who provide liaisons with the client's family, the community, and the reimbursement system; psychologists, who may be involved in client counseling; and vocational rehabilitation personnel, who are concerned with the client's eventual employment. Other team members who are called in if needed include the orthotist, who will make customized splints, and the prosthetist, who may evaluate the client's need for an artificial limb and then fabricate or adapt one. The supplier of durable medical equipment may also be asked to join the team to advise on suitable equipment (wheelchair, walker) to meet the client's needs. Long-term rehabilitation demands a strong team effort because the problems confronted are often complex and affect so many areas of the client's life. Good communication between team members greatly enhances the effectiveness of the total treatment program, and team members often resemble an institutional "family," all working together for the maximum benefit of the client.

SECONDARY EFFECTS OF PHYSICAL DYSFUNCTION

A disease or injury that causes severe physical or mental impairment can be devastating to an individual and to the individual's family. When the condition is the result of a sudden occurrence such as an accident, the physical and emotional shock is especially great. Although usually the patient's condition is nonprogressive, the disruption of the individual's life is so extreme that the physical injury can result in serious psychological disturbances as well. Patients may need to face not only changes in their physical abilities but also changes in their family and social relationships, temporary or permanent loss of work roles, and dependence in the most basic areas of self-care. Patients may have been disfigured by the injury or may have lost their ability to communicate with others. All of these losses combine to overwhelm the client who is suddenly disabled (2). Sometimes clients in this situation retire into the "sick role," giving up individual control of their daily life and retreating into invalidism. Clients may withdraw from social interactions and be unable to maintain their former family and social relationships. These psychological reactions are not unusual in people who must face severe physical impairment; the OTR and COTA must be prepared to deal with the patient's psychological reactions just as much as with his or her physical limitations. Versluys (3) has noted that normal emotional reactions to severe illness or injury may include depression, mourning, denial, regression, and anxiety. The OTR or COTA working with physically disabled clients needs to understand these reactions as part of the adjustment process. Sensitivity to the feelings of clients as they move through a long period of adjustment enables the therapist to know when the clients can be safely "pushed" toward further achievement and when their occasional refusal to participate in treatment activities must be accepted.

When the condition is progressive, such as in multiple sclerosis or arthritis, clients may experience alternate periods when they feel well and when they feel pain and experience limited function. These clients must be helped to accept the continuing nature of their disability and adjust to the changing status of their health. Often the emotional reactions of clients influence their physical condition. Clients may need to learn to reduce stress and express their frustration and anxiety in nondestructive ways.

Many injuries or illnesses lead to secondary complications that make the treatment process even more complex. The therapist may need to consider multiple problems when developing an intervention plan. The therapist works with the client to establish priorities and organizes treatment in a logical progression. Some problems may demand immediate attention, whereas others can legitimately be postponed until a later phase of treatment. By making the client a member of the treatment team, these issues can be discussed and resolved in a way that everyone can accept.

Family involvement is often an important part of the treatment program. To make treatment as relevant as possible to individual client needs, the therapist must be aware of the client's life-style, family relationships, home and work responsibilities, and personal goals. The family can be extremely helpful in sharing information and can also actively participate in treatment activities. The OTR and COTA may teach family members some of the therapy procedures so that they can provide additional practice for the client in treatment activities. Families often need encouragement and emotional support throughout the client's recovery and may wish to remain in contact with the OTR or COTA for a period of time after the therapy program has been completed. The therapeutic relationship among the therapist, the client, and the client's family is critical to success in the treatment process.

The occupational therapy process is the same for treatment of physical disorders as for other types of client problems. In a long-term rehabilitation program, however, therapy may continue for months before adequate functional abilities are restored. Because the delivery of health care services is rapidly changing in the United States, more and more rehabilitative care is being provided through nursing homes, outpatient programs, home health care, and community agencies. Good coordination is needed between agencies involved in rehabilitation services to ensure continuity of care to meet changing client needs.

BODIES OF KNOWLEDGE

Neurodevelopmental Approaches

One group of treatment approaches (Rood, Bobath, Ayres) is directed at facilitating changes in the central nervous system that will result in improved neuromotor control and function for the client. To use these methods effectively, therapists must have a comprehensive understanding of the anatomy and physiology of the nervous system, the sensory systems, the neuromuscular system, and the mechanisms that underly motor control. Therapy follows a developmental sequence, progressing gradually toward more complex motor patterns and skills.

Neurophysiological Approaches

Two treatment approaches (Brunnstrom, proprioceptive neuromuscular facilitation) focus on rebuilding basic movement patterns in the client and utilize sensory stimulation to elicit motor activity. Functional patterns of movement are developed while abnormal muscle tone and movements are reduced. There is less emphasis on developmental sequence in these two approaches. Positioning and manual pressure may be used to help the client approximate the desired movement patterns, and relaxation techniques are used to increase range of motion. As with the neurodevelopmental methods, these approaches demand a solid knowledge of anatomy, physiology, and the principles of motor control.

Biomechanical Approach

This approach focuses on the mechanical principles of movement as they are applied to the human body. The goal is to improve the client's range of motion (ROM), muscle strength, sensory awareness, and endurance.

Treatment may include the use of active or passive stretching of muscle groups, traction, resistance, and graded exercise. Orthotic devices (splints) may be applied if needed. Eventually clients are encouraged to participate in purposeful activities that provide practice in and reinforcement of the desired movement patterns. The biomechanical approach requires a knowledge of physics principles applied to human movement and an in-depth knowledge of human anatomy and physiology (4).

Hand Therapy

While not a separate treatment approach, hand therapy is a specialized type of rehabilitation for the restoration of hand function. An increasingly popular specialty area of occupational therapy, hand therapy concentrates on the prehensile and nonprehensile functions of the hand. Therapists work on sensory awareness, gross and fine motor control, prehension patterns, strength, and range of motion. Practitioners working as hand therapists develop close working relationships with surgeons, nurses, and family members when attempting to restore normal hand function.

TREATMENT GOALS

Goals in rehabilitation programs may include the restoration or improvement of functional abilities, the maintenance of a client's abilities at an acceptable level, the prevention of further disability, the improvement of the client's ability to function in the home and work environment, appropriate environmental adaptations, the adjustment of the client to temporary or permanent limitations, the exploration of the client's vocational or avocational potential, and resumption of a work role. Goals will vary with the nature of the illness or injury, the stage of recovery, and the client's developmental level and personal circumstances. Goals will be changed frequently as the client progresses in the rehabilitation program, and the OTR or COTA will need to reevaluate the client's status often to upgrade treatment goals and activities.

CHANGING PATTERNS OF CARE

One of the most notable changes in adult rehabilitation is that the client population is changing. Many of today's rehabilitation clients have experienced a whole series of problems that affect their ability to function in society. A patient may come into the hospital emergency room with a gunshot wound, but a serious drug addiction is the root cause of the injury. A middle-aged woman on welfare is unable to afford treatment for her alcoholism and falls down a flight of stairs, suffering multiple fractures. Clients are not only more culturally diverse but their health is directly influenced by poverty, poor nutrition, poor educational background, substandard housing, social disorganization, and a lack of access to health services. Therapists must increasingly consider these factors in looking at the client's overall needs and cannot simply focus on the physical limitation (5).

Therapists today are seeing more severe levels of disability in their practice. Due to advances in surgical technique and medical technology, patients with very severe disabilities are surviving and are posing a challenge to occupational therapists and therapy assistants.

Due to financial constraints, clients are usually staying for shorter periods of time in long-term rehabilitation facilities. A 1987 study reported an average length of stay of 26 days for all disability categories (6). Apparently rehabilitation facilities were little affected by the economic recession of the early 1990s. The Commission for the Accreditation of Rehabilitation Facilities (CARF) reported that there were a total of 8246 accredited rehabilitation programs in 1991 and new programs were continuing to develop (7).

Adults make up 90% of the clients seen in rehabilitation programs. In 1990, 11.4% of all OTRs and 10.9% of all COTAs were employed in rehabilitation facilities.

The use of outpatient programs is increasing in adult rehabilitation as inpatient costs continue to escalate. There is increased use of community support groups, and some groups are using disabled peer advisors to provide clients with emotional support and to answer questions about living with disability. The use of groups led by COTAs has declined in some areas because of difficulties with reimbursement.

PRACTICE ISSUES AND TRENDS

The rise of work assessment and retraining programs has been a major trend in recent years. The American Disabilities Act of 1990 protected the rights of individuals with disabilities and laid down criteria for the accessibility of public buildings and workplaces as well as prohibiting discrimination in hiring workers. OTRs and COTAs have developed and implemented programs to evaluate work capacity and tolerance, to conduct work-hardening training, to provide work simulations and on-the-job training, to evaluate job sites, and to lead injury prevention programs (8). This rapidly expanding area of practice has programs located in hospitals and rehabilitation centers, community facilities, private practice settings, mental health centers, and schools.

New treatment modalities have appeared that are increasingly being used in rehabilitation settings. Biofeedback, using the electronic monitoring of neuromuscular responses, has aided in relaxation training, pain management, and neuromuscular reeducation. Advances in biomedical technology have led to the development of myoelectric prostheses that require only minimal muscle function to operate the devices. New techniques have been developed in the treatment of burns, and innovative functional seating systems have made life in a wheelchair much more comfortable for many disabled people. Functional electrical stimulation (FES) and the transcutaneous electrical nerve stimulator (TENS) are being used in some facilities.

The use of physical agents (hot packs, paraffin, electrical stimulation, etc.) by OTRs has given rise to considerable controversy in the field. Some believe that such modalities belong within the realm of physical therapy and argue that occupational therapists are not educated in their use. However, many therapists working in rehabilitation programs point out that physical agent modalities are often needed early in treatment to prepare for later functional activity. In 1992 the AOTA Representative Assembly passed a revised modalities policy that sanctioned the use of physical agents by qualified practitioners when used to prepare for or as an adjunct to purposeful activity (9).

Technology has expanded occupational therapy services in many ways. Computer-assisted rehabilitation is now commonplace and OTRs and COTAs now need basic computer skills in order to appropriately use the technology. The development of new equipment for the disabled—robotic arms, lightweight wheelchairs, high-tech prostheses for amputees—is making daily life a lot easier for many people with limited function.

OTRs and COTAs are becoming more highly specialized in rehabilitation practice. We are seeing the continued development of chronic pain management programs, cardiac rehabilitation programs, specialized rehabilitation for breast cancer patients, driver reeducation programs, and visual rehabilitation. Therapists have become more active in preventive programs and many hospitals and clinics now have programs to prevent back injuries and other frequently occuring problems. OTRs and COTAs are also becoming involved in patient education, conducting classes on learning to live with diabetes, arthritis, chronic obstructive pulmonary disease, or the residuals of a stroke.

SUMMARY

New roles for occupational therapists and therapy assistants are developing rapidly in rehabilitation specialty areas. Practice in adult rehabilitation offers constant challenges to the practitioner and continues to be a strong area of occupational therapy practice. As the health care system continues to change, occupational therapy services may be modified or take new forms but will continue to provide vital services to physically disabled clients.

Case Study: Spinal Cord Injury

Mark is an example of a typical case seen in a long-term rehabilitation program. Mark is a 27-year-old man who was employed as an air traffic controller at the airport of a large midwestern city. He was married but had no children. On a summer Sunday, Mark and his wife were attending a family picnic in a country park beside a large lake. Mark joined other family members who were swimming and dove into the lake from a pier. When he did not come up, family members dove for him and recovered his body in three feet of water. He was quickly brought to shore, where he was found to have no pulse or respiration. While someone called an ambulance, Mark's cousin began cardiopulmonary resuscitation and was able to restore Mark's breathing. Mark was taken to the emergency room of a small rural hospital, where he was found to have a spinal cord injury. He was put into cervical traction and later underwent surgical resection of bone fragments at the level of cervical vertebra 5. Mark remained in this acute care hospital for a month and was then transferred to a larger hospital. Here a pulmonary embolism was diagnosed and treated. Mark continued to develop medical complications that required ongoing medical attention. When these conditions were stabilized, Mark was again transferred, this time to Lakeland Rehabilitation Hospital, a 96-bed private rehabilitation facility in his home city, for an extensive rehabilitation program.

The physiatrist who was supervising Mark's care referred him to occupational therapy for evaluation and treatment early in his stay. He was seen by the OTR on his treatment team, who completed a preliminary evaluation and found that Mark had the following problems:

1. Paralysis and loss of sensation below the level of cervical vertebrae 5 and 6. Mark had no movement or feeling in his legs or lower trunk.
2. Deficiencies in strength and sensation of the arms at the level of the lesion and lack of functional use of both arms.
3. Poor endurance and upper body balance.
4. Frequent dizziness and faintness due to blood pressure problems.
5. Dependence in all self-care activities: feeding himself, caring for his own hygiene, and dressing. Mark was unable to carry out any home or work tasks.
6. Impairment in bowel and bladder functions.
7. Occasional depression and sense of hopelessness about the future.

Five days after Mark's admission to Lakeland Hospital, the occupational therapist completed a comprehensive assessment. She found that Mark was unable to perform any independent living activities. He could tolerate only 20 minutes of sitting with his hips and trunk at a 90° angle. He could move his arms partially through their range of motion, but was unable to hold objects. He could partially extend his wrists, but had no adequate grasping action of his hands. He could communicate orally, but could not write because of his motor impairment.

At this point in his recovery, the resumption of his home and job responsibilities were long-term goals. A great deal of improvement in his physical abilities was needed before these could be realistic objectives. Fortunately, Mark's high level of intelligence, his emotional health, and his positive self-concept gave him many strengths to build on in working toward these end goals.

Biofeedback techniques were used for muscle reeducation, and some positioning splints were made to prevent further disability. The occupational therapist recommended that a dynamic (movable) wrist-driven flexor hinge splint be made for Mark and fitted him when he had developed strong enough wrist movements to be able to use it. The immediate goals were for the improvement of performance components that would enable him to move toward independent living. They included strengthening Mark's wrist extensor muscles, increasing his ability to sit in his chair for up to 30 minutes at a time, teaching him substitute patterns of movement for those he had lost, compensating for some of his sensory losses, developing increased independence in self-care tasks, improving his ability to use his hands for functional activities, and helping him adjust to his disability.

Treatment sessions were conducted on a daily basis, with frequent reassessment of abilities. Twice a month the treatment team met to discuss Mark's progress. Mark's team consisted of a physiatrist, who was in charge of the total treatment program, an occupational therapist, a physical therapist, a recreational therapist, a social worker, a nurse, and a psychologist. Mark also attended the team meetings and contributed to the development of new goals.

After a month of intensive treatment, Mark had achieved the short-term goals, and the emphasis of the occupational therapy program had changed to focus on lower extremity dressing, homemaking skills, bathing, and the bowel and bladder program. These areas required a longer training period. Mark's general muscle strength and endurance were assessed weekly by the COTA who was in charge of group sessions to increase muscular strength and power. The COTA also worked with Mark in two treatment groups. A strength- and power-building group was used that incorporated progressive resistive exercise to build physical endurance and muscular strength. An adaptive hand skills group was also led by the COTA; this group concentrated on developing the hand skills needed for performance of self-care and work tasks. The COTA also fabricated equipment adapted for Mark's use, including a hairbrush, shower handle, phone cuff, and knife.

Mark's family became involved in his treatment program as well. Because the staff encouraged communication, the family felt comfortable asking questions of the team and often came with Mark to his therapy sessions when they were visiting. At first Mark was uncertain of what to expect in the rehabilitation program but, as he became familiar with the philosophy of the staff and the institution, he began to take an active part in team decisions about his program. He was able to express his thoughts and feelings well and helped solve some of the difficult problems in his own program.

In addition to the individual treatment programs, an education group was conducted for patients with spinal cord injuries by the nursing staff, occupational therapist, and psychologist. Topics such as bowel and bladder care, muscle spasms, sexuality, and assertiveness were discussed and explored. An evening recreational program, jointly coordinated by the occupational therapist, physical therapist, and recreational therapist, offered daily living and recreational activities, such as homemaking class, wheelchair football, and trips to the shopping mall, laundromat, and miniature golf course.

Mark made steady improvement and was discharged from Lakeland Rehabilitation Hospital after four months of intensive rehabilitation. A home visit was made by the occupational and physical therapists along with Mark to see if environmental modifications were necessary. A similar visit that included the vocational counselor was made to Mark's work site. A few minor alterations were recommended, and additional practice was given with the wrist-driven tenodesis splint so that Mark would be able to accomplish his tasks at work.

At the time of discharge, Mark was able to feed himself independently, take care of his own hygiene, put on his own shirt and jacket, and use his splint for typing and writing. He still needed some help with putting on his pants and leg bag (a urinary drainage system), performing some homemaking tasks, and carrying out his bowel program. He was discharged to his parents' home, since he was in the process of a divorce. Home health services were initiated to offer him continued therapy in specific problem areas. He returned to Lakeland Hospital one month after discharge for outpatient help with work skills and some daily living skills. A customized wrist-driven flexor hinge splint had been made for him, and with some practice Mark was able to use this to accomplish fine motor tasks.

After his discharge, Mark completed a driver's training program, passed his driver's test, and purchased a customized van with a lift and hand controls. He returned to work part time in his old job as an air traffic controller and worked up to full-time employment. His fellow workers and employer are supportive and have confidence in his ability to perform his work tasks satisfactorily. Mark has served as president of his local spinal cord injury association and helped to develop an annual "Heels and Wheels" run in his community. He enjoys taking part in it each summer and is proud of a national award that he received for his contributions to the disabled community.

Discussion Questions

1. What special personal qualities do you think an occupational therapist or therapy assistant would need to work with physically disabled clients?
2. Were Mark's personal relationships affected by his injury?
3. If Mark had been unable to return to his old job, what additional services might have been needed in his rehabilitation program?
4. Discuss the role of the COTA in Mark's rehabilitation. How did the OTR and COTA share responsibilities in Mark's treatment program?
5. How much did Mark's positive attitudes contribute to the success of his rehabilitation program?
6. How important was the early treatment of Mark's injury to his eventual recovery?
7. Is there a hospital specializing in rehabilitation of physical dysfunctions in your area? What kinds of disabilities are treated there?
8. Consider the implications that a similar injury would have on your life. What does "coping with a disability" mean to you?

References

1. AOTA 1990 Member Data Survey. Special Insert. *OT Week* 5(22):6, 1991.
2. Spencer A: Functional restoration—theory, principles, and techniques. In Hopkins H, Smith H, eds. *Willard and Spackman's Occupational Therapy*, ed 6. Philadelphia, JB Lippincott, 1983, pp. 353–380.
3. Versluys H: Psychological adjustment to physical disability. In Trombly C, Scott A, eds. *Occupational Therapy for Physical Dysfunction*. Baltimore, Williams & Wilkins, 1977, pp. 10–27.
4. Trombly C, Scott A: The treatment planning process. In Trombly C, Scott A, eds. *Occupational Therapy for Physical Dysfunction*. Baltimore, Williams & Wilkins, 1977, pp. 3–9.
5. Boyle MA: The changing face of the rehabilitation population: a challenge for therapists. *AJOT* 44(10):941–945, 1990.
6. Length of stay is stable but costs increase. *OT Week* 1(12):4, 1987.
7. Egan M: Is rehabilitation growth restricted by the recession? *OT Week* 6(3):12–13, 1992.
8. AOTA Draft Statement: Occupational Therapy Services in Work Practice. *OT Week* 6(5):13–16, 1992.
9. AOTA Position Paper: Physical Agent Modalities. *OT Week* 6(5):12–13, 1992.

Suggested Readings

American Occupational Therapy Association: *Technology Review '90: Perspectives on Occupational Therapy Practice*. Rockville, MD, AOTA, 1990.

American Occupational Therapy Association: *Work in Progress: Occupational Therapy in Work Programs*. Rockville, MD, AOTA, 1989.

Bedbrook G: *The Care and Management of Spinal Cord Injuries*. New York, Springer-Verlag, 1981.

Ford J, Duckworth B: *Physical Management for the Quadriplegic Patient*. Philadelphia, FA Davis, 1974.

Nixon V: *Spinal Cord Injury: A Guide to Functional Outcomes in Physical Therapy Management*. Chicago, Rehabilitation Institute of Chicago, 1985.

Special issue on spinal cord injury. *Am J Occup Ther* 39:11, 1985.

Tator C: *Early Management of Acute Spinal Cord Injury*. New York, Raven Press, 1982.

Umphred D: *Neurological Rehabilitation*. St. Louis, CV Mosby, 1985.

Wyrick JM, Niemeyer LO, Ellexon M, Jacobs K, Taylor, S. Occupational therapy work-hardening programs: a demographic study. *AJOT* 45(2):109–112, 1991.

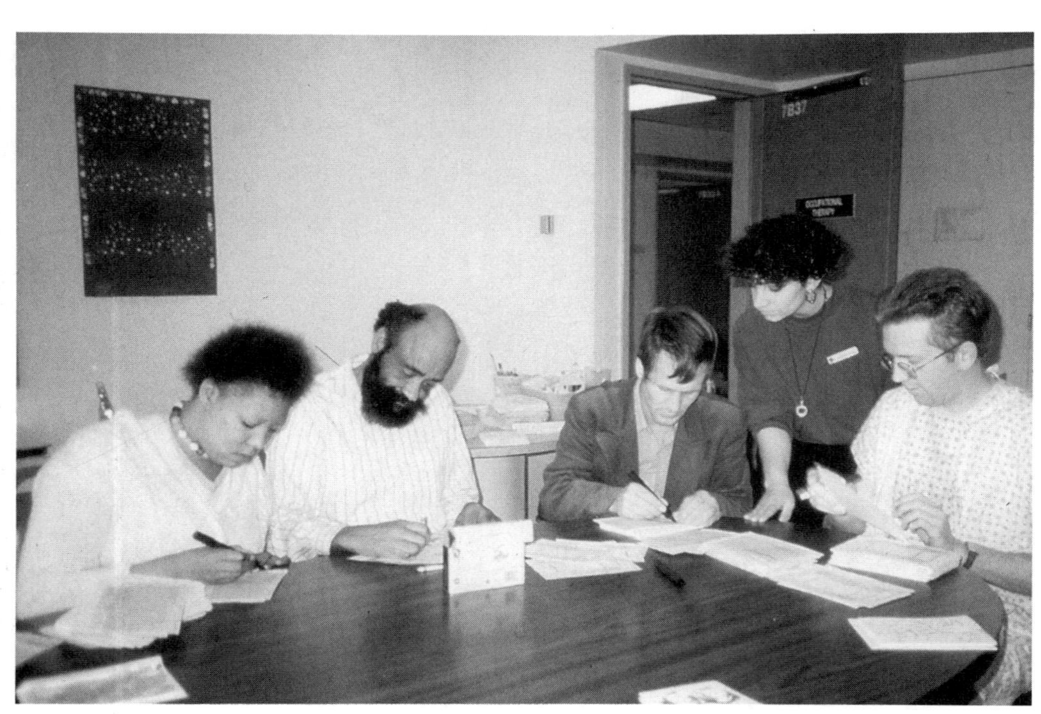

12 Adult Psychosocial Practice

As we saw in Chapter 3, occupational therapy had its origins in the treatment of the mentally ill. Today the treatment of psychosocial disorders is still the focus of practice for 16.6% of OTRs and 28% of COTAs according to the AOTA 1990 Member Data Survey (1). The percentage of the occupational therapy workforce employed in programs dealing with psychosocial dysfunctions has been declining for the past 20 years and has affected OTRs more than it has COTAs. Factors contributing to this decline are discussed later in this chapter.

There is in the 1990s a critical shortage of occupational therapy personnel working in mental health. The AOTA in 1992 formed a mental health task force to come up with a plan for increasing the number of practitioners in this practice area and for encouraging the retention of those now employed in mental health programs (2). Table 9.3 shows some of the mental health problems that OTRs and COTAs were treating in 1990 (1).

Tiffany (3) has identified three levels of mental health services. Primary care or prevention is the first level and is a relatively recent concern of mental health professionals. Through education and counseling, attempts are made to head off serious psychological disturbances. Early intervention for relatively minor disorders helps to prevent more severe problems from developing. Secondary care is the direct intervention in a psychological dysfunction that has developed. Tertiary care is concerned with maintaining an optimum level of function in chronically ill clients and with providing them with the necessary support services to prevent regression or deterioration. Occupational therapists in the past have been involved mainly with secondary and tertiary care. Preventive services are now receiving more attention, and increasing numbers of OTRs and COTAs are working in preventive programs.

PRACTICE SITES

There are multiple settings for occupational therapy practice in psychosocial dysfunction. Large public institutions for the mentally ill used to be the major source of care for this population. These institutions still exist, but their purpose has changed to that of providing services for specialized populations: psychotic and severely disturbed children and adolescents, persons with chemical addictions, and court-committed persons who have been judged to be criminally insane. Such institutions are usually residential and clients remain in treatment for an extended period of time. Occupational therapy departments in these settings tend to be large and may include other activity therapies as well as occupational therapy. Group treatment approaches are often used, although individual therapy goals for clients are usually identified.

Acute care hospitals in local communities usually provide the most immediate care for psychologically disturbed people. Many hospitals have a small inpatient psychiatric unit that admits persons who are experiencing a psychotic episode or a psychological crisis that requires intervention. The average length of stay in these units is short and is growing shorter as the cost of medical care escalates. Treatment is usually focussed on diagnosing the client's problem, prescribing appropriate medication, and stabilizing his or her condition. When these goals have been achieved, clients are usually discharged and referred to an outpatient or community-based program for further treatment and follow-up care.

The largest proportion of treatment services for the mentally ill and those with psychological disturbances is available in community mental health centers. These programs have been designed to offer psychiatric care to clients close to their home community and may include outpatient therapy, crisis intervention, group homes and geriatric programs, specialized services for children and adolescents, family therapy, drug and alcohol abuse programs, and outreach services.

Barris, Kielhofner, and Watts (4) have pointed out that work in community clinics is quite different from working on an inpatient hospital unit. There is often less structure in community programs, fewer physical boundaries, and less control of the treatment process by physicians. Community clinics tend to be more egalitarian, with coworkers sharing in the decision-making responsibilities and taking an active part in program planning. The occupational therapist in a community mental health clinic is more likely to work with clients in a friendly, collaborative relationship rather than in a directive one. It is important that the community-based therapist have a good working knowledge of community resources and services so that they can refer clients to appropriate related programs. They also need to be aware of local standards and cultural patterns so that clients can be helped to adapt their behavior to fit in with community norms and customs. Community-based treatment programs offer great advantages to clients since they can participate in treatment without leaving their homes, their families, or their employment. Treatment can be better adapted to their personal needs and environments, and mental health workers can better judge when to fade out their support as clients are able to assume more control of their own lives.

Day hospitals and day care programs are another site for mental health services and may be part of the overall program of a community mental health center or a local hospital. Day hospitals are a transitional stage between hospitalization and community living. They offer a full range of treatment services and maintenance programs for chronically mentally ill clients who are at risk for repeated hospitalizations. Occupational therapy is an important part of the therapeutic program. A balanced schedule of daily activities may include training in self-care and independent living, development of work habits and skills, and participation in leisure time activities. The end goal is stabilization of the client's status so that he or she can live in the community with some assistance (5, 6).

In addition to the settings already mentioned, there are other specialized treatment facilities that deal with a single type of psychosocial problem. Drug and alcohol abuse programs are one example, with some being part of a larger institutional setting and others operating as free-standing community agencies. Group therapies are usually a major part of the treatment effort and clients may spend an extended period of time in a program. Occupational therapy can provide useful insights into the effects of substance abuse on occupational performance and can help clients regain performance skills that may have been neglected or lost during periods of addiction. Constructive use of leisure time is another contribution that occupational therapy makes to the overall treatment program. Prevention is usually emphasized in these programs, with efforts made to educate the public about substance abuse and the need for early intervention (4).

Home treatment programs for psychosocial dysfunctions have not been frequently used but could become more prominent if they become a reimbursable health service. Occupational therapists could play an important role in such programs just as they now do in home care for the physically impaired.

A small number of occupational therapists have pioneered work in correctional institutions as a part of a general program of rehabilitation for convicted criminals. Occupational therapy concepts and methods could be of great value in such settings and we may well see more OTRs and COTAs employed in such programs within the correctional system in the future.

Nursing homes have begun to identify the need for more occupational therapy personnel to work with residents who show psychosocial disturbances. With the increasing numbers of elderly persons who develop dementias such as Alzheimer's disease, occupational therapy personnel could make substantial contributions to nursing home programs. The AOTA has projected that the community mental health programs and nursing homes hold the greatest growth potential for psychosocial occupational therapy in the future (7).

TREATMENT TEAM

The treatment team in mental health programs varies with the practice site for service delivery. In the psychiatric unit of an acute care hospital the team would be likely to include psychiatrists, nurses, social workers, psychologists, recreational therapists, occupational therapists, and COTAs. In a community mental health center some of the same health professionals would be found, but they might be joined by lay workers and members of the community. In specialized programs for drug and alcohol abuse, a variety of health care workers contribute to the treatment program. Counselors and representatives of the criminal justice system may be on the team. Many programs also employ former addicts as lay counselors to assist clients to gain control of their chemical dependencies.

BODIES OF KNOWLEDGE

In their text, *Psychosocial Occupational Therapy: Practice in a Pluralistic Arena*, Barris, Kielhofner, and Watts (4) offer a review of the bodies of knowledge that occupational therapists have applied to psychosocial dysfunctions. They include the psychoanalytic approach, existential-humanistic treatment methods, behavioral approaches, cognitive strategies, reality therapies, communications/interactions theories, social ecological approaches, community mental health concepts, and deviance or labeling theory. The OTR or COTA working with psychosocial dysfunctions needs to have a broad theoretical background in many of these approaches. Even more important, however, is the knowledge of how to apply concepts of human occupation and purposeful activity to the problems of the mentally ill or psychologically disturbed client. People with psychological disorders frequently have difficulty performing their everyday work, leisure, and self-care activities. It is in these occupational performance areas that the OTR and COTA can make their most meaningful contributions to the treatment program. Barris, Kielhofner, and Watts see the role of the OTR or COTA working in mental health as "an environmental manager, a problem-solver, and a co-planner together with the client, as one who uses his or her own personality as a therapeutic agent and directly engages the client in occupations as treatment, and as an organizer and leader of task-oriented therapeutic groups" (4).

Grossman in 1991 identified the need for a prevention model of practice in mental health occupational therapy. She reviewed social stress research and suggested that the maternal stress research model offered a feasible foundation for occupational therapy prevention programs (8).

Gage has proposed that the appraisal model of coping be the basis for occupational therapy intervention in mental health programs. She points out that differences in coping style lead to different outcomes in treatment and suggests that occupational therapists adopt this model's concepts in assessing a client's coping style and in developing a coping plan for dealing with the stresses of daily life (9).

As new knowledge is gained in occupational therapy theory, new bodies of knowledge may be applied to mental health practice. Therapists must remain open to innovative concepts that may enhance or improve their practice in psychosocial dysfunction.

CHANGING PATTERNS OF CARE

Around the turn of the century, state governments assumed the major responsibility for providing care for the mentally ill in the United States. Large state institutions were built to house those persons who were believed to be dangerous to society or unable to function in their community settings because of a mental disorder. Institutional care continued to be the main approach to dealing with the problems of mental illness until the 1950s when several factors combined to cause a rethinking of this policy.

Increasing numbers of mentally ill persons were causing severe strains on institutions, resulting in overcrowding and a declining quality of care. States could no longer afford to fund the increasing costs of institutional care, and the introduction of psychotropic drugs had made new treatment approaches possible. At the same time, the federal government had become more aware of the problems created by larger numbers of mentally ill people in the United States. In 1963 the Community Mental Health Centers Act was passed, which was intended to develop a network of preventive and treatment services within local communities and thus decrease the costs of mental health care. Public Law 88–164 followed in the late 1960s and early 1970s, funding the community mental health centers.

As a result of this shift in policy, large numbers of patients (some say as many as 75% of the total) were discharged from state mental hospitals. Unfortunately no linkages had been built between the state hospitals and the new community-based mental health programs. When patients were discharged from a state hospital, they were not necessarily referred to a community program, and when they were, the community programs often lacked services to meet their needs. Since their emphasis was on prevention and the treatment of acute episodes of mental illness, they were unprepared to deal with the problems of the chronically mentally ill.

Another factor in the 1960s was the increasing advocacy for the civil rights of the mentally ill. They should have the right to be treated in the least restrictive environment, their advocates asserted, and should not be deprived of their liberty in order to receive appropriate treatment. In a period when the civil rights of minority groups was high on the national agenda, this argument won support, and court rulings created a strong demand for community-based care.

In 1977 the National Institutes of Mental Health developed the Community Support Program. It provided funding for states to set up community support systems for those with chronic mental illness. Based on concepts from medical rehabilitation and social models of care, it included 10 components:

1. Identification of the target population;
2. Assistance in applying for entitlements;
3. Crisis stabilization in the least restrictive environment;
4. Psychosocial rehabilitation services;
5. Supportive services of indefinite duration;
6. Medical and mental health care;
7. Back-up support for families, friends, and community members;
8. Involvement of concerned community members;
9. Protection of client's rights; and
10. Case management.

Each state was allowed to implement this act in its own way. Public concern was mounting over the poor living conditions of persons with chronic mental illnesses (many were homeless), their low level of public benefits, and the failures of deinstitutionalization and community-based care. Legal rulings had supported restrictive civil commitment laws, the right to treatment in the least restrictive environment, and the right of clients to refuse treatment.

The Omnibus Budget Reconciliation Act of 1981 established block grants to the states to fund mental health care, increasing funding levels by 25%. Community programs increased their attention to the needs of the chronically mentally ill population, and improvements in care were seen. Problems continue to be felt, however; and the need for mental health services continues to increase. In 1992 there were estimated to be from 3 to 5 million persons with severe, persistent mental illness in the United States. From 15 to 20% of them were homeless and were easy prey for criminals and abusers. It was estimated that only from one-third to one-half of the mentally ill were receiving psychiatric treatment (10, 11).

In the late 1980s and early 1990s, health care in the United States was shifting to a profit orientation. Length of stay for patients in psychiatric units of acute care hospitals was becoming briefer—an average of 30 days or less in 1990. With shorter hospital stays, diagnosis, control of acute symptoms, and early discharge planning were given highest priority, and there was little time available for occupational therapy intervention. This same period saw an increase in the number of private, for-profit psychiatric hospitals. These hospitals hired occupational therapy personnel but limited their services to a standard treatment package in order to control costs (12, 13).

CURRENT PRACTICE ISSUES AND TRENDS

The decline in the numbers of occupational therapists working in mental health settings has been a source of concern to the AOTA and its members. Several factors have contributed to this situation. Changes in the health care industry have had an influence. The reimbursement of mental health services is restricted by most forms of health insurance and covers only limited care. As we have seen, government funding has gone into community-based care, but most OTRs and COTAs have been employed in hospital-based programs. The slowness of occupational therapy to adapt to community-based services has delayed its full participation in the new therapeutic programs. Some therapists also believe that adherence to the medical model of practice has prevented OTRs and COTAs from investigating alternative practice models that show promise in community-based programs (2).

Robinson and Avallone have proposed an activities health approach that is less concerned with diagnosis and symptoms of the client's disorder than with helping him or her perform necessary daily tasks in an organized and comfortable way. In the acute care hospital where length of stay is short, they recommend that OTRs and COTAs put their efforts into helping clients to quickly re-establish their usual daily routines so that they will be able to resume them at home after the hospitalization (12).

Kleinman has suggested that OTRs and COTAs consider a psychosocial rehabilitation model of practice. This is a community-based service model that focuses on helping clients learn to function in the community. It usually includes vocational and personal adjustment services as well as social and educational components. Practical aspects of daily living are emphasized: taking one's medications regularly, managing stress, and developing problem-solving skills. This approach appears to be a good fit with occupational therapy's basic philosophy, but Kleinman notes that, to fully participate in psychosocial rehabilitation, occupational therapists will have to adopt a social model of service provision and clearly delineate what their contributions could be to the total program (2).

In Chapter 11 we saw that the client population in adult rehabilitation was becoming much more culturally diverse. The same phenomenon is being seen in psychosocial practice. San Francisco General Hospital has developed some model programs with an ethnic and cultural focus in their inpatient psychiatric unit. Their staff points out that concepts of normality and deviance can vary considerably from one culture to another and that self-concept and insight into one's personality and actions are also culture-bound. The staff of the occupational therapy department has developed five special focus units for specific populations: Asian/Pacific Islanders, Latinos, African Peoples, Women, and HIV (human immunodeficiency virus) clients. Each focus program is designed to promote cultural sensitivity and awareness including languages, lifestyles, and history. Staff members are recruited for their cultural diversity and cultural competence and are encouraged to critically analyze their own culture as well as that of their clients. A self-evaluation tool, the Cultural Competence Questionnaire (Fig. 12.1), is used to help staff members assess their cultural competence (14). This model shows good potential for meeting the mental health needs of an increasingly diverse population.

The Americans with Disabilities Act of 1990 (ADA) has been described as a civil rights act for the disabled. Its provisions apply to persons with mental health impairments and mental retardation as well as to those with physical disabilities. The ADA prohibits job discrimination and supports inclusion of the disabled in employment as well as providing access to public accommodation and services. The emerging trend of supported and transitional employment is encouraged by this legislation. Supported employment assumes that all people are capable of productive employment if they are given supports or accommodations appropriate to the setting. Such programs are developing for the chronically mentally ill as well as for persons with less severe mental disorders. Occupational therapists and therapy assistants can play an important role in helping clients to develop appropriate attitudes, work habits, and skills that will lead to supported or transitional employment. In addition, occupational therapy personnel can serve as advocates for their clients, design appropriate work environments, and provide liaison between employers and disabled employees. The ADA will have far-reaching consequences on the employment of the disabled, and OTRs and COTAs will be directly involved in its implementation (15).

As new medical and social problems have emerged in the United States, occupational therapists have found themselves working in new areas. The problem of homelessness for 15 to 20% of the mentally ill has given rise to new community outreach programs that attempt to provide support services, protection from street violence, and case management services (16).

Eating disorders (anorexia, bulimia, obesity) have increased in frequency, particularly among young women, and new programs have evolved to help clients improve their self-image and learn new methods of coping (17). A new practice site is the medical detoxification unit, where some OTRs are consulting and bringing an activity orientation to the treatment program for recovering addicts (18). Other therapists are working in forensic psychiatry, dealing with persons who have been convicted of a crime but found to be not guilty

1. Are you open to the cultural experience?
2. Do you acknowledge that culture is an important consideration in teatment?
3. Do you recognize that there is cultural bias from both the therapist and the patient?
4. Have you explored your feelings about culture and how these feelings affect interactions with patients?
5. Do you understand how Euro-American culture affects the treatment setting?
6. Are the patients utilized as a resource in understanding cultural beliefs, family dynamics, and patients' views of illness?
7. Are the patients encouraged to utilize resources commonly used within their own culture that they see as important?

Figure 12.1 Seven questions that will help you think about the role of culture within treatment.

by reason of insanity. Forensic units have tight security but provide a treatment focus. Occupational therapists often organize task groups designed to improve work skills, communication skills, and management of life situations (19).

The stress level appears to be rising in American society as many people face increased job demands, unemployment, financial reversals, child rearing problems, marital problems, responsibility for caring for ill or elderly relatives, and lack of adequate leisure time. Stress management programs have proliferated in recent years to help people learn to cope more effectively with stressful events. OTRs and COTAs have been actively involved in stress management programs. Exercise, assertiveness training, task groups, and relaxation methods have been used as adjuncts to stress management training. As society becomes more complex and the pace of daily life increases, these programs will be needed by larger numbers of people (20).

The awareness of the problems resulting from co-dependency has increased in recent years. Co-dependency is a mental, emotional, spiritual, and behavioral disorder that can result from living with or being raised by an addicted family member. It is estimated that 28 million United States citizens grew up in alcoholic families. Many others were the victims of abuse or neglect. Co-dependency can be manifested as a fear of abandonment, involvement in destructive relationships, compulsive or perfectionistic behaviors, or neglect of one's own needs. OTRs and COTAs can contribute to the treatment of co-dependency by helping clients look at their feelings, values, and behaviors to analyze how their history of life in a dysfunctional family has influenced the way they respond to life events and situations. As it becomes more acceptable to discuss negative life experiences openly, more people are participating in co-dependency programs and are being helped to lead a healthier and more satisfying life (21).

Although many areas of mental health practice have expanded for occupational therapists, some areas appear to be in need of further development. Florey has identified child psychiatry as an underdeveloped specialty area of occupational therapy. While it is not a new area of practice, it does not appear to have developed expanded programs to meet increased needs for service. Florey points out that there is greater public awareness of the emotional problems that can result from child abuse, the emotional overlay that often accompanies learning disorders, and problems that are related to living in a dysfunctional family. Children with emotional disturbances comprise the fourth largest group of disabled children in the public schools, but few of them are referred for occupational therapy services. School therapy services tend to be concentrated on children with physical limitations and Florey questions the rationale behind this reality. Occupational therapy services to emotionally disturbed children seem to have lagged behind other areas of practice, and Florey urges OTRs and COTAs to correct this deficiency (22).

SUMMARY

OTRs and COTAs working in mental health settings have seen massive changes in their practice as health care delivery has changed in the United States. They are in the process of redefining their services and moving toward new practice settings in the community. Psychiatric illnesses are complex and affect many aspects of clients' lives. The challenge to occupational therapy staff members is to focus on the daily life needs of clients from diverse ethnic and cultural backgrounds. There is a severe shortage of occupational therapy personnel in mental health programs, and opportunities exist for many types of nontraditional practice in this specialty area (23, 24).

Case Study: Major Depressive Disorder

Let's look at a community-based program to see how occupational therapy services are provided in this type of setting. Hillside Hospital is an acute care hospital in a metropolitan area and has a psychiatric adult day treatment program as an extension of its inpatient psychiatric services.

The program is staffed by a consulting psychiatrist, nurses, and occupational therapists. It is located in a separate wing of the hospital and is open from 7:30 AM to 4:00 PM on weekdays. Program components include one-to-one counseling, medication monitoring, verbal and practice groups aimed at developing a variety of personal and job-related skills, individual occupational therapy sessions, task groups, and liaison services. The program is funded through a combination of private insurance reimbursement and state or county funding.

Clients are referred to the program by a physician or other health care professional. When clients are accepted in the program, they must agree to attend regularly, maintain confidentiality, maintain regular contact with their referring physician, actively participate in the program, get themselves to the program each day, and meet the financial obligations of their treatment. Clients are not permitted to attend if intoxicated. The length of client involvement varies considerably.

Laura is a 32-year-old divorced woman who has held jobs in the past but lost them due to poor work skills, depression, and withdrawal. She was referred to the program by her psychiatrist and was diagnosed as having a major depression disorder and a dependent personality disorder. Laura has had a history of psychiatric problems over the past 5 years and has had several hospitalizations. One hospitalization followed a suicide attempt in which Laura had taken an overdose of her prescribed medication.

When the occupational therapist first interviewed Laura, she was showing poor coping skills. She spent most of the day worrying about her problems, crying hysterically, and hyperventilating. She was extremely anxious and would withdraw to her bed rather than go out of the house. At night she had difficulty sleeping because she was so inactive during the day. Her motivation was poor and so were her communication and interaction skills. Her high anxiety level prevented her from relaxing.

Laura had tried living in her own apartment but had trouble coping with the day-to-day challenges of independent living. She could not manage her money, often spending money on unnecessary items rather than on paying her bills. She had little knowledge of nutrition and had become obese. Her self-confidence was low. At the time of her initial interview she was taking both an antidepressant and an antianxiety medication.

Laura's history indicated that she had experienced a difficult childhood. She described physical and sexual abuse by a stepfather at an early age. As an adolescent she became rebellious and was placed in a series of foster homes. Intellectually she was in the low normal range. She was married to a construction worker, but the marriage lasted only 3 months. She had tried to support herself by working as a maid and as a kitchen worker, but her poor attitude, lack of motivation, and inability to assume responsibility led to her being fired by each employer. Her physical health was generally good, although she had sustained a back injury while doing heavy lifting.

The Framingham Functional Assessment Scale was completed by the treatment team when Laura entered the adult day treatment program and was readministered every 3 months that she remained in treatment. The results of the initial evaluation showed that Laura had minimal concentration. She required constant guidance in performing tasks and her functioning broke down under the slightest stress. Her social functioning was extremely limited. She would rarely initiate contact with others and expressed discomfort and anxiety when among a group of people. She tolerated only limited interaction with staff members.

On an Allen Cognitive Level Test she scored 4.5, which indicated that her cognitive abilities were very limited. She could perform a familiar activity but required supervision. Her total attention span was about 10 minutes. She was oriented to person and place but frequently confused the date and time of day. She often missed scheduled sessions and was late for appointments, but showed little awareness of being late.

Laura's ability to care for her personal needs was poor. She neglected her grooming and hygiene and needed feedback to perform these tasks. She had trouble budgeting her money and needed help with meal planning and preparation as well as with shopping for and maintaining her clothing.

A Leisure Skills Inventory was performed and indicated that Laura had once enjoyed activities like crocheting, knitting, needlepoint, volleyball, and exercise classes. Recently, however, she had been unable to motivate herself to participate in any of them. She said that she had friends but refused to contact them. Her verbalizations were often child-like and whiny. In a group situation she would often interrupt others and would speak only to the therapist, avoiding eye contact.

The occupational therapist evaluated Laura's current behaviors and identified several priority areas for intervention. These were discussed with the treatment team, and an intervention plan was developed and discussed with Laura. The occupational therapy objectives included:

1. Helping Laura to build confidence in her own abilities and to improve her self-esteem,
2. Teaching Laura more effective methods of coping with stress,
3. Helping Laura to develop improved work habits,
4. Encouraging more appropriate group interaction and communication skills, and
5. Helping Laura to improve her physical health.

Laura's involvement with the program had to be limited due to the limited funding available to cover treatment costs. Laura was scheduled to attend occupational therapy treatment sessions twice a week to work on the above objectives.

Initially the therapist spent time getting to know Laura better and to establish a good relationship with her. The next step was for Laura and the OTR to work toward improving Laura's self-confidence by completing familiar activities and gradually introducing new leisure activities that Laura could continue at home. She was taught methods of stress reduction and was helped to see that some of her physical symptoms were stress-related. Laura began to attend a relaxation group led by the OTR twice a week for a 6-week period. She was encouraged to use relaxation techniques when she felt stressed and to practice them regularly at home.

Laura also attended a work skills group once a week to help her develop job-related skills and to improve her work habits. During these sessions, communication and group interaction skills were worked on. Laura was beginning to feel more comfortable in group situations and could now express some opinions appropriately. She received help with grooming and personal hygiene. A weekly exercise schedule was developed by the OTR, and Laura's progress on a weight loss diet was monitored along with her caloric intake. She was taught how to plan and prepare nutritious low-calorie meals for herself, to budget her money, and to take care of her clothing.

Laura's progress was reviewed weekly by the treatment team and the consulting psychiatrist. Her intervention plan was updated regularly. After several months in the day program, Laura had established positive relationships with the OTR and other staff members. Her attendence had become regular. She was better able to handle stressful situations and was developing leisure time interests that she enjoyed. She gradually began to sleep better at night.

Laura now lives in a group home and shares the daily chores with other residents. She is able to reach out to others socially, can initiate conversation and maintain eye contact. Her conversation is more adult and appropriate. Her appearance has markedly improved. She has lost 20 pounds, feels better physically, and has few physical complaints.

Her involvement in the day treatment program was gradually replaced by volunteer work at a children's day care center. She now works there 3 half-days a week and gets a lot of positive feedback from the staff. She enjoys the children and works well with them. Recently she was referred to a transitional work program that will offer her 3 months of paid work experience with a job coach for support. Eventually Laura would like to work as a teacher's aide in the local school system. Plans have been made for Laura to continue her individual sessions with the OTR on a once-a-week basis. The occupational therapist will continue to offer her support and will assist with any problems that arise. Laura continues to see her psychiatrist but less frequently than before. Her medications appear to be well-regulated and her mood is stable. Laura feels pleased with what she was able to achieve in the day treatment program and says that things are much better than before.

Discussion Questions

1. Does your health insurance cover psychiatric care? How much is allowed, and for what kind of care?
2. Visit a community-based mental health program in your area. What kind of programs are offered and what kind of clients are seen?
3. What role should the government play in mental health care?
4. If there is a private, for-profit psychiatric hospital in your area, find out what services are offered. How does their program compare to those of non-profit hospitals?
5. Although no COTA was employed in the day treatment program described in this chapter, were there parts of the occupational therapy program that could have been carried out by a COTA? Discuss the potential contributions of a COTA to this type of program.
6. How did the occupational therapist help Laura make the transition from the day treatment program to the community?
7. What kind of personality traits do you think that an OTR or COTA needs to work successfully in a mental health program?

References

1. AOTA 1990 Member Data Survey. *OT Week* 5(22):1–8, 1991.
2. Kleinman BL: The challenge of providing occupational therapy in mental health. *AJOT* 46(6):555–556, 1992.
3. Tiffany E: Psychiatry and mental health. In Hopkins H, Smith H, eds. *Willard and Spackman's Occupational Therapy*, ed. 6. Philadelphia, JB Lippincott, 1983, pp. 267–333.
4. Barris R, Kielhofner G, Watts J: *Psychosocial Occupational Therapy: Practice in a Pluralistic Arena*, Laurel, MD, Ramsco, 1984, pp. 3–172, 262–280.
5. Gabriel J: Day treatment. *Mental Health Special Interest Newsletter*, AOTA, 3(4), 1981.
6. Day treatment services. *Mental Health Special Interest Newsletter*, AOTA, 3(3), 1980.
7. Ad Hoc Commission on Occupational Therapy Manpower: *Occupational Therapy Manpower: A Plan for Progress*. Rockville, MD, AOTA, 1985, pp. 55–59.
8. Grossman J: A prevention model for occupational therapy. *AJOT* 45(1):33–41, 1991.
9. Gage M: The appraisal model of coping: an assessment and intervention model for occupational therapy. *AJOT* 46(4):353–361, 1992.
10. Ellek D: The evolution of fairness in mental health policy. *AJOT* 45(10):947–951, 1991.
11. Estroff S: Pills, Policy, and Purposeful Lives: Community Care for Persons with Enduring Mental Illnesses, an address to the Madison Civics Club, 3/4/89.
12. Robinson AM, Avallone J: Occupational therapy in acute inpatient psychiatry: an activities health approach. *AJOT* 44(9):809–814, 1990.
13. Bonder BR: Occupational therapy in mental health: crisis or opportunity? *AJOT* 41(8):495–499, 1987.
14. Dillard M, Andonian L, Flores O, Lai L, MacRae A, Shakir M: Culturally competent occupational therapy in a diversely populated mental health setting. *AJOT* 46(8):721–725, 1992.
15. Crist P, Stoffel V: The Americans with Disabilities Act of 1990 and employees with mental impairments: personal efficacy and the environment. *AJOT* 46(5):434–443, 1992.
16. Brack C: Pathways—community outreach: the road to a new life for the homeless mentally ill. *Occupational Therapy Forum* III(24):1–6, 1988.
17. Saltz DL: Breaking through the control barrier. *OT Week* 4(41):4–7, 1990.
18. Schroff JT: The role of an occupational therapy consultant in a medical detoxification unit. *Occupational Therapy Forum* VII(7):6–11, 1992.
19. Melanson M: New horizons for occupational therapists in forensic psychiatry. *Occupational Therapy Forum* VII(13):4–6, 1992.
20. Courtney C, Escobedo B: A stress management program: inpatient to outpatient continuity. *AJOT* 44(4):306–310, 1990.
21. Adair J: The role of occupational therapy in the treatment of co-dependency. *Occupational Therapy Forum* XI(24):9–10, 1991.
22. Florey LL: Treating the whole child: rhetoric or reality? *AJOT* 43(6):365–369, 1989.
23. Dickie VA: The changing world of mental health practice. *OT Week* 5(17):14, 1991.
24. Palmer F: Job options in psychiatric occupational therapy. *OT Week* 4(9):2, 1990.

Suggested Readings

Barris R, Kielhofner G, Watts J: *Bodies of Knowledge in Psychiatric Practice*. Thorofare, NJ, Slack, 1990.

Custer VL, Wassink KE: Occupational therapy intervention for an adult with depression and suicidal tendencies. *AJOT* 45(9):845–848, 1991.

Devereaux E, Carlson M: The role of occupational therapy in the management of depression. *AJOT* 46(2):175–180, 1992.

Estroff S: *Making It Crazy: An Ethnography of Psychiatric Clients in an American Community*. Berkeley, CA, University of California Press, 1981.

Hemphill B, Peterson C, Werner P: *Rehabilitation in Mental Health*. Thorofare, NJ, Slack, 1991.

Ostrow P, Kaplan K (eds): *Occupational Therapy in Mental Health: A Guide to Outcomes Research*. Rockville, MD, AOTA, 1987.

Szasz T: *The Therapeutic State: Psychiatry in the Mirror of Current Events*, Buffalo, NY, Prometheus Books, 1984.

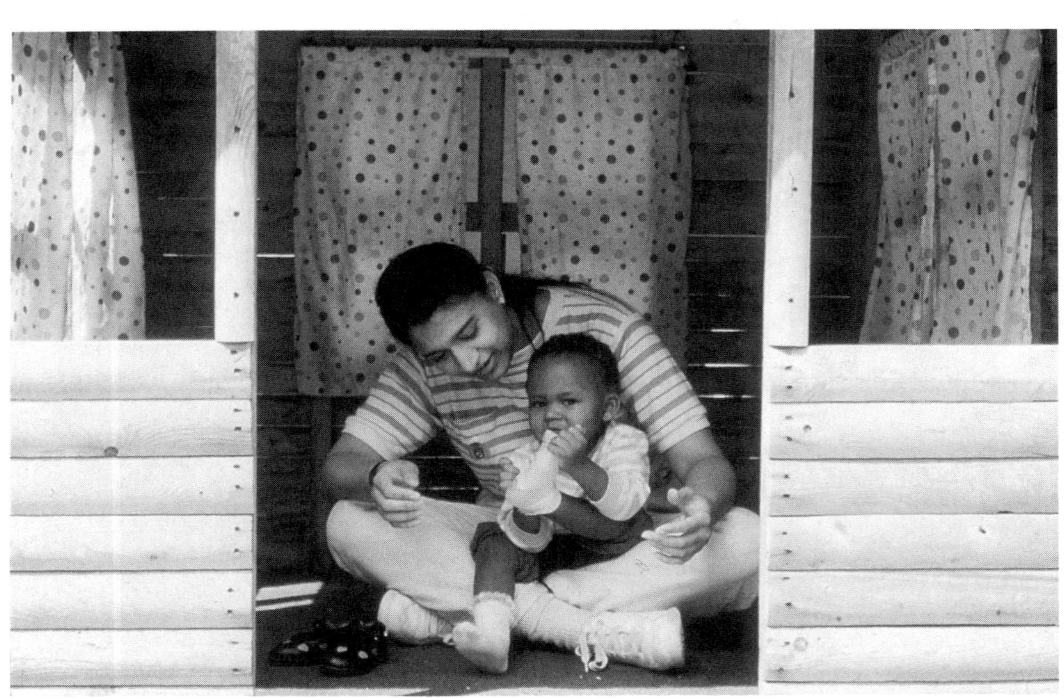

13 Practice with Developmental Disabilities

Occupational therapy has a long tradition of involvement with clients who have lifelong disabilities. The early literature in the field had many references to occupational therapy interventions for clients with cerebral palsy, birth defects, and multiple handicaps. Many of these lifelong disabilities are now grouped under the general term of *developmental disabilities*. Federal funding, beginning in the 1960s, helped to support the development of new therapeutic programs for this group of disabled people and gave rise to many new opportunities for occupational therapists and therapy assistants to work with this population.

According to the AOTA's 1990 Member Data Survey, 34.7% of OTRs and 25.5% of COTAs reported that they were working with children or adolescents (1). The AOTA's Developmental Disabilities Special Interest Section was the organization's second largest specialty group in 1991 with a membership of 7729 (2). Developmental disabilities practice is complex, covering a wide range of conditions and serving a diverse clinical population. Conditions most frequently seen include cerebral palsy, mental retardation, Down's syndrome, developmental delays, neuromuscular disorders, failure to thrive and the effects of prematurity, congenital disorders, head injury/trauma, and multiple disabilities (3).

DEFINITION OF DEVELOPMENTAL DISABILITIES

The Developmentally Disabled Assistance and Bill of Rights Act of 1975 provided a broad definition of developmental disabilities that is still in general use today. A developmental disability is a severe, chronic disability of a person, which

1. Is attributable to a mental or physical impairment, or a combination of mental or physical impairments;
2. Is manifested before the person attains the age of 22 years;
3. Is likely to continue indefinitely;
4. Results in substantial functional limitations in three or more of the following areas of major life activity:
   a. Self-care,
   b. Receptive and expressive language,
   c. Learning,
   d. Mobility,
   e. Self-direction,
   f. Capacity for independent living, and
   g. Economic self-sufficiency; and
5. Reflects the person's need for a combination and sequence of special, interdisciplinary, or generic care, treatment, or other services that are individually planned and coordinated (4).

The law intentionally did not list diagnostic categories because it wished to avoid the labeling of clients. It also tried to focus attention not on the causes of the disabilities but rather on their effects. Limitations in functional performance and adaptive living skills were the areas in need of training and development, and the federally funded programs were aimed at helping developmentally disabled persons develop their optimum potential for living a full and satisfying life. Developmental disabilities have their onset early in life, are chronic in nature, and cannot be cured. They persist for the lifetime of the individual and interfere with the person's ability to acquire and perform basic life skills. For these reasons, developmentally disabled people require the help of many care providers and need a continuum of services throughout their lives.

PRACTICE SITES

Today OTRs and COTAs work in a variety of programs that deal with developmentally disabled people. The first facility to serve them is often the neonatal intensive care unit (NICU) of the acute care hospital. Once developmental problems have been identified, families may receive services from infant intervention programs (usually seeing children from 0 to 3 years of age) or family support and home care programs. In these programs the OTR or COTA may teach the family how to promote the optimum growth and development of the disabled child during the preschool years. When the child reaches school age, public or private schools become involved, and these usually include occupational therapy services. At a later point, sheltered workshops and vocationally oriented programs may be utilized, along with community living arrangements, institutional care programs, if needed, and medically based programs (skilled nursing facilities, intermediate care facilities). During the 1980s a new type of facility developed: the intermediate care facility for the mentally retarded. Such programs provide active treatment and developmental training specific to the needs of the mentally retarded. Recently there has been renewed interest in work-related programs for the developmentally disabled.

Lawlor and Henderson studied the clinical practice patterns of occupational therapists who worked with infants and young children in 1989 and found that early intervention programs had greatly expanded. Over 37% of their respondents were working in schools. Twenty-two percent were located in hospitals, 17.8% in community intervention programs, 12.7% in outpatient clinics, 5.1% in private practice, and 4.2% in other types of facilities. More than half of the therapists surveyed said that they provided their services in children's homes. Direct treatment was the service most frequently provided, although consultation services were also often provided to parents, other agencies, and related disciplines (3).

TREATMENT TEAM

Because developmental disabilities are complex conditions that require a multidisciplinary approach, a treatment team is generally employed in service delivery. The OTR or COTA in this practice area is likely to be working with physicians, nurses, psychologists, educators and school administrators, physical therapists, speech and language therapists, social workers, workshop personnel, and vocational rehabilitation specialists. The OTR and COTA must clearly outline their contributions to the total program. Often the OTR is viewed as an equipment specialist and is consulted when the client has need of special assistive technology. Training in activities of daily living is another major focus for occupational therapy personnel and is often the core of a training program.

Lawlor and Henderson found that 67.8% of the therapists they surveyed worked as part of a team effort. Multidisciplinary teams were the most common (48.1%), followed by interdisciplinary teams (27.8%) and transdisciplinary teams (16.5%). Team composition varied with the practice setting. Most therapists acknowledged that there was some overlap between their services and those of other disciplines; however, some unique occupational therapy services were identified. They included feeding and oral-motor intervention, prescribing adaptive equipment, improving activities of daily living, sensory integration intervention, parent training, splinting, working on fine motor development, and positioning (3).

KEY CONCEPTS

Models of Service Delivery

At least five different models of practice have been used by professionals who provide service to developmentally disabled persons. The most traditional is the **medical model**, which views the developmentally disabled person as one who has suffered a physiological insult that has resulted in reduced functional capacity. The medical model has helped to provide information on some of the causes of developmental disability and has contributed to the assessment of impairment but has been unable to provide many cures or intervention strategies for some disabilities such as mental retardation. The medical model concepts of "illness" and "normality" are not very useful when applied to chronic conditions. Diagnostic labels have helped to stigmatize some groups of developmentally disabled clients by identifying them as subnormal and by implying that they are incapable of improvement. Although the medical model has made valuable contributions to the origin of some of these disabilities, it has failed to offer solutions to the broad range of functional limitations that are seen in this client population.

The **child development model** has also been applied to the education and treatment of the developmentally disabled. This model assumes that the physical, social, and emotional development of a person goes through certain recognizable stages. Failure to achieve certain developmental milestones is viewed as preventing or interfering with the development of more advanced skills. This model helps care providers focus on the progress of the individual through his or her own developmental stages and provides a realistic frame of reference when looking at the functional abilities of the developmentally disabled. It is less useful when the client is an adult. Adult stages of development have not been emphasized to the extent that childhood stages have, and there is less basis for comparison.

A third model in current use is the **social-ecological model**. This model looks at disabled individuals in relation to their social ecology and considers their habits, modes of life, and relationship to their surroundings. The principle of **normalization** is derived from this model. It holds that it is beneficial to provide a lifestyle for the disabled person that is similar to that of the normal population and favors getting clients out of institutional environments and into community living arrangements. This model focuses less on the disability than on an appropriate and satisfying lifestyle for the individual.

The **behavioral model** has been a dominant influence in programs for the developmentally disabled for the past several decades. This model, based on the concepts of Skinner and other behaviorists, considers that human behavior is learned according to well-established principles. It asserts that abnormal or deviant behavior can be changed through the systematic application of basic learning principles. Operant conditioning methods are used, including reinforcement and extinction procedures, shaping techniques, modeling, and precision-teaching methods. This model has been successful in teaching new skills to the mentally retarded and in extinguishing undesirable behaviors. It has been criticized for ignoring intrinsic motivation and failing to develop self-direction in individuals, but the model is widely used and has been particularly helpful in working with clients of low intellectual levels.

The **psychoeducational model** is a synthesis of some of the previous models. It focuses on learning and attempts to assess the individual's skill deficits and then sets target goals to be achieved. A course of programmed instruction is then designed to lead the individual systematically toward goal achievement, with the end result of increased competence. An educational orientation is used, with prescriptive teaching as the method. This model has value for prevention and early intervention programs as well as for education (5).

The choice of a practice model depends on the philosophy of the staff and the program. Occupational therapy has its own frames of reference, and some of them are particularly applicable to developmental disabilities. In the sample of therapists surveyed by Lawlor and Henderson, OTRs said that they were using developmental, neurodevelopmental, neurophysiological, sensory integrative, biomechanical, psychodynamic, and occupational behavior frames of reference in their practices. Of these, the first two were considered the most essential to pediatric practice (3).

Principles of Practice

An important concept for the occupational therapist working in developmental disabilities is that of **habilitation**. In Chapter 11 we discussed **rehabilitation**, by which we usually mean the relearning or restoration of skills and functions that have been lost or impaired due to an illness or an injury. Clients who have a developmental disability, however, have never developed some of the basic skills that are needed to function in society. Their need is for **habilitation**: the acquisition of abilities that were not previously present and that need to be learned "from scratch." This fundamental difference is important when working with developmental disabilities. One cannot build on a client's memory of how it felt to move her arm if she has never experienced normal movement. Rather, the therapist must provide the client with opportunities to feel and experience normal patterns of movement so that she can eventually achieve them more independently. Basic skills must be built rather than rebuilt, and the OTR or COTA needs a good background in normal growth and development to provide guidance for the treatment program.

The principle of **normalization** is another important one in developmental disabilities practice. This is based on the idea that quality of life increases as access to culturally typical activities and settings increases. A related concept is that of **deinstitutionalization**, which holds that a developmentally disabled person should be able to live and work in the least restrictive environment compatible with his or her functional limitations. These two ideas have been a strong influence on promoting the integration of the mentally retarded and other disabled groups into the mainstream of society. In 1967 the mentally retarded population in public institutions in the United States had reached an all-time high of nearly 200,000. By 1984 that figure had fallen 45% to about 110,000. Deinstitutionalization for the mentally retarded began about 12 years later than for the mentally ill and proceeded more gradually. As a result there were fewer failures in the transition.

Landesman and Butterfield (6) identified three things that were critical to successful deinstitutionalization:

1. Alternative community care and training programs,
2. Predischarge preparation of residents for community living, and
3. A community environment protective of the rights of the retarded and sensitive to their needs.

Follow-up studies of residents discharged from institutional settings suggest that even severely and profoundly retarded individuals can progress in community settings if they are given adequate support systems. Probably a diversity of programs and living arrangements is the best approach since the needs of the developmentally disabled are so varied (6).

CHANGING PATTERNS OF CARE

In the early 1960s, President Kennedy formed a special panel to investigate the needs of the mentally retarded population. The report of this panel led to the enactment of Public Law 88–164, which provided for the development and construction of research and treatment facilities for the mentally retarded and established a network of university-affiliated facilities to conduct research and educate students who work in the disciplines relevant to mental retardation. During this period, care of the retarded was beginning to shift from large institutional settings to community-based programs. There was renewed concern over the civil rights of retarded persons and an interest in seeking alternatives to institutional living. The Developmental Disabilities Services and Facilities Construction Act of 1970 (P.L. 91–517) broadened the mental retardation law to include a wider range of disabilities, including cerebral palsy and epilepsy. Later, the Developmentally Disabled Assistance and Bill of Rights Act of 1975 (P.L. 94–103) expanded the 1970 law even further to include autism and dyslexia (when related to a neurological condition).

The Developmental Disability Act of 1970 (amended in 1975) established a planning council in each state and required that states draw up a plan for services to their developmentally disabled citizens. Federal funds were allocated to help support a wide range of services: diagnosis, evaluation, treatment, personal care, day and residential care, special living arrangements, training, education, sheltered employment, recreation, counseling, protective and other social and legal services, information and referral, follow-through services, and transportation. These pieces of legislation provided both incentive and funds to support major improvements in the care of developmentally disabled people in the United States. For the first time a network of services was developed specifically to meet their needs. It was increasingly recognized that developmentally disabled citizens were not only children but also adults who had their own set of needs and wants: better housing arrangements, vocational training and employment, recreational programs and facilities, and integration into their communities as fully participating citizens. The concept of a continuum of services was proposed, because the needs of the developmentally disabled varied as they moved through their life stages. The need to educate professionals who could function in the multidisciplinary environment was apparent, and a variety of educational programs were developed to train the additional personnel needed. Professionals working with the developmentally disabled also needed to act as advocates for their clients in many situations to ensure that their rights were protected and that their best interests were being served. Developmental disabilities includes an extremely large client group, and these clients have a primary need for occupational therapy services. Job opportunities for OTRs and COTAs have vastly expanded for this clientele and are expected to continue to do so.

In 1986, Public Law 99–457, the Education of the Handicapped Amendments, was passed by the U.S. Congress. This act provided the states with funding to develop and implement statewide interagency programs of early intervention services for developmentally delayed or disabled children from birth through 2 years of age. It also strengthened special education programs for children from 5 to 18 years. The emphasis on early intervention services was of particular importance for identifying children with developmental delays who needed multidisciplinary services. Services included family training and counseling as well as direct treatment of physical, cognitive, speech and language, psychosocial, and self-help abilities. States were given the authority to come up with their own definitions of developmental delay, and family service plans were to be developed by interdisciplinary teams that could include occupational therapists. Case management services were also required by this legislation. This act greatly improved the chances for early diagnosis and treatment of developmental disorders and expanded available services to the families of developmentally disabled children. As a result, occupational therapy services in neonatal intensive care units have increased as well as those in home care programs (7, 8).

Another federal act, the Early and Periodic Screening, Diagnosis, and Treatment

Program (EPSDT) was passed in 1989 as part of the 1989 Budget Reconciliation Bill. This legislation provided children who were Medicaid recipients with screening, vision, dental, and hearing services under state Medicaid programs. Occupational therapists were among the health professionals authorized to provide services under this act, and they were encouraged to apply for participation in the program (9).

The Americans with Disabilities Act of 1990 (ADA) was a further piece of legislation that opened up employment opportunities to thousands of developmentally disabled persons by mandating physical accessibility of worksites and public transportation services and the provision of job-related accommodations and supports. Transitional and supported employment services were expected to greatly increase the numbers of disabled persons in the workforce and to allow them to contribute productively to their local community and to society as a whole (10).

In 1992 eight states received authorization to begin Medicaid funding of Community Supported Living Arrangements (CSLAs). The purpose of this program was to assist developmentally disabled persons to develop the daily living skills necessary to live in the community. The goal was to enable individuals to live in their own homes, a family home, or a rental unit. Services included the provision of assistive technology and adapted equipment, 24-hour emergency assistance, personal assistance, training, and rehabilitation. If these pilot programs prove to be successful, we can expect to see expansion of the program to other states under the Medicaid umbrella of services (11).

The concepts of supported living and supported employment come from a shift in thinking about the needs of the developmentally disabled. In order to make them work, service providers need to change their focus from providing lifetime care and support to providing choices for the disabled population. The current idea is to put the disabled client in control of what services and programs he or she wishes to receive rather than giving them services that caregivers think are appropriate. Supported living does not mean that care providers do something for their clients, but rather that they do something *with* them. Empowering the disabled to make their own decisions is an entirely different approach to service delivery. Will it work? It's too soon to say, but these concepts may bring about a revolution in how society views and cares for its disabled members (12).

CURRENT PRACTICE ISSUES AND TRENDS

Neonatal ICU

As medical advances are made in sustaining high-risk pregnancies, more babies are surviving with mild-to-severe developmental disorders. Occupational therapists are working in NICUs in greater numbers and are seeing newborns with a variety of problems. The experienced OTR can contribute toward solving the feeding problems of newborns, influence the sensory environment, teach parents how to handle and bond with their baby, and evaluate neuromotor status. The NICU is a high-tech environment and demands a high level of clinical expertise. It is not an entry-level job. An AOTA Task Force is currently working to determine the roles and functions of occupational therapy in neonatal care (13).

Drug-Exposed Infants

As early intervention programs have expanded, occupational therapists are seeing more babies who have been exposed to cocaine, alcohol, and other high-risk substances. These babies are often developmentally delayed and may also be subject to environmental risks and parental neglect. An addicted mother may be unable to care for her infant, and if the baby is irritable and easily upset, it may provoke further abuse on the part of the mother.

The problem of drug exposure is no longer confined to cities but is widespread throughout the United States. Because of the complexity of the problems seen, a team approach is usually employed. This is a challenging new area for occupational therapy intervention and requires good skills in dealing with families, a nonjudgmental attitude, and awareness of cultural influences on drug use and lifestyle (14).

Case Management

Just as in adult rehabilitation, case management is becoming an important service for the developmentally disabled and their families. Occupational therapists are beginning to fill this role, particularly in early intervention programs. The case manager tries to serve as an enabler, helping families to prioritize their needs and seek appropriate services and coordinating the care provided by various agencies. This new role for occupational therapists will become more common as community systems of care evolve (15).

Long-Term Care for the Developmentally Disabled

Better living conditions and improved care have led to longer life spans for many developmentally disabled clients, with some living into their 80s and 90s. Many will outlive their parents and will require some type of long-term care. In 1988 the aging segment of the developmentally disabled was estimated to be from 200,000 to 500,000. A 1985 survey conducted by Janicki, Ackerman, and Jacobson (16) found that only 34% of state agencies for the aging had a state plan for the care of aging developmentally disabled clients. A unified approach by state agencies is needed to solve this problem. Most of this group will have no pension plan or retirement income to support them in old age.

Because of long waiting lists in many nursing homes and group homes, some states are exploring new alternatives. Ideas like home sharing and family foster care may be practical solutions. The Older American Act may be a vehicle for the integration of developmentally disabled persons with their nondisabled age-peers in a variety of community programs and residential living arrangements (17). Occupational therapy personnel need to advocate services for this group and encourage the development of local programs in their communities.

New Technology

The use of technical aids to help disabled children and adults achieve a degree of independence has increased in recent years. New types of switches and controls allow even severely disabled individuals to operate electric wheelchairs, and microcomputers have been adapted to enable people to communicate, operate environmental controls, and participate in educational and work activities. The cost of such equipment is still high, but often public or private funds can be found to cover basic costs. Technology has also opened the door to employment for many disabled people, and early training in the use of these systems is often carried out by the OTR or COTA. Consultation in equipment selection and application continues to be an important function for clinical occupational therapy personnel (18).

Cultural Diversity of Clients

As we have seen with other disability groups, the developmentally disabled are also showing greater cultural diversity. African-Americans and Hispanics were the two fastest-growing minority groups in the early 1990s, and OTRs and COTAs were finding it more and more necessary to become knowledgeable about minority life-styles, beliefs, and values so that their intervention would not conflict with the client's cultural background (19).

SUMMARY

Due to increased federal funding and a shift in thinking about how to best meet the needs of developmentally disabled people, some innovative programs have evolved to improve early diagnosis and intervention, education, residential living, and employment for this client group. Occupational therapy roles and services continue to expand in this specialty area, and it is a growth area of occupational therapy practice.

Case Study: A Multiply Handicapped Child

Jesse was a normal, healthy infant until the age of 19 months, when he was involved in an automobile accident. He was not in a car seat and was thrown from the vehicle. Immediately after the accident, as he was being rushed to a hospital, he stopped breathing. He suffered multiple cuts, fractures, and bruises to the head, particularly to the right side of the skull. A CT scan revealed a subdural hematoma, which was removed. Jesse remained in an unresponsive state, and 2 months later a feeding gastrostomy was performed. After a craniectomy, Jesse showed some response to light touch, verbal stimuli, and colored objects. Other problems that were evident were a seizure disorder, spastic quadriplegia, and blindness. Retardation was believed to be in the profound range.

Three months after the accident, Jesse entered a rehabilitation hospital, where he remained for 6 weeks. Then followed a period of therapy at home. At the age of 2 years, he began attending the preschool program at Belle Harbor School for half days. When a sibling was born, Jesse's parents placed him in residential care at the school. He now lives in a group home at Belle Harbor School and attends school full-time in a class for the multihandicapped.

Jesse continued to have severe physical impairment. His movement was limited to primitive reflex responses. There was overall muscle spasticity (tightness) that was greater on the right side. He had facial weakness on the lower right side and diminished right lip closure. After a time he no longer needed the gastrostomy tube for feeding and could eat soft foods. His overall level of functioning was estimated at 7–8 months of age and his level of retardation was now thought to be in the severe to profound range. (A decrease from the original estimate.)

When assessed by the occupational therapist, Jesse was found to be dependent in all areas of self-care. He could assist minimally in feeding by helping bring a spoon to his mouth. In dressing, he was almost totally dependent. He was unable to walk and required an adapted wheelchair with special supports to keep him properly positioned. Jesse communicated his basic needs by crying, vocalizing, using body language, and making facial expressions. He was unable to manipulate objects, except for batting at objects with his left hand.

When performance components were analyzed, Jesse was observed to be more severely limited on his right side. He was functioning at the brainstem level of reflex development and was dominated by primitive postural reflexes that controlled his movement. He could not perform isolated movements but moved in total body patterns. He got most of his information about the external environment through touch and hearing. He enjoyed movement sensations such as rocking, swinging, and riding on the bus.

According to the psychological evaluation, Jesse had a tested IQ of about 25. He was functioning in the severe-to-profound range of mental retardation. He was able to anticipate familiar events and to discriminate between familiar people. He had little awareness of bowel and bladder function. Jesse enjoyed physical contact with his adult caretakers and peers. He was attentive toward familiar voices and would become quiet and turn toward a recognized voice. His grandparents became his only family contacts, and he occasionally went on overnight visits to their home.

Because of the severity of his handicaps, Jesse required a number of pieces of adapted equipment. He now uses an adapted wheelchair for positioning and transportation that is equipped with trunk supports, a head support, adductor pads, footrests, and a tray. He uses a flexion sidelying device and a prone kneeler to help align his hips for weight-bearing. A supine position helps to relax his muscle tone and align his body. Jesse wears ankle-foot orthoses (splints) on both feet to reduce muscle tone and to prevent contractures. He also uses a cone splint on his right hand. A built-up handled spoon is used to assist in hand-over-hand feeding, and various toys have been adapted so that they can be operated by only gross hand movement.

To prevent further limitations, range of motion exercises were performed three times a day. Various pieces of adapted equipment and positioning devices were used to inhibit Jesse's high muscle tone and to position him properly. Relaxation methods were also used to reduce muscle tone.

The overall goals for Jesse's school program are included in an Individual Education Plan that is written annually and revised three times during the year. The occupational therapy treatment plan is part of the Individual Education Plan and contains several objectives for the current school year. They include increasing his ability to communicate through vocalizing or facial expression, increasing his responses to external stimuli, maintaining the present range of motion in all of Jesse's joints, improving his ability to drink liquids, and increasing his ability to feed himself with a spoon.

To help Jesse achieve the treatment objectives, a daily session with the COTA was scheduled. She was responsible for carrying out activities recommended by the OTR for each objective listed. Behavior modification methods were used to elicit greater communication, and a variety of sensory stimuli were presented to elicit responses from Jesse. The COTA ranged all of Jesse's joints daily so that their mobility would be maintained. The OTR worked with the classroom aide who fed Jesse his meals so that consistent feeding and positioning methods would be used. The COTA reported her results weekly to the OTR so that modifications in the program could be made if needed.

In addition to supervising individual therapy, the OTR consulted with classroom teachers and aides to ensure consistent programming and carryover. She also monitored orthopedic and equipment needs. In consulting with the classroom staff, she instructed them on the use of equipment, positioning and handling techniques, lifting and carrying techniques, and methods for carrying out the occupational therapy objectives.

Jesse is 12 years old now and has made only limited progress over the past 3 years. The continuing occupational therapy goals are to maintain his passive range of motion, prevent further deformity, maintain his body alignment, break up abnormal muscle tone, and try to elicit more voluntary movement. Adaptive switches are being used to encourage him to actively use his left arm. Jesse enjoys swimming, listening to music, and roughhousing with staff members. He will always have severe physical and mental limitations and will need supportive services for the rest of his life. Since Jesse's parents do not visit him, the residential school staff has become his family. They try to see that he has a reasonable quality of life and that he remains as active as he is able to be.

DISCUSSION QUESTIONS

1. More severely developmentally disabled individuals are surviving today because of medical advances and improvements in care. Their needs for a continuum of care throughout life place a heavy financial and social burden on society. Is it ethical to discontinue life support for multiply handicapped individuals if they or their families wish it? Who should make this decision?
2. As this chapter shows, the trend is toward services being located in the community rather than in institutional settings for developmentally disabled clients. Do you think Jesse could be adequately cared for by community programs? If so, what kind of support services would he be likely to require during his lifetime?
3. Jesse's parents cut off contact with him and no longer visit him. Do you think that this is typical behavior for parents of a severely disabled child? Why might they feel unable to visit him?
4. Take a look at your state's development disabilities plan. What priorities does it set for the care of developmentally disabled individuals? What services are available? Do they provide for a continuum of care throughout the lifetime of a client?
5. What facilities are available in your area for the aging developmentally disabled person? Are nursing home personnel given additional training for dealing with this population? Are there special housing facilities available?
6. Have you had any personal experiences with developmentally disabled individuals? Discuss these with your classmates. What are your feelings and reactions when trying to communicate

with and relate to a severely handicapped person?

7. Largely in response to the demands of families for improved services, the federal government has established more adequate facilities and services than existed prior to the 1960s. In the light of increasing cost-containment efforts in medical care, can we continue to afford the amounts we are spending on programs for the developmentally disabled? Should the federal government continue its involvement in this aspect of health care?

References

1. AOTA: *1990 Member Data Survey, Summary Report*, AOTA, Insert in *OT Week* 5(22):1–8, 1991.
2. AOTA: Personal communication, Research Information & Evaluation Division, AOTA, March 25, 1992.
3. Lawlor MC, Henderson A: A descriptive study of the clinical practice patterns of occupational therapists working with infants and young children. *AJOT* 43(11):755–764, 1989.
4. Summers J: The definition of development disabilities: a concept in transition. *Ment Retard* 19:259–265, 1981.
5. Baldwin S: Models of service delivery: an assessment of some applications and implications for people who are mentally retarded. *Ment Retard* 23:6–12, 1985.
6. Landesman S, Butterfield E: Normalization and deinstitutionalization of mentally retarded individuals: controversy and facts. *Am Psychol*, in press.
7. Case-Smith J: Federal early intervention: PL 99–457, *Developmental Disabilities Special Interest Newsletter* 10(3):6–7, 1987.
8. Hanft B: The changing environment of early intervention services: implications for practice. *AJOT* 42(11):724–731, 1988.
9. Staff: EPSDT amendments present opportunity for occupational therapists. *OT Week* 4(13):5, 10, 1990.
10. Schelly C, Sample P, Spencer K: The Americans with Disabilities Act of 1990 expands employment opportunities for persons with developmental disabilities. *AJOT* 46(5):457–460, 1992.
11. Bergman AI: HCFA awards CSLA to eight states. *AAMR News & Notes* 5(1):2, 1992.
12. Karan OC, Franfeld JM, Furey EM: Supported living: rethinking the rules of residential services. *AAMR News & Notes* 5(1):5, 1992.
13. Saltz DL: Special care for special babies. *OT Week* 5(1):4–5, 1991.
14. Lane SJ: Prenatal cocaine exposure: a role for occupational therapy. *DDSIS Newsletter* 15(2):1–3, 1992.
15. Case-Smith J: Case management in early intervention. *DDSIS Newsletter* 13(4):5–8, 1990.
16. Janicki M, Ackerman L, Jacobson J: State development disabilities/aging plans and planning for an older developmentally disabled population. *Ment Retard* 23:297–301, 1985.
17. Saltz DL: The graying of persons with developmental disabilities. *OT Week* 5(10):4–5, 1991.
18. Brandenburger SG: Integration of assistive technology in the classroom. *DDSIS Newsletter* 14(3):1–3, 1991.
19. Vergara ER; Guest Editor, Special Issue on Cultural Diversity. *DDSIS Newsletter* 15(1):1–4, 1992.

Suggested Readings

Bazyk S: Changes in attitudes and beliefs regarding parent participation in home programs: an update. *AJOT* 43(11):723–728, 1989.

Kibele A: Occupational therapy's role in improving the quality of life for persons with cerebral palsy. *AJOT* 43(6):371–377, 1989.

Powell NJ: Supporting consumer-mandated programming for persons with developmental disabilities. *AJOT* 46(6):559–562, 1992.

Treffler E: The funding challenge for pediatric technology. *The AOTA Practice Symposium, 1989, Program Guide*, Rockville, MD, AOTA, 1989, pp. 38–42.

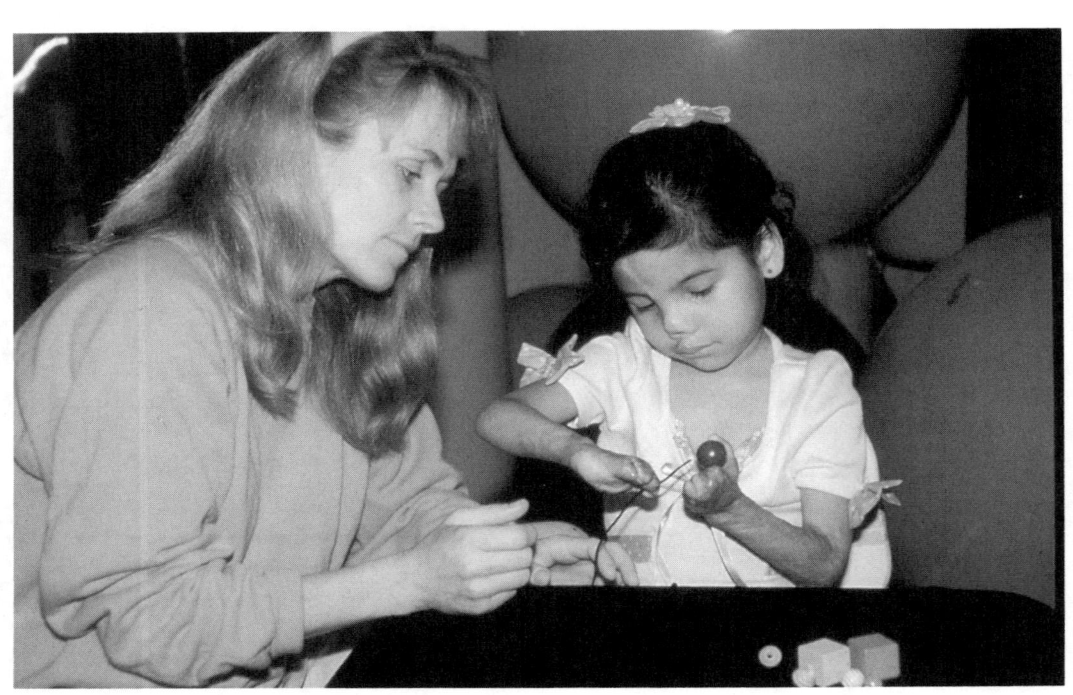

14 Public School Practice

One of the most dramatic changes in occupational therapy practice in recent years has been the rapid growth of services in public and private schools. The 1985 AOTA Manpower Report showed that schools had become the second most common employment setting for OTRs and the third for COTAs (1). This trend has remained stable. The AOTA 1990 Member Data Survey showed the same proportions as the 1985 study (2). Occupational therapists have long worked in schools for handicapped children, but the impetus for increased services in schools came from two pieces of federal legislation. The Education of All Handicapped Children Act of 1975 (Public Law 94–142) and Section 504 of the Rehabilitation Act of 1973 permanently changed the kind of education and services available to handicapped children in the United States.

Public school occupational therapy is not a specialty area in itself, but the setting is sufficiently different from those that occupational therapists have traditionally worked in that it merits special consideration. In this chapter we look at how occupational therapy services are delivered in public schools and how this type of practice differs from medically oriented service delivery.

PRACTICE SITE

In the school setting, the chief concern is the education of the child. Occupational therapists and therapy assistants function as support personnel in the educational environment to assist teachers in providing a quality education for children who have functional limitations. OTRs and COTAs are usually responsible to the school principal or to a special education coordinator. In some school districts a local educational agency may hire occupational therapy personnel on a contract basis to provide services to a number of schools in the area. Since public schools are tax supported institutions, each state has its own set of regulations governing school policies and procedures. Local districts also have a voice in the operation of their schools and keep a close eye on annual budgets. In 1989 Carr surveyed the education departments of all U.S. states and territories and found that only 18 of the 50 states (36%) had guidelines for school-based occupational therapy. Carr suggested that occupational therapists volunteer to assist state education departments in developing such guidelines to ensure uniform service provision and student access to services (3).

Therapy personnel may be assigned to one school or may work on an itinerant basis, serving a number of schools in the district. Treatment activities may be conducted in a separate therapy room or may be incorporated into the classroom program. Itinerant therapists must carry much of their equipment with them and may be expected to work in unused offices, classrooms, or the school gym. OTRs and COTAs are hired on an annual contract basis just as teachers are, with salaries and benefits often negotiated through collective bargaining. Some states require separate certification for public school practice, so OTRs and COTAs may be expected to hold a school certification granted by the state department of education in addition to state licensure.

A variety of private schools also exist to serve the needs of disabled children. Most of them are specialized to deal with one group of disabilities: mental retardation, physical handicaps, emotional disturbance, or learning disabilities. These programs are also supervised by the state department of education and must meet educational standards similar to those of public schools. Some private schools are residential, with students remaining at the school for the entire year or for several years. Occupational therapy services may be available, along with a range of special education services.

Stephens (4) and Ottenbacher (5) have pointed out that occupational therapy personnel are usually educated according to the medical model. This may make for some conflicts and misunderstandings when they practice in educational settings because the models of practice are quite different. The medical model focuses on identification of disease or dysfunction and the development of treatment or intervention strategies to halt the disease process or reduce the dysfunction. The educational model is concerned with the normal growth and development of the child and with helping children achieve mastery of the skills needed to function in society. Teachers and therapists may view the needs of a disabled child differently because of these different orientations and philosophies. Ottenbacher believes that these differences can be minimized if therapists and educators try to put aside their biases and put their differences in perspective. He suggests that therapists try to merge their goals with those of educators and develop cooperative and mutually supportive relationships with them. Because occupational therapy has often found the medical model limiting, the educational model may offer new opportunities to become fully involved with the needs of disabled students (5).

TREATMENT TEAM

Unlike medical settings, the school includes largely educational personnel who will function as team members when dealing with children's educational needs. The school-based OTR and COTA are likely to be working closely with special education teachers, school and program administrators, psychologists, speech and language therapists, physical therapists, social workers, school nurses, counselors, and classroom aides.

A study conducted in 1988 by Traylor and Graham found that the occupational therapists in their sample spent an average of 20.3 hours a month with special educators. Most of their collaboration took place in team meetings, classroom work, case conferences, consultation sessions, and program planning meetings. These therapists reported that misunderstandings between themselves and special educators often centered around the educators' lack of knowledge about the education and competencies of occupational therapists, issues of professional status, threats of encroachment on professional domains, and insufficient use of one another's capabilities (6).

Coutinho and Hunter have emphasized that occupational therapists need to effectively communicate their areas of competence to other members of the educational team and be willing to share their skills with teachers and school staff. Avoiding the use of medical jargon and learning the language of educators will also make collaboration more effective. Taking part in schoolwide activities such as faculty meetings, school assemblies, and afterschool activities will help to establish the OTR or COTA as a full participant in the school's program and will help to build positive relationships with other school team members (7).

KEY CONCEPTS IN SCHOOL PRACTICE

Occupational Therapy Process in Schools

The occupational therapy process follows many of the same steps in school settings that it does in medical settings. The differences center around specific procedures that are mandated by Public Law 94–142. Children are not eligible for occupational therapy or other related services unless they have been judged to need special education. The assessment of a child's educational needs is the first step in service delivery in schools. The occupational therapist may or may not be a part of the initial referral/assessment process.

According to Rourk and her colleagues (8), two types of screening occur in the educational setting. The first is type 1 screening, in which high-risk children are identified who may need special education. An example of type 1 screening is the routine prekindergarten assessment that is conducted to determine readiness for entry into kindergarten. A child who is found to have visual problems, motor impairment, or a hearing loss during this initial screening is referred for a more complete assessment. The in-depth assessment is type 2 screening and is conducted by a multidisciplinary team. The occupational therapist and other related service personnel may be asked to evaluate the child and contribute data to this more detailed assessment. The child's family may also be asked to contribute information. When all of the relevant data have been collected, the multidisciplinary team meets to analyze findings and determine the child's total educational needs. If the child has a need for special education, the team prepares an individualized educational program (IEP), which outlines the child's present level of function, sets annual goals and short-term objectives, identifies the special education and related services that need to be provided, establishes the date for starting service, estimates how long services are expected to continue, and sets the criteria for measuring the achievement of goals and objectives. The IEP becomes the blueprint for the child's educational program for the school year. If occupational therapy is recommended as a related service, the child is referred to the OTR attached to the school program. A physician's referral for occupational therapy services in schools is needed in some states, and the therapist is responsible for following whatever referral procedures are required by the state and by local education agencies.

An occupational therapy intervention plan is then developed, but the objectives in this plan must relate to the overall IEP objectives. The occupational therapy plan includes short-term objectives, strategies to be used to achieve the objectives, relevant treatment concepts, a statement of how frequently the child will be treated and for how long, and a statement of the predicted outcome. The COTA may assist in developing the intervention plan. The plan is then initiated, and results are regularly assessed. Implementation is the responsibility of the OTR, but some intervention activities may be delegated to the COTA, the classroom teacher or aide, the family, or a combination of these individuals. Changes that are seen in the child's abilities must be documented objectively. Each child's IEP is reviewed annually, and a comprehensive assessment by the multidisciplinary team is required at least every 3 years.

Models of Service Delivery

Occupational therapists and therapy assistants work in school settings in three major ways.

1. In *direct service delivery*, therapists or assistants carry out occupational therapy interventions with children on a regular basis. Children may receive occupational therapy either individually or in small groups. Some problems may require one-to-one intervention, and this is built into the child's weekly schedule. Other therapy interventions may be scheduled in small groups to work on common objectives. This method has the advantage of saving time for the OTR or COTA and is comparable to groupings used for classroom instruction.
2. The OTR may *monitor* therapy programs being carried out by others. In this type of service delivery, the OTR directly supervises nonoccupational therapy personnel who implement all or part of the therapy program. The therapist is responsible for teaching correct procedures to the assistants, maintaining regular contact with them to ensure proper implementation of the program, and reassessing to determine whether ade-

quate progress is being made or whether adjustments are needed in the program.

3. Through *consultation* the OTR may offer services to classroom teachers, families, and colleagues in the school setting. The occupational therapist may be able to offer expertise to the school system as a whole when new programs are being planned or systemwide changes are being considered (9).

OTR and COTA Roles

In the public or private school, as in other practice settings, the OTR is legally responsible for all aspects of occupational therapy services and supervises the work of COTAs who are part of the service staff. OTRs must establish the service competency of those they supervise and may delegate therapy tasks, providing that the quality of the service is not compromised. In general, the same roles and functions that were described in Chapter 6 apply to the school setting. The primary difference is that in schools the OTR is responsible for contributing to the development of team goals and objectives for the IEP and for preparing the occupational therapy intervention plan for each student to be served. Implementation of the intervention plan may be delegated in part to the COTA but the OTR remains responsible for its outcome (10, 11). There may be fewer administrative responsibilities for the OTR in a school setting since most management functions are assumed by educational personnel.

CHANGING PATTERNS OF CARE

By the early 1970s some states had already passed legislation requiring free public education for all handicapped children, but many states still refused to accept some types of disabled children into special education classrooms. Those with the most severe handicaps were frequently excluded. In an effort to establish a uniform national standard, Public Law 94–142 was passed, guaranteeing a free public education to all children regardless of type or severity of handicap. The law also required that the effectiveness of educational programs for disabled children be monitored. Among the provisions of this law was the inclusion of occupational therapy as one of the related services that might be required to enable a disabled child to benefit from special education. Occupational therapy was described as

> *. . . services directed at improving, developing, or restoring functions impaired or lost through illness, injury, or deprivation; improving ability to perform tasks for independent functioning when functions are impaired or lost; and preventing, through early intervention, initial or further impairment or loss of function. (12)*

The legislation applied to children from 3 to 21 years of age, although states were required to provide special education only to children from 3 to 5 years and from 18 to 21 years if educational programs were offered to nondisabled children in these age groups as well.

In 1986, amendments to the law were added (P.L. 99–457) that required all states, if receiving federal funds, to provide education and related services to children from 3 to 5 years (13). This act added new services for preschool children and their families and extended services to children under the age of 3 years who had developmental delays or disabilities (14).

A third law, Section 504 of the Rehabilitation Act of 1973, had prohibited discrimination against handicapped persons in any programs that received federal funding and mandated that disabled children be educated in the least restrictive environment possible for each individual. This meant that children with limitations did not need to remain in segregated special education classrooms. Those who could participate in regular classes for all or some instruction were to be mainstreamed into the regular educational program. Schools were required to provide learning environments that were fully accessible to disabled students and that contained facilities for instruction that were equal to those provided for nonhandicapped children (15).

Colman has pointed out that, with each successive piece of federal legislation, governmental responsibility has increased until now it extends to providing special education and related services to children from birth to 21 years of age. The effect on occupational therapy has been to greatly increase the number of OTRs and COTAs employed in school and preschool programs. Public schools have become the chief site of services for disabled children and adolescents, and in that role they have had to develop cooperative relationships with other health and social service agencies. School occupational therapists must merge the concepts of medicine, rehabilitation, and education in order to bring the best of each practice model to the children they serve (14).

The most recent legislation to affect disabled children and adults is the Americans with Disabilities Act of 1990 (ADA). Although not directed specifically at children, it addressed environmental factors that each disabled individual will encounter at some point in their lives. Kalscheur has identified ways in which this legislation relates to children and their families. She believes that deficit-reduction models of practice will have to give way to environment-centered models of service provision, requiring a change in how occupational therapists think about disability and how they perceive their role as service providers.

CURRENT PRACTICE ISSUES AND TRENDS

Technology Explosion

Computers are here to stay in educational programs and are heavily used to assist disabled students to participate in educational activities. Even students with severe limitations can learn to use computers if provided with appropriate switches and control units. Language development, reading, math, sequencing, fine motor skills, visual perception, and composition skills have been improved through use of computerized instruction. Lightweight electric wheelchairs allow students independent mobility, and electronic communication aids enable students to "talk" and interact with their peers. Occupational therapists and therapy assistants are in the forefront of technology applications for disabled students and must keep up-to-date on new software, new devices, and new applications.

Ethical Issues

With tighter school budgets, administrators are looking at ways to cut corners and save money in therapy programs as well as in educational programs. Many therapists were becoming concerned in the early 1990s that direct occupational therapy services were being replaced by consultation and monitoring types of service delivery. The ideal of "treating the whole person" is being overridden by reimbursement realities in the school just as it is in many other clinical settings. Therapists frequently see children who could benefit from occupational therapy services but who do not meet the eligibility requirements for special education. In 1992, school therapists were being urged to unite in order to seek solutions to these dilemmas. Another problem in some schools was a too-heavy caseload. Because of personnel shortages or budget constraints, fewer therapists were being expected to treat more children, and this also negatively affected the quality of service (18).

Huebner has argued that children's developmental needs vary considerably at different stages and believes that different service delivery models are appropriate at different developmental periods. For the very young child, direct service from a small team is very effective. A child in elementary school has much more contact with a variety of school personnel, and scheduling multiple therapy sessions can become an overwhelming problem. Huebner suggests setting some priorities. One or two disciplines could carry out the most important parts of a child's program, and other team members could be available on a consultation basis. All team members do not have to be involved with every child, Huebner asserts. She advocates flexibility in service delivery so that most needs of most children can be met (19).

Fee-for-Service in Public Schools

In 1988, Congress clarified that schools could bill Medicaid for "health services" to eligible recipients and could also ask parents to allow the school to bill their private insurer for health-related services. This meant that school therapists were confronted with all of the paperwork that goes along with fee-for-service reimbursement. Although the availability of reimbursement should not determine whether a student receives needed services, it is becoming more of a factor in some schools. Direct therapy services are the most difficult to justify in the school setting and there is a risk that a medical model of service provision could replace the educational model if fee-for-service becomes a common practice. Private insurers vary greatly on coverage of services. Each state has the option of whether to pursue Medicare reimbursement of school-based services. In the early 1990s, state occupational therapy associations were becoming involved in this issue, and it is uncertain how far this trend will go (20).

Integration of Therapy and Educational Programs

Because both therapy time and instructional time are limited, more schools are integrating their therapy programs into the classroom. When a teacher is familiar with a child's therapy goals, treatment activities can often be incorporated into daily classroom activities. This implies that teachers and therapists must meet to discuss goals and methods and find out what they can realistically expect of one another. Parents too can become involved in carrying over treatment methods at home, giving additional practice in needed skills and extra reinforcement of successes. Integrated therapy takes a lot of cooperative effort but is proving successful in many school settings (21).

Mobile Therapy Units

In some school districts, space limitations have forced occupational therapy personnel to become creative about finding new work areas. In Louisiana a group of therapists converted a donated school bus into the "Therapy Express"—a mobile clinic that traveled throughout the district providing occupational therapy services to 10 outlying schools. Local fundraising provided the necessary materials and equipment, and students were enthusiastic about their special therapy bus (22).

Itinerant therapists in Florida were also frustrated by a lack of workspace in the schools they served. Their solution was a remodeled motor home, purchased second-hand and adapted to serve as a clinic on wheels. The mobile unit has been used for several years and has provided efficient therapy services to students in widely scattered areas (23).

Independent Living Programs

For high school students in special education programs, independent living skills and vocational preparation are important components of the educational program. Bober has described an independent living training program that was implemented by special education teachers, assisted by an OTR who served as a resource person to the project. Students' individual needs for independent living skills were identified and prioritized, and a highly structured training program was then implemented. Students' progress was carefully monitored and documented, with students expected to achieve a skill level consistent with their probable future living environment (24). This program was a good example of coordination between an occupational therapist and special education teachers and resulted in a most successful program.

SUMMARY

Schools are likely to continue to be the primary site of therapy services for children and adolescents in the 1990s, although there may be changes in the way services are paid for and delivered. More school-based practitioners will be needed to serve this very large population. The school setting offers both challenges and opportunities to OTRs and COTAs who wish to contribute to the education and development of disabled children. School occupational therapy personnel must be prepared to deal with a diverse range of disabilities and to provide a variety of services to students enrolled in school and preschool programs.

Case Study: Cerebral Palsy

Erin is 4 years 7 months of age and is enrolled in a preschool program for hearing-impaired children. Her diagnosis is cerebral palsy, athetoid type, and is moderate to severe in degree. She has a 50% hearing loss in both ears that is corrected to 30% with hearing aids.

Erin was born prematurely at 32–34 weeks gestation and weighed only 3 pounds 4 ounces. At birth she was found to have severe hyaline membrane disease, a respiratory disorder in which there is inadequate development of the lungs. Erin had also suffered a ventricular hemorrhage that resulted in hydrocephalus; a mechanical shunt was installed to ensure circulation of cerebrospinal fluid. Despite these problems, Erin appears to have normal intelligence and is an outgoing, well-adjusted child.

In the state where Erin lives, children are eligible for special education services at the age of 3 years. Erin entered the preschool program at that age and will continue to be eligible for school services until the age of 21. Her current educational program focuses on language development, learning total communication (the use of both signed language and speech), and the development of self-help skills.

When initial screening showed that Erin was likely to need special education services, she was referred for a type 2 screening by a multidisciplinary team. Her problem areas were identified, and the team developed an individualized educational program that established annual goals and short-term objectives. Among the related services that were recommended for Erin were physical and occupational therapy.

The assessment conducted by the multidisciplinary team revealed several areas of dysfunction that occupational therapy could address. Erin had fluctuating muscle tone, causing her movement patterns to be uncoordinated and unreliable. She tended to appear floppy, with overly flexible joints. When she reached for a toy, she had difficulty holding her head and trunk steady to allow her to reach accurately and smoothly. Sometimes her muscles tightened, contributing to her incoordination. She had excessive range of motion in her elbows, wrists, and fingers. Because sign language was expected to be her major form of communication, it was especially important that Erin develop adequate fine motor skills.

Erin was strongly motivated to master developmental tasks. Her normal level of intelligence promoted a strong desire for independence, and she had been known to give helpful adults a swat when they offered to help her with a task she would prefer to do alone. She fell frequently while walking, but this did not discourage her. The OTR made knee pads for her to wear to protect her sensitive joints. Erin enjoyed her preschool program and tried hard to keep up with the other children. Although all were hearing-impaired, none had movement problems as severe as Erin's.

Erin's family was warm and supportive and offered her many opportunities for independence in her daily routine. They gave her extra time to dress in the morning and overlooked spills at the dining table so that her independence in everyday tasks would be encouraged.

The occupational therapy intervention plan for Erin focused on helping her to develop self-care skills, on providing environmental adaptations to enable her to function at school and at home, and on improving her physical stability while working toward coordinated movement. It was also important to assess her need for computer technology to assist in communication and writing.

A COTA was assigned to see Erin for twice a week occupational therapy sessions. The OTR conferred with Erin's classroom teacher and parents to discuss therapy objectives and suggested related activities that could be carried out in the classroom and at home. During the treatment sessions the COTA used a variety of activities (most of them in the form of play) to help Erin achieve her objectives. A therapy session might involve a game of "push me over, push you over" or "ride the wild therapy horse" (a suspended bolster) to help Erin develop better ability to stabilize her neck and trunk during movement. Sometimes the COTA and Erin would play "hanging out the wash," with Erin hanging weights on a line with clothespins, or have "turtle races" down the hall. (The "turtle" is a riding toy powered by arm movement, which required Erin to contract her shoulders and rotate her trunk to make it go.) On other days the COTA and Erin played dress-up games to work on dressing skills. Sometimes Erin was allowed to make a Cheerios necklace that she could later eat as a reward for good work. In all of these activities, the goal was to help Erin develop adequate body stability so she could move more easily from a fixed position. Later the emphasis would move to better fine-motor coordination. The classroom teacher carried out counting and writing activities and everyone helped with signing practice.

As the COTA continued to work directly with Erin, the OTR recommended the following environmental adaptations that would make classroom participation easier for Erin:

1. Installation of plastic pipe grab bars in the toilet stall so that Erin would have enough stability to safely use the toilet by herself.
2. Use of a cut-out table with raised edges. This allowed Erin to rest her arms on the table while using her hands and prevented objects from falling off the table when knocked about by Erin's flailing arms.
3. Use of a prone stander for some classroom activities and in therapy sessions. This piece of equipment allowed Erin to stand in a supported position and helped her develop stability around her weight-bearing joints.
4. Use of a well-fitting and supportive chair with a footrest during classroom activities. This provided better stability for Erin while seated and allowed her to participate more easily in tabletop activities.
5. Use of a keyguard and special software to enable Erin to write simple words.

Erin has been seen in occupational therapy for 2 years and has carried over her therapy activities in the classroom and at home. She has made considerable gains in several areas of function. The most notable has been her increasing independence in self-care and her developing communication skills. Her use of signing and the number and quality of signs used has increased considerably. Self-help and fine-motor tasks are now achieved in less time and with greater ease. Her improved body stability is reflected in improved gait while walking and in an overall improvement in posture and movement skills.

The occupational therapy program directly contributed to Erin's performance in the classroom and at home. Because her teachers and parents assisted with the therapeutic program, gains occurred faster and with greater consistency than if Erin had been seen only by the COTA. Although long-term predictions cannot be made, her therapist and teachers expect that Erin will be able to master most educational tasks and should be able to lead a productive adult life.

Discussion Questions

1. How does your local school district provide occupational therapy services to children such as Erin? At what ages are children eligible for services?
2. As school services for disabled children evolve, eligibility requirements for special education services may become more restrictive. What should a therapist or COTA do if he or she believes that a child needs occupational therapy services but the educational team does not agree?
3. Does your state require any special certification for OTRs and COTAs who work in public schools? If so, what are the requirements for certification?
4. What kinds of programs are available in your area for handicapped persons beyond the age of school eligibility who

have a need for further training or sheltered work?

5. Invite a school-based OTR or COTA to visit your class and share their experiences with you. What personal rewards or frustrations have they encountered in public school practice?
6. Should OTRs and COTAs who plan to work in school settings take additional classes in education to better understand this practice environment? Should a pediatric fieldwork experience be required in a school setting?

References

1. Ad Hoc Commission on Occupational Therapy Manpower: *Occupational Therapy Manpower: A Plan for Progress*. Rockville, MD, AOTA, 1985, pp. 6–7, 55–59.
2. AOTA: 1990 Member Data Survey, Summary Report, Special Insert in *OT Week* 5(22):108, 1991.
3. Carr SH: State guidelines for school-based occupational therapy: 1989 survey. *AJOT* 44(8):755–757, 1990.
4. Stephens L: Occupational therapy in the school system. In Pratt P, Allen A, eds. *Occupational Therapy for Children*. St. Louis, CV Mosby, 1989, pp. 593–611.
5. Ottenbacher K: Occupational therapy and special education: some issues and concerns related to Public Law 94–142. *AJOT* 36:81–84, 1982.
6. Traylor MD, Graham GT: School-based occupational therapists' perception of their involvement in special education teams. *DDSIS Newsletter* 14(4):3–4, 1991.
7. Coutinho MJ, Hunter DL: Special education and occupational therapy: making the relationship work. *AJOT* 42(11):706–712, 1988.
8. Rourk J, Andrews J, Dunn W, Stephens L, Wendt, G: *Guidelines for Occupational Therapy Services in Schools*. Rockville, MD, AOTA, 1986, pp. 12–23.
9. Dunn W: Models of occupational therapy service provision in the school system. *AJOT* 42(11):718–723, 1988.
10. AOTA: Roles of occupational therapists and occupational therapy assistants in schools. *AJOT* 41(12):798–803, 1987.
11. AOTA: Standards of practice for occupational therapy services in schools. *AJOT* 41(12):804–808, 1987.
12. Government and Legal Affairs Division. American Occupational Therapy Association. Final regulations, PL 94–142, Education of all Handicapped Children Act. *Federal Report* 77–5.3–17, 1977.
13. DeBello L: New law provides occupational therapy for preschoolers. *Occup Ther News* 40(12):6, 1986.
14. Colman W: The evolution of occupational therapy in the public schools: the laws mandating practice. *AJOT* 42(11):701–705, 1988.
15. Nondiscrimination on basis of handicap: programs and activities receiving or benefitting from federal financial assistance: *Fed Reg* 42:86, 1977.
16. Kalscheur JA: Benefits of the Americans with Disabilities Act of 1990 for children and adolescents with disabilities. *AJOT* 46(5):419–426, 1992.
17. Prestigiacomo G: School therapists go high-tech. *OT Week* 3(27):16–17, 1989.
18. Fox S: School-based therapists grapple with thorny issues. *Adv Occup Ther* 7(30):6–7, 1991.
19. Huebner R: Occupational therapy in the schools. *Occup Ther Forum* V(13):1–5, 1990.
20. Chandler B: Fee-for-service: a new reality. *OT Week* 4(36):9, 1990.
21. Hackbart P: Integrated therapy can really work. *Adv Occup Ther* 8(20):34, 1992.
22. Fox S: Schools solve space crunch. *Adv Occup Ther* 6(20):1–2, 1990.
23. Cruz AS, Swal S: Occupational therapy creates and constructs mobile therapy unit. *OT Week* 3(9):4, 32, 1989.
24. Bober P: Independent living training in public schools. *Occup Ther Forum* May 1, 1989, pp. 10–14.

Suggested Readings

Dunn W (ed): *Pediatric Occupational Therapy: Facilitating Effective Service Provision*. Thorofare, NJ, Slack, 1990.

Logigian MK, Ward JD (eds): *Pediatric Rehabilitation: A Team Approach for Therapists*. Waltham, MA, Littlt, Brown & Co, 1989.

Pratt P, Allen A (eds): *Occupational Therapy for Children*. ed. 2. St. Louis, CV Mosby, 1989.

Special Issue on Occupational Therapy in the Schools. *AJOT* 42:11, November, 1988.

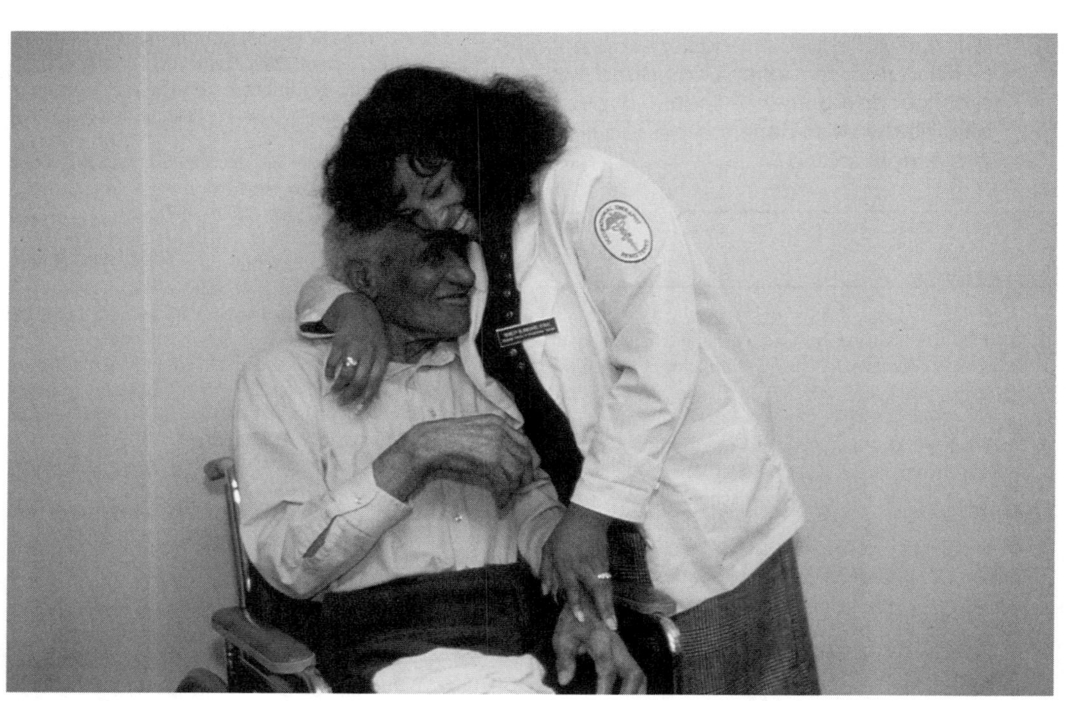

15 Practice with Elderly Populations

Old age is not a disease, but older people in our society are often viewed in terms of diminished physical capacity, mental competency, and status. The general public tends to have some fixed beliefs about aging that often influence public policies relating to care of the elderly. How accurate are your ideas about the elderly population of the United States? Take the following quiz to find out.

T F 1. Mental confusion is an inevitable consequence of old age.
T F 2. Sexual urges and activity normally cease around the ages of 55–60.
T F 3. Older workers are more careless and unsafe than younger workers.
T F 4. The numbers of old people in the U.S. population have stabilized and are expected to hold steady well into the next century.
T F 5. Automobile accidents are the most common cause of injury among the elderly.
T F 6. Creativity tends to decline with advancing age.
T F 7. Most elderly people eventually require nursing home care.
T F 8. More men than women survive to old age.
T F 9. The aged are typically preoccupied with death and fear its approach.
T F 10. American families have by and large abandoned their older family members.

If you marked all of the above statements false, you have a better than average awareness of aging and the elderly population. Each statement in the quiz represents a common myth about aging. Now let's look at the facts.

Mental confusion and forgetfulness in old age can be caused by Alzheimer's disease or other dementias, but over 100 other conditions can cause the same problems. Many are easily correctable, so mental confusion is not inevitable.

Most older people are capable of leading an active and satisfying sex life well into their 80s and 90s. It is a myth of the young that the sex drive subsides or disappears sometime in middle age.

Today 12% of the U.S. population is 65 or older. By the year 2030 one in five people will be over the age of 65. The elderly population is growing rapidly, and more are surviving to advanced ages.

The most common cause of injury among the elderly is falls, many of which are preventable. Adequate lighting, nonskid carpets, and an obstacle-free environment could prevent many of the serious falls that elderly people experience.

Picasso painted until his death in his 90s, and Grandma Moses kept painting until her death at the age of 101. Many older adults begin new careers or hobbies late in their life. Once a creative person, always a creative person.

Only about 5% of the older population require nursing home care and this is usually necessitated by the effects of a serious illness. The majority of older people can live safely and comfortably in the community with the aid of some support services. Over the age of 85, however, about 22% of the elderly live in nursing homes.

Most elderly people do not fear death but accept its inevitability. In healthy adults a fear of death is actually more common in middle age. Depression or a terminal illness can lead to a preoccupation with death at any age.

The American family is still the number one caretaker of older adults today. Most older people live near their children and see them often. Today about eight of ten older men and six of ten older women live in family settings (1, 2).

While Americans are living longer, they are also retiring earlier. Many retirees can look forward to 20 or 30 years of retirement. Being elderly doesn't have to mean being poor, but one-fifth of all older adults live under or near the poverty line. The very old, members of minority groups, and women tend to be poorer than other groups of elderly people (3).

PRACTICE SITES

When we think of care of the elderly, our first thought is usually of nursing homes. Although only a small proportion of older people need skilled nursing care, there will always be some who require the comprehensive services and protective environment of a skilled nursing facility. Ellis (4) has predicted that the need for such facilities will increase as more and more Americans live to advanced ages. The long-term residential care facility is the most restrictive living environment for the elderly, but it can provide programs designed to meet the elderly client's needs for personal safety, healthy nutrition, environmental comfort and security, and curative or palliative treatment. Ellis has proposed greater use of work-oriented activities for nursing home residents and an increased attention to improvement of residents' abilities in work, leisure, and self-care tasks.

Frequently COTAs are employed in long-term care facilities as activity directors. Activity programs are important in promoting and maintaining the physical and psychological health of residents and offer social opportunities to residents as well. Today, with shorter hospital stays, the nursing home has become a primary site for rehabilitative services, with occupational, physical, and speech therapy being mandated by law. These services are sometimes provided by therapists working on a contract basis and who are called in when a resident is in need of their services (5).

More and more, occupational therapy services to the elderly are being provided through community agencies rather than in institutional settings. The results of the AOTA's 1990 Member Data Survey showed that OTRs and COTAs were working in residential care facilities, retirement or senior centers, skilled nursing homes and intermediate care facilities, home health agencies, day care programs, and hospice programs (6).

TREATMENT TEAM

Since both the problems seen and the sites of service delivery are so varied, it is difficult to describe all of the potential team members that might contribute to elder care. Medical problems require the ongoing services of physicians, both in primary and specialized care practices. Fortunately physicians today are better educated in the special needs of the elderly and more primary care physicians have some background in gerontology.

In hospitals and skilled nursing homes one would expect the involvement of nurses and nurse practitioners, physician assistants, social workers, nursing assistants, and a variety of medical technologists. Senior centers and residential care facilities are less likely to have medical personnel on board but may have lay workers and volunteers working under the direction of a program manager. Home health agencies may have nurses and occupational, physical, and speech therapists on their staff. Day care programs often include OTRs or COTAs, social workers, and volunteers to help run the program. In hospice care, volunteers or lay workers may assist nurses, social workers, and therapists in providing supportive care to the terminally ill and their families.

Because elderly persons may need several types of health care services, it is often desirable to have one person responsible for coordinating care. This is usually a family member who assumes responsibility for scheduling appointments, supplying the necessary transportation, filling prescriptions, and seeing that recommendations are carried out. In the absence of an involved family member, a case manager may be needed to provide these services.

Family members are an important part of the care team for elderly individuals. They know the elderly person well and can often supply needed information about his or her habits, behavior, and physical limitations. If the family member is the elderly person's chief caregiver, he or she may need support services too. Full-time care of an aging spouse or relative is stressful. We are seeing many more elderly men and women trying to provide care for a disabled spouse and having a difficult time coping with day-to-day needs. Burnout can and does occur, and health care professionals need to tune in to caregiver needs as well as those of the client.

KEY CONCEPTS

Theories of Aging

Theories of aging attempt to explain the aging process and to identify factors that account for individual differences in how people age. Aging theories can be grouped into three major categories: **psychosocial**, **developmental,** and **biological.**

Psychosocial theories look at psychological characteristics and how they change as the individual ages. The activity theory of aging holds that by maintaining a high level of activity the effects of the aging process can be minimized and life can be made more fulfilling for the older person. The disengagement theory hypothesizes that as people age, their social systems also decline and they tend to withdraw from social interaction. The continuity theory of personality development assumes that the personality remains consistent over time and that during aging individuals become "more" of what they already are. Lifelong patterns of behavior continue as the individual grows older.

Developmental theories look at the aging process as a phase of normal human development. Erikson's stages of ego development theory view old age as a time in which spiritual values predominate and the individual develops feelings of acceptance, fulfillment, and respect for the life cycle. Havighurst divides adulthood into three periods: early adulthood, middle age, and old age. During old age, people are expected to adjust to retirement, the death of spouses and friends, and declines in health and strength. Kohlberg's theory of moral development proposes that in the third and final stage of development the individual accepts the standards of society, values universal ethical principles, and formulates his or her religious beliefs.

Biological theories are concerned with the physical manifestations of aging. Physical changes associated with aging have been well documented. The immune system begins to decline at about age 30, and its gradual weakening makes it harder to fight off illnesses. The metabolism slows down gradually after the age of 25 and fewer calories are needed to maintain body weight. The kidneys lose up to 50% of their efficiency between the ages of 30 to 80 years. Liver function declines and the lungs lose from 30 to 50% of their capacity between the ages of 30 to 80 years. Bone mass peaks in the 30s and then declines about 1% a year, and even faster in postmenopausal women. The senses lose their sharpness, and taste, smell, hearing, vision, and body awareness decline. Changes in the skin make it a less efficient regulator of body temperature. Sleep needs change, with a greater frequency of insomnia. The brain loses about 20% of its weight and the speed of recall and mental performance slow down.

One of the oldest biological theories of aging is the wear-and-tear theory, which holds that body parts and systems simply run down during aging, leading to physical deterioration and death. Genetic theories hypothesize that certain genes may be responsible for built-in defects that interfere with function and shorten life. The free radical theory proposes that unstable free radical chemicals produce physical changes that over time interfere with cellular processes and lead to illness and death. Stress and adaptation theories identify life stresses as the origin of physical damage and deterioration of bodily functions.

As the various theories of aging are tested, we will probably find that a combination of theories may explain many of the changes that occur during aging. Aging is a complex process and extremely variable, with changes occurring at many different levels of function. The study of aging is a fast-growing discipline, and health professionals working with the elderly should keep informed about the new developments in theories of aging. As we try to deal with the disabilities and disorders of the elderly, we need answers to the mysteries of aging (7, 8).

Goals of Occupational Therapy with the Elderly

Because the older person is likely to have multiple physical or psychological disorders, it is particularly important that a holistic approach be taken in treatment. The herontic occupational therapist must be able to deal with independent living needs, physical limitations, cognitive changes, and psychological adjustment. The leading causes of death in the elderly continue to be cardiovascular disease, malignant neoplasms (cancer), and cerebrovascular disease. Physicians report that arthritis is seen in over half of all females over the age of 65. Other common disorders include hypertension, diabetes mellitus, and visual and hearing impairment. The occupational therapist and therapy assistant will need to carefully assess the elderly client's status in all three functional areas. Care must be taken to consider any secondary conditions that may affect the client's total function; prevention of further disability is an additional consideration. Just as with other age groups, the therapist or therapy assistant should encourage the client to help with the identification of personal goals and priorities so that the treatment program can be individually tailored to the client's needs. In the last few years many acute care hospitals have developed outpatient geriatric assessment clinics to provide comprehensive evaluation of the physical, cognitive, and psychosocial status of elderly persons. This team effort to identify multiple problems of the aging has been a major improvement in the care of older clients. An OTR may contribute to the team results by looking at the occupational performance of clients and at specific performance components that may limit function.

Solomon has pointed out that the elderly are at high risk for developing serious psychopathology. An estimated 30% of persons over age 65 develop at least one major depressive disorder and many more experience depression symptoms. Alcohol and drug abuse occur in 25% of the elderly, with the addiction frequently being to prescription medications. Approximately 6% suffer from cognitive impairment, and another 5% have diagnosable personality disorders. Solomon believes that the multiple stresses that impact upon the elderly frequently lead to the phenomenon of "learned helplessness." Individuals give up their control of personal affairs and become dependent on others to care for them and fulfill their needs. Some environments tend to foster this dependence by maintaining tight control of all aspects of the individual's daily life and offering few or no choices (9).

Trace and Howell have emphasized the importance of offering older clients some measure of autonomy in their daily life. Often even small changes such as enlarged telephone buttons or use of a compartmentalized medication box can help an individual live independently at home for a while longer. These writers point out that chemical and physical restraints have been used more often with the elderly than with any other group. Recent legislation has curtailed this practice, but practitioners should be aware of any attempts to limit the activity and self-direction of elderly persons. Group activities have been particularly successful with older client groups since they promote socialization as well as maintain physical and mental abilities. Safety is always a concern with the impaired elderly, and assessment of functional performance is critical to judgments about a client's ability to live safely at home (10).

The mental health needs of the elderly are attracting more public attention, and efforts are being made to better serve the mental health needs of this population. Many elderly persons do not seek help for mental health problems, and when they do, they are often handed a prescription for medication. Improved mental health services are a major need of this client group.

In the elderly client, many of the goals of therapy center on improving cognitive awareness and psychological adjustment. For clients who have been institutionalized for a period of time, mental confusion and disorientation may be a problem. Therapeutic programs that help the client maintain contact with reality are often helpful. *Reality orientation* provides a structured method of improving cognitive awareness in clients. *Remotivation groups* are aimed at helping clients become more interested in their immediate surroundings and in encouraging them to share their past experiences. *Life review groups* offer opportunities for elderly clients to reminisce about their life, review unresolved conflicts, and integrate their experiences into an acceptance of their life as it draws to a close.

Physical needs are another focus of occupational therapy intervention. Physical fitness is a concern of people of all ages, and the elderly, although subject to some physical limitations, can continue to benefit from mild exercise. *Exercise groups* help clients to maintain joint range of motion and general flexibility as well as provide some social stimulation. Clients who have major physical dysfunctions may need a rehabilitation program to restore as much function as possible and to help compensate for physical limitations. Most older clients will show some degree of sensory loss. Low vision may necessitate the use of magnifiers for reading, large-print reading materials, special lighting, and other environmental adaptations. Hearing loss may prevent some elderly clients from participating fully in social activities and may contribute to the development of paranoid behavior, depression, and social isolation. Telephone amplifiers, use of a hearing aid if feasible, and use of special methods when communicating with hard-of-hearing clients may make it possible to communicate more effectively. Programs of sensory stimulation are sometimes used with elderly clients to maintain their perceptual skills and increase their awareness of internal and external sensory cues. Some elderly persons may be aphasic (language-impaired) as a result of a stroke. These clients will have difficulty understanding spoken or written language and may also have trouble expressing themselves. A multidisciplinary treatment approach can be designed to help clients relearn appropriate language patterns and develop functional communication with those around them.

Daily living skills are an important area of occupational therapy intervention. The occupational therapist or therapy assistant is the most relevant member of the treatment team to assist the elderly client who is having trouble performing the ordinary tasks of daily life. Occupational therapy treatment in this realm may include teaching grooming and dressing techniques, working on feeding skills, teaching the client to transfer safely from wheelchair to toilet or chair, working on bathing and daily hygiene needs, helping the client to master cooking and meal planning, teaching work simplification techniques to relieve stress on joints and to avoid fatigue, and helping the client to develop or maintain avocational interests (7).

CHANGING PATTERNS OF CARE

Legislative Influences

Social security retirement benefits came into being in 1935 and were intended to provide a minimum income for retired workers. Benefits are paid through a trust fund that is supported by payroll taxes paid by workers and employers. Although never intended to be a sole source of income, today 55% of retirees say that social security is their biggest source of income, and 20% say that it is 90% of their retirement income.

In 1965 the Older American Act was passed, establishing state and community grants for programs on aging and funding senior centers, senior volunteer programs, nutrition programs, and other services designed to increase job opportunities and enhance life for America's elderly citizens.

In the same year Medicare and Medicaid were added to the social security system. Medicare included compulsory hospital insurance and voluntary health insurance for persons over the age of 65. Medicaid provided federally funded medical assistance for the poor, administered by the states. It was hoped that these programs would enable the elderly and the poor to "buy into" the private U.S. health care system. In 1972 Congress passed a Social Security Income Bill (SSI) that was intended to offer a minimum monthly income to the blind, the aged, and the disabled. In the same year Congress added an annual cost-of-living adjustment (COLA) to the social security program to ensure that the minimum income of retirees kept pace with inflation.

During the 1990s the United States is facing increasing problems with maintaining the social security funds as the workforce grows smaller in proportion to the aging population. In addition, some administrations have "borrowed" from social security funds to finance the cost of other programs and to reduce the national debt. The costs of Medicare and Medicaid have increased annually, and cost containment measures such as Diagnostic Related Groups (DRGs) have worked only to a degree. There is serious doubt in the 1990s as to whether this system of benefits can be maintained at its present level.

Even though it is a costly program for workers to support, Medicare pays only 80% of physician and hospital charges and fails to cover a whole range of needed services. People must pay the remaining 20% from their own pockets or from supplementary private insurance plans.

During 1983 and 1984, Medicare had begun a new reimbursement policy for hospitals that treated Medicare patients. It established DRGs for 472 different medical disorders or procedures. Each was assigned an average length of hospital stay, and Medicare paid a fixed cost for each DRG. The system was intended to provide an incentive for earlier discharge of patients from the expensive hospital setting, thus saving Medicare money. The result was that hospital stays were reduced by about 20%, and more people were referred to nursing homes or to community care programs for convalescent and rehabilitative services.

These changes were not necessarily bad. The problem was that Medicare coverage for nursing home care and home health care did not expand to replace the reduced length of hospital stays. Patients were being discharged "quicker and sicker" and needed care outside the hospital. Nursing homes were finding that Medicare and Medicaid reimbursement didn't come close to covering the actual costs of care.

Some nursing homes began to refuse to admit Medicaid patients and discharged those they already had. Others raised their private-pay rates in order to partially subsidize Medicare and Medicaid patients. Nursing homes' inability to pay acceptable wages to workers resulted in a large turnover of nursing assistant staff, and quality of care suffered because of chronic staff shortages and inadequate training of staff.

The Nursing Home Quality Reform Act of 1987 (part of the Omnibus Budget Reconciliation Act) did much to improve nursing home care. The act took effect in 1990 and protected the rights of nursing home residents, raised standards of care, tightened up staffing requirements, and reinforced the concept of maintaining as much functional independence as possible for residents. It also provided Medicare reimbursement for outpatient services needed by patients recovering from hospital procedures. Occupational, physical, and speech therapy were covered under this act, and nursing homes were required to provide these services for residents who needed them. If a nursing home could not provide full-time therapists, it was permitted to hire them on a contract basis. These changes helped nursing homes and home health agencies become active providers of care to Medicare recipients.

Currently Medicare covers only 100 days of extended care annually for its recipients. Hospice care is covered, but only if the recipient agrees to waive his or her right to all other Medicare benefits. In 1988 the Medicare Catastrophic Coverage Act was passed by Congress. This act provided insurance to cover the costs of major illnesses and was funded through premiums assessed to Medicare recipients. Older Americans were infuriated that this mandatory coverage duplicated coverage that many already had through private insurers. The outcry was so great that Congress was forced to repeal this act in 1989. The real need, senior citizens told their elected representatives, was for coverage for long-term care of chronic illnesses and disabilities. Elderly voters urged their congressional representatives to fund this kind of coverage instead.

Some authors have advocated setting limits on elder care since the resources of society are limited and care of the elderly is an expensive proposition. Medical ethicist Daniel Callahan has argued for spending American medical resources on the young and productive members of society rather than on artificially prolonging life for the old (11). This debate will continue as health care resources become more and more costly. American legislators hope to avoid an intergenerational conflict between the young workforce who are the chief support of the social security programs and the retired elderly who live in fear that their hard-won benefits will be reduced.

New Models of Service Delivery

In response to changes in health care and the funding of health services, nursing homes are assuming a greater share of the responsibility for rehabilitative care. Rehabilitation goals are being recognized as important in restoring older persons to a reasonable level of health and well-being. Since occupational therapists and therapy assistants are educated to focus on function, they are important contributors to elder care.

Since family members provide so much of the care for the elderly, it is important that they have the resources they need. Home health services, geriatric day care programs, and respite care can relieve the burden on family caregivers and can help them to cope. Support groups for the families of Alzheimer patients and others can alleviate feelings of isolation and helplessness and can often offer practical advice on how to handle the day-to-day problems that arise.

Information and referral services help families locate the kind of services they need and may provide counseling on aging and family issues. Transportation services allow elderly people to do their shopping and keep medical appointments. Case managers can provide coordination of care for elderly persons without family resources. New concepts in retirement living have broadened the housing options available and include such ideas as boarding homes, low-income housing developments, and retirement communities that offer a continuum of living arrangements. Packages of housekeeping, home maintenance, and health monitoring services are being offered by some community agencies. Work activity programs help elderly people to remain productive and useful during their retirement years. Hospice programs that provide direct care for terminally ill patients and support services for their families are becoming more widespread.

Most of these services have a community orientation and are intended to help elderly persons avoid institutionalization and enable them to continue to live comfortably and safely in the community. Occupational therapy services have followed this trend and are increasingly located in community agencies, private practices, and outpatient programs.

PRACTICE ISSUES AND TRENDS

Staff Shortage

A 1987 study showed that there had been a 50% increase in the number of occupational therapists working in gerontology since 1982 (12). With the aging population increasing rapidly, many more OTs are needed to serve the needs of this client group. The 1990 Member Data Survey conducted by AOTA found that 28.2% of OTRs and 37.2% of COTAs were working with clients over the age of 65 (6). Although these figures look impressive, still more personnel are needed. In order to increase the numbers of occupational therapy practitioners working with the elderly, Haselkus and Kiernat have suggested encouraging optional fieldwork experiences in geriatric programs, working to overcome students' biases and stereotypes about the elderly, and increasing the geriatric content in OTR and COTA educational programs. Occupational therapy, they argue, needs to prepare more practitioners to work in this specialized area of practice whose clients need their services so much. They predict a marked expansion of occupational therapy services for the elderly providing that the needed staffing is available (13).

Need for Long-Term Care Funding

Americans are becoming aware that Medicare and most private health insurance policies do not cover the cost of long-term care. As more elderly people live to advanced ages, this need is growing critical. The financial resources of most elderly people run out long before their care needs do. In recent years some health insurers have been marketing nursing home insurance, but costs are high, coverage is limited, and home health care is not included. A number of proposals have been introduced into Congress for federally funded long-term care insurance, but as of this writing, none have been passed. Nursing home care in 1990 cost an average of $30,000 a year, and about half of those costs come from direct client payment. Home health services would be less costly and more appropriate for most people.

Somers, writing in 1991, stated that the cost of long-term care was the most significant threat to the security of elderly Americans (14). Crabtree and Caron-Parker have described some of the ethical issues involved in long-term care. They support a partnership model between the family and the health care team for planning optimum long-term care services (15).

Elder Abuse

In 1991 an elderly man in a wheelchair was found abandoned in the parking lot of a dog-racing track. He was unable to identify himself and was clutching a bag of adult diapers. All of the identifying labels had been removed from his clothes. Police eventually learned that he had been abandoned by a daughter who had embezzled his pension and social security funds and then had left him in a public place to fend for himself. The case was widely publicized through the news media, and fortunately he was recognized by other family members who took over his care.

This kind of problem is becoming more common. Elder abuse and "granny dumping" are on the rise, and a survey of emergency room physicians in 1992 showed that they saw an average of eight elderly patients a week who were brought to a hospital emergency room and left there. Most of those abandoned were frail and in poor health. Some had dementia, and families were apparently unable to cope with their need for 24-hour-a-day care.

Over half of all reported cases of abuse are really cases of self-neglect. An elderly person may live alone but be unable to provide his own food, clothing, or self-care. Other forms of abuse are misuse of the elderly person's property or financial resources, neglect by caregivers, physical abuse, and emotional abuse. The rising number of cases of elder abuse highlights the gap between social service programs and the needs of older people. Protective services are badly needed. By 1990, 42 states and the District of Columbia had adopted mandatory reporting of abuse situations; however, enforcement varied from state to state. More social agencies are trying to deal with the problem, but it continues to be a major concern (16).

Suicide

The suicide rate for persons over the age of 65 has increased each year since 1980. White males have the highest suicide rate. Longer life spans don't necessarily mean life satisfaction. Some experts believe that more older people are choosing to end their lives rather than face terminal illness and a lonely existence. The publicity in recent years about cases of "assisted suicide" has tended to support this hypothesis. Most of the persons who took their lives in this way did so because they did not wish to experience the helplessness and total dependence of a devastating illness. Here too, ethical arguments can be made on both sides of the issue.

New Housing Options

A number of creative solutions have been proposed to keep the elderly in community settings and out of residential care. One of the simplest is home modification. Some community agencies offer services that will install grab bars in bathrooms, replace door knobs with more easily grasped lever handles, and install walk-in showers. Such modifications can mean the difference between independent living and having to go to a nursing home.

Home sharing is another approach. In this program an elderly homeowner is paired with a younger person who needs a place to live in exchange for low rent or support services to the homeowner. Such arrangements work well when careful screening and matching is done and when each party has realistic expectations of the other.

Special communities are now being designed for the elderly that include independent living apartments, health care services, day care and activity centers, an equipment loan center, and food services. Such residential facilities are meant to be all-inclusive and are equipped to handle a full range of geriatric disabilities (17).

Greater Attention to Cognitive Impairments

Alzheimer's disease and other dementias have received much attention in recent years. Alzheimer's is a progressive dementia that impairs memory, thought processes, emotional responses, activities of daily living, and communication. Gradual deterioration may lead to incontinence, refusal to eat, agitated behavior, emotional outbursts, and hallucinations or delusions. Most families try to care for their demented family member at home, but many support services are needed. As these conditions have become better known and understood, health care providers have been able to teach families more effective ways of dealing with the unpredictable behavior and cognitive limitations that are typically seen. The effect on driving ability is particularly serious, and accidents can easily occur when a demented client is permitted to continue driving. These conditions require the help of a number of health care providers, and nursing home care may be needed toward the end of the disease process (18, 19).

SUMMARY

Gerontology is a growing specialty area of occupational therapy practice, and more staffing is needed to meet the needs of this rapidly expanding segment of the population. New community-based programs offer exciting opportunities for OTRs and COTAs to develop innovative services. The new role of the nursing home as a rehabilitation center means that restorative care can be given closer to the client's home environment and can be better geared to his or her daily living needs. If federal funding is approved for long-term care, older citizens will have access to a full range of health care services.

Case Study: Bilateral Hip Fractures, Arthritis

Katherine is a 75-year-old retired woman. She was admitted to a local hospital after a fall in her home in which she fractured her left hip. She had a central fracture dislocation of the left hip, and while in the hospital sustained a fracture of the right hip as well. Surgery was done first on the right hip, with a total hip arthroplasty being performed. Later she underwent a left total hip arthroplasty. Occupational and physical therapy services began in the hospital. After a period of recovery, she was discharged from the hospital to a skilled nursing facility in her community for continued rehabilitation. Her physician anticipated that a 1-month intensive program of rehabilitation would be needed before she would be able to return to her apartment and live independently.

Upon admission to the nursing home, she was found to have severe rheumatoid arthritis in addition to her other problems. She was on a variety of medications, and precautions were necessary to prevent dislocation of both artificial hip joints. Her endurance was poor. Movement needed to be gentle because of her severe arthritis.

When first seen by occupational therapy, Katherine was able to perform personal hygiene and grooming activities (except for bathing) and could dress and undress the upper half of her body. Areas of dependency included bathing, donning lower extremity clothing, and functional mobility, including transfers, bed mobility, and ambulation. Katherine could feed herself independently, but her arthritis made it difficult for her to grasp standard eating utensils. Before her hospitalization, she had been living alone in a one-bedroom apartment and was accustomed to preparing her own meals and managing her household activities independently.

Katherine's ability to use her hands and arms was extremely limited because of chronic rheumatoid arthritis. Her upper extremity strength was graded poor to fair, and her endurance, both in general and for specific upper extremity activity, was poor. She quickly became short of breath and needed to rest frequently. She had only half of the normal range of motion in her shoulders, and several of her finger joints had been fused to give her better stability. She could grossly manipulate objects but had poor fine-motor skill. Katherine complained of pain during movement and required assistance to get to a standing position from her wheelchair. In physical therapy she was able to use a walker and hoped eventually to be able to walk with crutches.

Katherine was aware of energy-conservation techniques and the need to protect her joints from further damage. She had also learned to use appropriate body mechanics and had incorporated these principles into her daily living activities. For example, to conserve her limited energy she sat on a stool when working in the kitchen and knew how to open containers in a way that would not cause further damage to her joints.

Katherine was alert and oriented. She had good short- and long-term memory and could concentrate for extended periods of time. She was highly motivated to regain the independent function that would allow her to return to her home. The occupational therapy intervention plan included: teaching Katherine hip safety precautions; teaching her adapted bathing and dressing methods; making adapted eating utensils for her to use; maintaining her present range of motion, strength, and coordination in her upper extremities; and insuring that she could perform her homemaking activities when she returned home. A COTA was assigned to help Katherine carry out her treatment activities on a daily basis.

After 1 month of treatment, Katherine was discharged from the nursing home, and home visits were made weekly by an OTR who worked with a local home health agency. The OTR conducted a home assessment to determine the accessibility and safety of Katherine's apartment and found that some additional modifications were needed in the bathroom. A raised toilet seat and toilet rails were installed, as well as grab bars on the walls. A tub bench was provided to allow Katherine to bathe in a seated position. Because her apartment had six steps at the entrance, the physical therapist assumed responsibility for teaching Katherine to negotiate the stairs using crutches. A home health nurse monitored Katherine's medications and served as the liaison to her physician. Until Katherine felt capable of preparing all of her meals, the social worker arranged for her to receive Meals on Wheels once a day. Family members assisted Katherine with shopping, laundry, and housekeeping until she was able to resume these tasks herself. Katherine was happy to return home and was confident that with time she would be able to resume most of her everyday activities.

Discussion Questions

1. Did you have a close relationship with a grandparent or elderly friend or neighbor? If so, did this relationship influence your attitudes about aging and elderly people? How?
2. What kind of resources are available in your community for elderly people? Are

the services adequate to meet the needs of the older people who live there?

3. Some states have mandated that all persons admitted to a hospital or nursing home must complete and sign a living will or a power of attorney for health care. This document spells out what level of emergency care the individual wishes to receive, and it may designate an agent to make health care decisions if the patient is unable to do so. If your state has such legislation, obtain a copy of the document and look at its provisions.
4. Have you visited a nursing home in your community? What kinds of programs does it offer to its residents? How much does it cost to live there? Is occupational therapy provided?
5. Did Katherine's occupational therapy intervention plan differ in any significant way from that that might have been prepared for a younger client?
6. Does your state have a Commission on Aging? If so, what services does it provide to elderly citizens?
7. Discuss the relative quality of life available in different kinds of living situations for the elderly. Consider institutional settings, retirement communities, low-income housing, and remaining in one's own home. What type of living situation would you prefer as an older person?
8. Should we be spending such large amounts of money for health care for the elderly? How can we balance our responsibility to older people and to the younger population of the United States?

References

1. National Institute on Aging: *What is your aging IQ?* Public Health Service/National Institutes of Health, U.S. Department of Health and Human Services, Nov. 1986.
2. Staff: What's on your mind? *OT Week* 6(6):8, 1992.
3. Joe B: The future—statistically speaking. *OT Week* 5(25):8, 1991.
4. Ellis N: The challenge of nursing home care. *AJOT* 40:7–11, 1986.
5. AOTA: *Long Term Care/Nursing Homes*. AOTA, Rockville, MD, 1985, pp. 1–86.
6. AOTA: 1990 Member Data Survey, Summary Report, Special insert in *OT Week* 5(22):1–8, 1991.
7. Lewis SC: *Elder Care in Occupational Therapy*. Thorofare, NJ, Slack, 1989, pp. 56–73.
8. Jones PW: Mysteries of aging continue to puzzle health experts. *OT Week* 1(29):12–13, 1987.
9. Solomon K: Learned helplessness in the elderly: theoretical and clinical considerations. *Occup Ther Ment Health* 10(3):31–51, 1990.
10. Trace S, Howell T: Occupational therapy in geriatric mental health. *AJOT* 45(9):833–837, 1991.
11. Callahan D: *Setting Limits: Medical Goals in an Aging Society*. New York, Simon & Schuster, 1988.
12. Peterson DA: Manpower study. *OT News* 43(1):3, 1989.
13. Hasselkus BR, Kiernat JM: Not by age alone: gerontology as a specialty in occupational therapy. *AJOT* 43(2):77–79, 1989.
14. Somers FP: Long-term care and federal policy. *AJOT* 45(7):628–635, 1991.
15. Crabtree JL, Caron-Parker LM: Long-term care of the aged: ethical dilemmas and solutions. *AJOT* 45(7):607–612, 1991.
16. Fox S: Abuse of elderly rising as living conditions deteriorate and social programs lag. *Adv Occup Ther* 6(27):1–2, 1990.
17. Egan M: Planning for the future. *OT Week* 6(24):12–13, 1992.
18. Nolinske T: Working with Alzheimer's disease. *OT Week* 3(38):1, 20–22, 1989.
19. Egan M: Drivers with Alzheimer's: hazardous conditions ahead. *OT Week* 6(5):12–13, 1992.

Suggested Readings

AOTA: Special issue on serving older adults. *AJOT* 45:7, July, 1991.

Kari N, Michels P: The Lazarus Project: the politics of empowerment. *AJOT* 45(8):719–725, 1991.

Kiernat JM (ed): *Occupational Therapy and the Older Adult, A Clinical Manual*. Frederick MD, Aspen Publishers, 1991.

Killeffer EH, Bennet R (eds): *Successful Models of Long-Term Care for the Elderly*. Binghamton, NY, The Haworth Press, 1992.

Lewis SC: *Elder Care in Occupational Therapy*. Thorofare, NJ, Slack, 1989.

Taira ED, Christenson MA (eds): *Aging in the Designed Environment*. Binghamton NY, The Haworth Press, 1990.

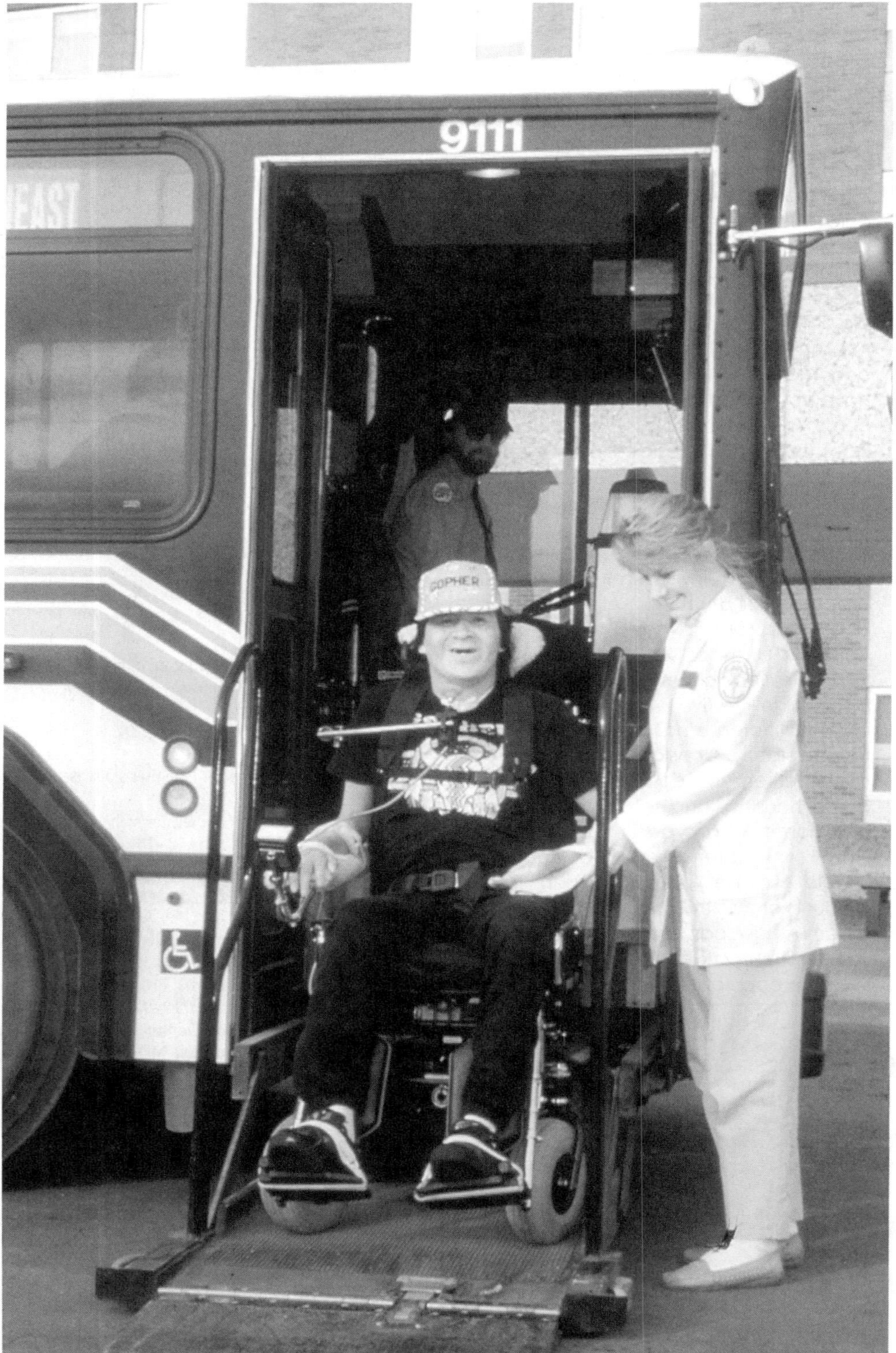
9111
GOPHER

16 Practice in Community-based Programs

The movement of occupational therapy services from traditional institutional settings into the community has been one of the biggest changes in the field in recent decades. As the Medicare prospective payment system began to take hold, there was a steady increase in the number of community-based occupational therapy programs that were intended to provide care to persons needing continued therapy after discharge from acute care hospitals and those who needed help to continue to live independently in their homes. According to the 1985 AOTA Manpower Report, there was a 4-fold increase in the number of OTRs working in home health agencies and a 2-fold increase in the number of therapists in private practice over a 9-year period (1). Data from the 1986 and 1990 AOTA Member Data Surveys confirmed these increases and showed steady growth in OTR and COTA employment in a variety of community settings. Table 16.1 shows the percentage of AOTA members working in community-based settings in 1990. According to the 1990 data, over 19% of OTRs and over 17% of COTAs surveyed were working in community care during 1990 (2).

According to AOTA data, private home health agencies (those not certified to provide service to Medicare patients) were the second fastest growing segment of the home health industry in 1989. Medicare-certified agencies had been developing rapidly until 1985, when funding cutbacks reversed the situation. In 1986 nearly 60% of all home health agencies provided occupational therapy services.

This chapter describes occupational therapy community-based services and introduces the student to concepts of community care. A variety of practice settings are described, and a case study is presented that illustrates occupational therapy home care with a home-bound client.

PRACTICE SITES

When we talk about community care, we are referring to a variety of practice settings that provide services to clients within their local community. Table 16.1 lists some of these settings, but the three that employ the largest numbers of OTRs and COTAs deserve special mention. They are home health agencies, independent living centers, and private practices.

Home Health Agencies

Much of the home care of clients receiving occupational therapy is coordinated by home health agencies. Medicare defines a home health agency as a public or private organization primarily engaged in providing skilled nursing care or other therapeutic services. To qualify under Medicare certification regulations, an agency must do the following:

Provide at least one therapeutic service besides skilled nursing,
Have policies developed by at least one physician and one registered nurse,
Maintain records for all clients seen,
Employ professional personnel who meet established qualifications, and
Provide for regular review of policies.

Under Medicare guidelines, any client services provided by a home health agency must be ordered by a physician. In the original reg-

Table 16.1. Community Practice Sites of OTRs and COTAs in 1990

Site	OTRs (%)	COTAs (%)
Community mental health center	1.1	1.7
Day care program	0.9	1.7
Home health agency	3.6	1.5
Hospice	0.0	0.0
Public health agency	0.9	0.6
Private industry	0.8	
Private practice	7.7	2.7
Residential care facility (includes group homes, independent living centers)	2.7	5.9
Retirement centers, senior centers	0.2	0.8
Sheltered workshops	0.4	1.6
Voluntary Agencies (Easter Seals, United Cerebral Palsy, etc.)	1.0	1.1
Totals	19.37	17.6

ulations, clients had to be homebound, and the services that were provided could not duplicate any other services. If a client is found to be in need of occupational therapy services, the therapist conducts an initial evaluation to determine the client's functional status and then prepares a written intervention plan to deal with the observed problems. Documentation is required for each home visit. According to an AOTA position paper, occupational therapy home care is intended to assist the client to attain a maximum level of functioning in his or her own home and community. Home treatment may focus on:

1. Improving daily living skills, work or leisure skills, sensorimotor skills, and cognitive or psychosocial skills;
2. Adapting the environment to allow for more effective functioning; or
3. Preventing further limitations in function (3).

Clients who are no longer making progress toward stated goals and those who do not comply with the program or who have achieved maximum benefit must be discharged from active treatment.

Home health agencies can provide therapeutic services by hiring the appropriate professionals as part of their staff or by contracting with private practitioners to provide therapy on an hourly basis. Because home health agency therapists travel from one client's home to another, they are limited in the kind of treatment equipment that can be used. COTAs working in home health agencies must be supervised by an OTR and may not accept referrals for service independently. In home care, on-site supervision is often not practical, but a system of supervision must be established. Working in a home health agency requires flexibility and creativity. The home health OTR or COTA needs a broad background of clinical experience since he or she will work with clients fairly independently and will address a great variety of problems. Home health agency work is not easy, but offers a challenging diversity to the skilled OTR or COTA.

Independent Living Centers

Independent living centers are another type of community program in which occupational therapy can play an active role. In the 1960s and 1970s the concept of independent living for the disabled gained momentum, and in 1978 Congress amended the Rehabilitation Act of 1973 to include provisions for comprehensive services to encourage independent living. This action was the result of increased awareness that disabled people needed more than vocationally oriented rehabilitation. The ability to enjoy a reasonable quality of life and to live independently or semiindependently in community settings was believed to be as important as employability for the disabled. This legislation supported a variety of self-help programs intended to promote independent living for disabled persons. One of the major provisions of the act was the establishment of independent living centers, defined as facilities offering a combination of services to encourage independence in family and community settings for the severely disabled population. State rehabilitation agencies were designated as the principal applicants for grant monies to establish and operate the centers. By 1987 there were 290 independent living centers nationwide. Some states had also developed local independent living programs funded through taxation, grants, fees for service, or third-party reimbursement sources.

Independent living programs vary considerably because they are intended to meet local needs. Some programs provide direct service, but a more common pattern is to utilize the services of existing community agencies. Independent living centers follow three basic patterns:

1. The free-standing center, providing services, giving adaptive housing assistance, and offering training in living skills;
2. Transitional living programs, where severely disabled clients are enabled to live in less-dependent or independent living arrangements; and
3. Residential programs, where several disabled individuals live in a group housing unit and share attendant care and services.

A key feature of all programs is a strong emphasis on consumer decision making. Disabled persons plan and often implement their own programs, making them more responsive to real consumer needs. AOTA takes the view that, where state regulations permit, COTAs should be able to work independently of OTRs in independent living programs. Roles that could be filled by an occupational therapy practitioner include those of consultant, advocate, director, case manager, and a provider of occupational therapy services. According to 1990 AOTA data, more COTAs than OTRs were working in independent living programs. Since the programs are complex, this is not considered an entry-level position. Practitioners respond directly to consumer requests for service if permitted by state regulations. Physician referral is usually not necessary in these programs (4).

Private Practice

A growing proportion of OTRs and COTAs are providing their services as private practitioners or are self-employed. Occupational therapy practices may be located in hospitals, medical centers, storefront clinics, or office buildings for health professionals. Private practitioners contract to deliver services for a fee and establish a small business to provide such services. A therapist might contract with a facility to provide its occupational therapy services, with agencies to see referred patients in their homes, or with individual clients whose doctors have requested occupational therapy services. Home care is generally on a fee-for-service basis. Contract therapy is usually based on units of time, for example providing 8 hours of therapy time a week at an hourly rate. Consultation charges are based on a completed project. A therapist might conduct a consumer satisfaction survey for a community agency, and would charge a lump sum for the entire project. Table 16.2 shows the percentages of OTRs and COTAs who were self-employed or in private practice during 1990.

Various types of private practice exist. An individual practice consists of a single therapist providing contracted services. An associate practice has one therapist who serves as director and who employs other professional and technical staff members of the same professional group. In a group practice, a va-

Table 16.2. Self-employment and Private Practice among AOTA Members, 1990

	OTRs (%)	COTAs (%)
Self-employed[a]	26.4	11.3
Private practice[b]	7.7	2.7

[a] Question asked: Are you paid either on a contractual basis or directly by your client or his or her agent?
[b] Identified as the primary employment setting.

riety of health professionals might be employed to offer more comprehensive services. A private practice may also be structured as a partnership between two or more therapists (5).

Private practitioners must be business-oriented because they must make a profit to remain in business. They need to set financial goals for their business just as they set treatment goals for their clients. The private practitioner establishes a set of specific services to be offered and then sets a fee schedule accordingly. Fees may be based on a set fee for each client visit, or units of time (15-minute or hourly units are common), or on the prevailing rate for the geographic area.

Private practitioners tend to make higher incomes than salaried practitioners make, but their expenses are also greater. They have direct control over their time and can work as many or as few hours as they wish in contrast to salaried employees. Tulanian, Hammond, and Tulanian (6) have identified a number of differences between private practitioners (contractors) and salaried therapists that are shown in Table 16.3.

These authors note that, while there is great independence of action in private practice, there is also great responsibility. Smith (7) confirms this in her discussion of private practice. She points out that the therapist has full control over the philosophy of the practice, the quality of care that is given, and the size of the practice. At the same time, the professional and financial success of the practice rests squarely on the shoulders of the therapist. It takes time and effort to build a reputation and a flourishing practice. The first few years may be difficult, and one must have sufficient capital to survive this establishment phase. Also, in private practice, if one is ill or takes a few days off, one earns no income.

Most private practitioners agree that a therapist or assistant should have several years of experience in clinical settings before entering into a private practice. The needs of the community should be thoroughly explored before setting up the practice. One must be willing to assume financial risks and be prepared to work hard to establish the business on a sound footing. Financial and legal advice may be needed, and knowledge of current business practices and procedures is as necessary to the private practitioner as is expertise in occupational therapy. The growth of private practice is expected to continue, and this type of practice is a major source of community-based occupational therapy service.

TREATMENT TEAM

Occupational therapists and therapy assistants working in community programs may work with public health nurses, physical therapists, speech and language therapists, home health nurses, social workers, and home health aides. Nonprofessionals provide 70% of the services in home health care (8). The home health aide who assists clients with bathing and daily care may have the most frequent contact with the client and can be a valuable ally for the OTR or COTA. Family members also contribute much to therapy programs and are valued members of the health care team.

Communication between team members is often difficult when working in the community since each may be visiting the client at a different time. Some team members may work for different agencies. Telephone calls help to keep team members in touch, and written reports are essential to keep the team informed of changes in the client's status. Time must be set aside for team meetings so that

Table 16.3. Differences between the Private Contractor and Employee

Contractor	Employee
Paid by the service (pay includes paperwork, preparation, travel)	Paid by the hour
Paid lump sum per day travel fees	Paid by the mile
Therapist maintains time records, calculates amount due, submits bill for reimbursement	Facility keeps time records, computes salary, and pays on designated paydays
Provides own equipment or pays for use of equipment	Equipment provided by employer
Provides own liability and property damage insurance	Facility provides liability and property damage coverage
No taxes are withdrawn from paychecks; responsible for state and federal taxes, social security	Facility computes and deducts payroll taxes
Chooses own hours	Hours set by facility
No vacation or sick leave; no health insurance or workers compensation provided	Vacation and sick leave; health insurance and workers compensation provided by employer
Therapist chooses type of treatment to be given	Supervisor can specify type of treatment
Therapist provides own continuing education	Continuing education may be provided by employer
Therapist provides own space or pays for use of space	Facility provides space
Therapist bills third parties or pays for facility's billing service	Facility provides all billing services
Therapist has no mail slot or bulletin board space unless facility is reimbursed for these	Therapist provided with mail slot and bulletin board space for messages
Therapist provides for own secretarial services	Therapist uses facility's secretarial services
Therapist provides own name tag and personal business cards; may not use facility business card	Therapist uses name tags and business cards of facility

cases can be discussed and mutual goals agreed upon.

It is usually best to keep the team small. Clients become confused when too many people are coming and going in their homes, and they may have trouble following up on multiple recommendations. One or two disciplines are usually enough to carry out most of the intervention while other team members take a less active role.

KEY CONCEPTS IN COMMUNITY CARE

Value of the Home Environment

Rowles has suggested that many people underestimate the importance of a person's environment as a source of identity and well-being. He conducted an ethnographic survey of elderly residents of a small town and found that each participant lived in a very individualized "lifeworld," with his or her own patterns of daily activity, social relationships, and feelings about the environment. Understanding the significant "lifeworld" of clients helps the OTR or COTA to better understand the individual and what's important to him or her. Intervention strategies can be tailored to clients and their customary environments in a more sensitive way. Awareness of a client's "sense of place" can be especially important in community care where the intervention takes place in the client's home (9).

Holistic Approach

The community-based therapist is in a good position to look at a client's total needs. By assessing physical, emotional, cognitive, and environmental status, a comprehensive intervention plan can be developed. Devereaux believes that therapists who have maintained their skills as generalists are most successful in community-based practice. They are able to move easily from one area of practice to another, giving clients good value for their money and making referrals for specialized service if needed (10).

The medical model that is usually the basis for hospital practice is less useful in community practice. Here function is the most important consideration, and a holistic approach that considers all aspects of the client's life is more practical. Prevention is often an essential part of home care. Clients must become aware of safety factors, must learn performance methods that will reduce the chances of reinjury, and must understand how to maintain their health and well-being. In community care, therapists must look at the big picture and try to meet a variety of client needs within a single intervention program.

Skills Needed in Home Care

When a health professional delivers service in a client's home, he or she must remember that they are on the client's turf. Respect for the client's ways of doing things and acceptance of his or her preferences is critical to the success of a therapeutic program. New ideas can only be suggested, not imposed.

Attention must be paid to the cost of needed services and equipment. Even a $20 bath bench may be too expensive for a client to purchase, and another approach may be needed to solve the problem. Flexibility is important, as the OTR or COTA is often confronted with unexpected situations or events. Daily schedules do not always work out as planned, and therapists must be able to quickly adapt to changes in caseload and visits that were more time-consuming than expected.

Imagination and creativity are needed in abundance as conventional therapy equipment may be too heavy or bulky to tote around in the therapist's car. The home health therapist must develop a knowledge of common, everyday items that can be pressed into service as therapy equipment. Cans of vegetables can serve as weights to help improve a client's strength, spring clothespins can help to develop pinch, and a broomstick may be used for bilateral arm exercises.

Home health therapists must sometimes deal with aspects of care outside their area of expertise. It may be necessary to put a client in touch with a social worker to help him or her figure out medical bills or with a community nutrition program if he or she is not eating properly. A working knowledge of community resources is especially helpful when working in community care (11).

Networking

Therapists working in community-based settings often feel isolated from their peers because so much of their work is done independently. Hurff and her colleagues have suggested networking with occupational therapy colleagues and other health care professionals in related agencies to form a mutual support system, share experiences, and solve clinical problems. When mutual give-and-take relationships are established with other colleagues, all will benefit, and it may be possible to establish some innovative services. As OTRs and COTAs move into more nontraditional settings, networking will become even more necessary to build professional alliances and gain acceptance and support (12).

CHANGING PATTERNS OF CARE

The concept of home and community-based care is not a new one to occupational therapy. Since the 1920s occupational therapy services have been available through visiting nurse associations, public health programs, and hospital and community-based home care agencies. A relatively small number of practitioners were involved in community care.

By the mid-1970s social and economic changes in the United States were creating growing pressure for community health and therapeutic services. The trend toward deinstitutionalization increased the pressure; however, few funding mechanisms were available to pay for community care. The enactment of Title XVIII (Medicare) and Title XIX (Medicaid) in 1965 was the beginning of funding to support the delivery of community-based services. These acts were followed by the amendments to the Social Security Act in 1983 that established the prospective payment system for hospital care of Medicare recipients. Under Medicare provisions, a client found to have continuing needs for therapy after a hospitalization could receive in-home services if a physician so ordered and if the client was homebound and was considered to have potential for further improvement. Other pieces of legislation also spurred the development of community services. The Architectural Barriers Act of 1968 and section 504 of the Rehabilitation Act of 1973 mandated that community facilities be fully accessible to the disabled, and Title VII (another amendment to the Rehabilitation Act of 1973) created comprehensive independent living services to aid severely handicapped persons to live more independently in their homes and communities. All of these laws combined to encourage the development of services on the community level and provided funding to assist in this effort.

Although the growth of community-based occupational therapy services has been rapid, it has not been without problems. For many years, occupational therapy was not covered by Medicare if it was the only therapeutic service being given. Reimbursement for occupational therapy services was sometimes questioned by Medicare and by other third-party payers, and there was increasing demand for documentation of the effectiveness of occupational therapy intervention.

As the introduction of DRGs produced shorter stays in the acute care hospital, home care services began to take up some of the slack. Between 1975 and 1984 there was a 100% growth rate of home care services (13). The restrictions on occupational therapy coverage were eased in 1986 with the passage of amendments to the Medicare Act that permitted extended occupational therapy services to inpatients in skilled nursing facilities, provided Medicare coverage of occupational therapy services in rehabilitation agencies even if that were the only service being given, and enabled occupational therapists to become independent service providers for Medicare recipients. The latter provision opened the door to private practitioners to offer services to individual clients covered under Medicare and to bill directly for their services. Clients no longer had to be homebound to qualify for occupational therapy services. These changes (effective July 1, 1987) increased the use of occupational therapy services for this client population (14).

By 1989 parts A and B of Medicare were paying for home health care if it was deemed medically necessary. In the same year the Health Care Finance Administration developed guidelines for outpatient occupational therapy that included cognitive assistance as well as physical assistance (13).

AOTA has made the reimbursement of occupational therapy home health services a high priority item and is now trying to get occupational therapy recognized as one of four primary providers of skilled home health services. If this can be achieved, the home care caseloads of occupational therapists and therapy assistants are expected to increase by 37% (13).

PRACTICE ISSUES AND TRENDS

Need to Increase Referrals and Reimbursement

Kelly and Steinhauer have suggested some new approaches to generating referrals for occupational therapy home health services. They made home visits with the nurses of a home health agency and suggested adaptations to make clients more comfortable. After seeing what occupational therapists could contribute to client care, the nurses made more referrals for occupational therapy services and made them earlier in the treatment process. Therapists also provided inservice education to nursing staff and intake coordinators, outlining potential occupational therapy services. Publicizing occupational therapy to the whole agency staff also helped to make the services known and understood. Agency therapists networked with hospital-based therapists to familiarize one another with their programs and established good working relationships that led to improved continuity of care. As a result, referrals increased 3-fold, and there was better staff awareness of occupational therapy services (15).

OTRs and COTAs have had to learn to work within Medicare regulations to be reimbursed for their services. Client progress must be documented; when progress stops, reimbursement stops. Some practitioners worried that by allowing reimbursement regulations to determine treatment, therapists were neglecting the holistic aims of occupational therapy. Psychosocial skills, preventive services, and family support services were often not considered reimbursable by Medicare (16). Devereaux has suggested that new sources of reimbursement for community-based care may develop from non-health-related payers. Consumers may also become a more important reimbursement source (10).

New Client Groups

Levine and Gitlin have observed that medically stable, chronically disabled persons may be an underserved group in community health care. They propose that occupational therapists and therapy assistants could provide environmental adaptations for this group of consumers and have described a student training program that attempted to do so. Students were able to learn about client problems and home care while clients were able to benefit from student adaptations (17).

Persons with mental health problems are another client group that could be served by home health agencies. Hospital stays for episodes of acute mental illness are growing shorter, and home care may be a way to maintain the gains achieved during a hospitalization and prevent regression when the client returns home. A mental health team within a home health agency can see not only psychiatric cases but also clients who present behavioral problems that the regular home health team has trouble dealing with. Therapists can assist in the transition from hospital to home and can continue the work on functional goals. Home health care may be a new mode of service delivery for OTRs and COTAs who work in mental health (18).

The numbers of homeless people were increasing in the United States during the early 1990s as the economic slowdown continued. Local programs usually provided temporary shelter for the homeless, but a few programs provided much more. Batty described a program that included an OTR and a COTA on its staff who taught homeless persons practical skills that would help them gain employment and find new housing options. Therapists worked with clients on cleaning and sewing skills, assertive communication, rights and realities, leisure activities, and housing search skills. When appropriate housing was found, a client was followed through weekly visits and helped with locating a job and integrating back into the community. This program achieved a good success rate and provided a model for improving the lives of the homeless (19).

Disabled farmers are another group that could benefit from extended occupational therapy services. Since 1979 Purdue University has operated a program called "Breaking New Ground" that has applied rehabilitation technology to agricultural work sites. Later, Easter Seal Societies in midwestern states joined this effort and distributed information about adapting tools, equipment, machinery, and buildings for disabled farmers. Rural occupational therapy personnel could assist by customizing the adaptations and making follow-up visits to ensure that they worked. Medicare and Medicaid would not fund such services, but funding is available through vocational rehabilitation agencies and agricultural organizations (20).

The 1990 AOTA Member Data Survey showed no significant proportion of OTRs or COTAs working in hospice programs even though a 1989 survey had identified 150 therapists that were involved in hospice care nationally. This is rather surprising, as hospice programs are becoming more widespread as a needed service for terminally ill persons and their families. Hospice care is paid for by Medicare and by some private insurance policies. Care involves physical, emotional, psychosocial, and spiritual care. Relief from pain, communication of feelings, and achievement of personal and family goals are the focus of intervention. Enabling the client to live fully until he or she dies is a priority of hospice personnel. Occupational therapists could contribute much to these programs, and it is hoped that more OTRs and COTAs will participate in these much-needed programs (21).

New Roles and Opportunities

Stoffel and Gwin reviewed the occupational therapy home health care scene in 1989 and concluded that there were some unfilled needs that occupational therapy personnel could fill. Companies selling durable medical equipment could use OTRs or COTAs on their staffs to assess client equipment needs and to teach the use of equipment to clients. Pediatric home care was another area in need of development, and case management was a further role that OTRs and COTAs could fill. These authors proposed that the following actions would help to increase the number of OTRs and COTAs working in community-based care.

1. More educational experiences for students in home and community settings,
2. More efficacy studies showing the cost-effectiveness of community-based services,
3. More publications describing community programs and providing data on their use, and
4. More continuing education on community care for OTRs and COTAs (13).

SUMMARY

Community-based occupational therapy is a rapidly growing area of practice with many opportunities for both OTRs and COTAs. It is a particularly suitable location for occupational therapy services because of the profession's focus on functional performance and the practical skills of daily living. As health care costs have forced shorter stays in the high-tech hospital, more of the long-term health and restorative care services will be delivered in the community.

OTRs and COTAs can also contribute to the development of community services in their area. Service on community boards, governmental committees, and the boards of local service agencies is one way occupational therapists can extend their skills to benefit the community at large. The community-based therapist of the future will be an individual who is able to accept new responsibilities, work with minimal supervision, and creatively apply occupational therapy theory and principles to new client groups and in new practice sites (22). The community will be where the action is in the health care of the future.

Case Study: Venous Ulcers and Obesity

Mary is a 70-year-old woman who worked as a candy wrapper in a large candy company prior to her retirement. Mary had 2 years of high school education and came from a lower middle income family. She never married; however, Mary raised her sister's daughter when the sister died shortly after the child's birth. Mary has lived with her niece ever since a hospitalization in 1985, and the niece is now Mary's primary caretaker.

A nurse from a home health agency originally saw Mary, who had chronic venous ulcers on both legs and was extremely obese. Her obesity caused valve incompetency, and blood tended to pool in her legs, causing swelling and ulcerations. Mary was first referred for physical therapy treatment, but after a month of treatment little progress had been made. As a last resort, she was referred to occupational therapy for evaluation of her functional status and her ability to perform self-care tasks.

The OTR performed an initial assessment that showed that Mary was independent in grooming, some hygiene tasks, and in dressing her upper body. She had difficulty with bed mobility and with all transfers. Her standing tolerance was limited, and she did not ambulate. Mary ate all her meals from a bedside table and performed her limited self-care activities in bed. She required a bedpan. Rolling to the left or right in bed required the use of bed rails. She was able to get from a seated position to standing only by having her bed raised to its highest level and having her niece stabilize a walker while Mary held onto it and pulled up to stand. Her standing tolerance was only 1 minute and 45 seconds. Mary was afraid of falling and did not initially trust the COTA who was assigned to her case.

Mary was self-conscious about her weight. She was aware that her obesity contributed to the development of her leg ulcers but was not on a diet and did not perform any exercise. The nurse had been unable to weigh her, as the scales did not register high enough for Mary's weight. Mary viewed herself as an invalid and seemed content to watch TV or look out of her large picture window. Mary showed adequate strength and range of motion in both arms and had no deficits in fine-motor function. No sensory limitations were present and she was cognitively intact.

The OTR developed an intervention plan for Mary that concentrated on promoting her ability to dress the lower part of her body independently, to use proper body mechanics so that she could rise to a standing position, to improve her ability to transfer, to increase her standing tolerance, to train the niece to assist in her program, and possibly to develop some ability to ambulate. Visits by the COTA were scheduled weekly, with the OTR to be kept informed of any changes in Mary's status. The OTR was also in communication with Mary's home care nurse regarding her program. A commode was obtained for Mary's room. The COTA taught Mary correct body mechanics for rising from sitting to standing, and each week her bed was lowered by a half inch until it reached a height of 20 inches (the height of the commode). Work on ambulation with a walker was begun so that Mary could eventually walk to the commode and back to her bed. Her ability to rise to a standing position improved, but she continued to have trouble lowering herself down to a sitting position.

Eventually Mary could stand using the walker for up to 7 minutes at a time. She began to practice slight movement while standing, shifting her weight and stepping from side to side. Her niece helped her practice these skills and monitored her standing time. Mary had begun to show an interest in dressing and began to put on her shoes and a dress rather than spending the day in a hospital gown. She was now able to walk 4 feet to the sofa and back with assistance. Gradually she began to walk to the commode, which was 18 feet from her bed. She began to show increased socialization and started to take an interest in community events. The COTA now taught her to walk with a side step into the kitchen. Once there she was able to walk to the sink, operate the stove, remove items from the refrigerator, and make herself a cup of coffee. Her niece encouraged her by placing a sturdy bench near the kitchen door so that she could rest and by asking her to help with light chores. Occupational therapy services were terminated. Mary was now independent in getting to a standing position, could ambulate the length of her apartment with supervision, could use most kitchen appliances safely and independently, and could transfer onto the bed, the commode, and the kitchen bench without assistance. Her standing tolerance had reached 10 minutes. She was able to dress her lower body independently and no longer required her niece's help for most self-care tasks. Her mental attitude had improved, and she took a more active interest in neighborhood happenings. Mary's niece was grateful for her aunt's increased ability to care for her own needs and for her improved motivation to participate in daily homemaking activities.

Discussion Questions

1. What kinds of community services are available in your area for the home-

bound, the severely disabled, or the chronically ill? How are these services supported?
2. Invite an OTR or COTA who works in a community-based program to visit your class. What are some of their rewards or frustrations in this type of practice setting?
3. Interview an elderly or disabled person in your community and find out what support services he or she might find most useful.
4. Collect newspaper clippings that describe new community health programs. How could occupational therapists and therapy assistants contribute to these programs?
5. Are any occupational therapists in your area engaged in private practice? If so, how did they get started? What is the scope of their practice? Why do they prefer private practice over traditional employment?
6. A therapist working in the community needs to be tuned in to local politics and issues in order to be sensitive to community needs. How could a therapist become acquainted with the political issues of a community that is new to him or her?
7. When working in home care, it is often important to have the client practice skills between the therapist's visits. How can the OTR or COTA ensure that the client correctly carries out the therapy activities?

References

1. Ad Hoc Commission on Occupational Therapy Manpower: *Occupational Therapy Manpower; A Plan for Progress*, Rockville, MD, AOTA, 1985, pp. 55–59.
2. AOTA: 1990 Member Data Survey, Special Insert. *OT Week* 5(22):4–5, 1991.
3. AOTA: Home health, part I. *OT News* 39(10):7, 1985.
4. AOTA: *Draft Statement on the Role of Occupational Therapy in the Independent Living Movement*. Commission on Practice, Rockville, MD, AOTA, June 18, 1992.
5. Frazian B: Establishing and administrating a private practice in a hospital setting. In *Private Practice Information Packet*, Rockville, MD, AOTA, 1986, pp. 26–30.
6. Tulanian M, Hammond S, Tulanian S: *The Business Management of Private Practice: Occupational Therapy, Physical Therapy*. Middletown, CA, Applied Educational Systems, 1985, pp. 1–39.
7. Smith S: Private practices, home care, and consultation for the occupational therapist. In *Private Practice Information Packet*. Rockville, MD, AOTA, 1986, pp. 55–58.
8. AOTA: Home health, part II. *Occup Ther News* 39(11):7, 1985.
9. Rowles GD: Beyond performance: being in place as a component of occupational therapy. *AJOT* 45(3):265–271, 1991.
10. Devereaux EB: The issue is: community based practice. *AJOT* 45(10):944–946, 1991.
11. Jahnke PO: Developing a workable attitude in the home care setting. *Occup Ther Forum* V(29):7–8, 1990.
12. Hurff JM, Lowe HE, Ho BJ, Hoffman NM: Networking: a successful linkage for community occupational therapists. *AJOT* 44(5):424–430, 1990.
13. Stoffel SA, Gwin CH: Home health care revisited: challenges for the future. *AJOT* 43(8):499–502, 1989.
14. Staff: Provisions of Medicare amendment expand coverage for occupational therapy. *Occup Ther News* 40(12):4, 1986.
15. Kelly PA, Steinhauer MJ: Strategies for increasing referrals for occupational therapy in home health care. *AJOT* 45(7):656–658, 1991.
16. Kunstaetter D: Occupational therapy in home health care. *AJOT* 42(8):513–519, 1988.
17. Levine RE, Gitlin LN: Home adaptations for persons with chronic disabilities: an educational model. *AJOT* 44(10):923–929, 1990.
18. Javernick JA: Delivering psych services in the home: do OTs have a role? *OT Week* 6(35):14–17, 1992.
19. Batty J: Homeless offered a new beginning at transitional center. *OT Week* 2(30):16–17, 1988.
20. Nolinske T: Programs help disabled farmers reap benefits of new technology. *OT Week* 2(35):18–19, 35, 1988.
21. Brennan P: Hospice: a special way of caring. *OT Week* 3(36):20–21, 1989.
22. Taira E: After treatment what? New roles for occupational therapists in the community. In *The Roles of Occupational Therapists in Continuity of Care*. Binghamton, NY, Haworth Press, 1985, pp. 13–23.

Suggested Readings

Anderson H: *The Disabled Homemaker*. Springfield, IL, Charles C Thomas, 1981.

AOTA: *Draft Statement on the Role of Occupational Therapy in the Independent Living Movement*. Commission on Practice, Rockville, MD, June 18, 1992.

AOTA: Special issue on home health care. *AJOT* 38:11, 1984.

Crewe N, Zolak K: *Independent Living for Physically Disabled People*. San Francisco, Jossey-Bass,1983.

McClain L, McKinney J, Ralston J: Occupational therapists in private practice. *AJOT* 46(7):613–618, 1992.

Special on home health care. *Gerontology Special Interest Section Newsletter* 8:1–6, 1985.

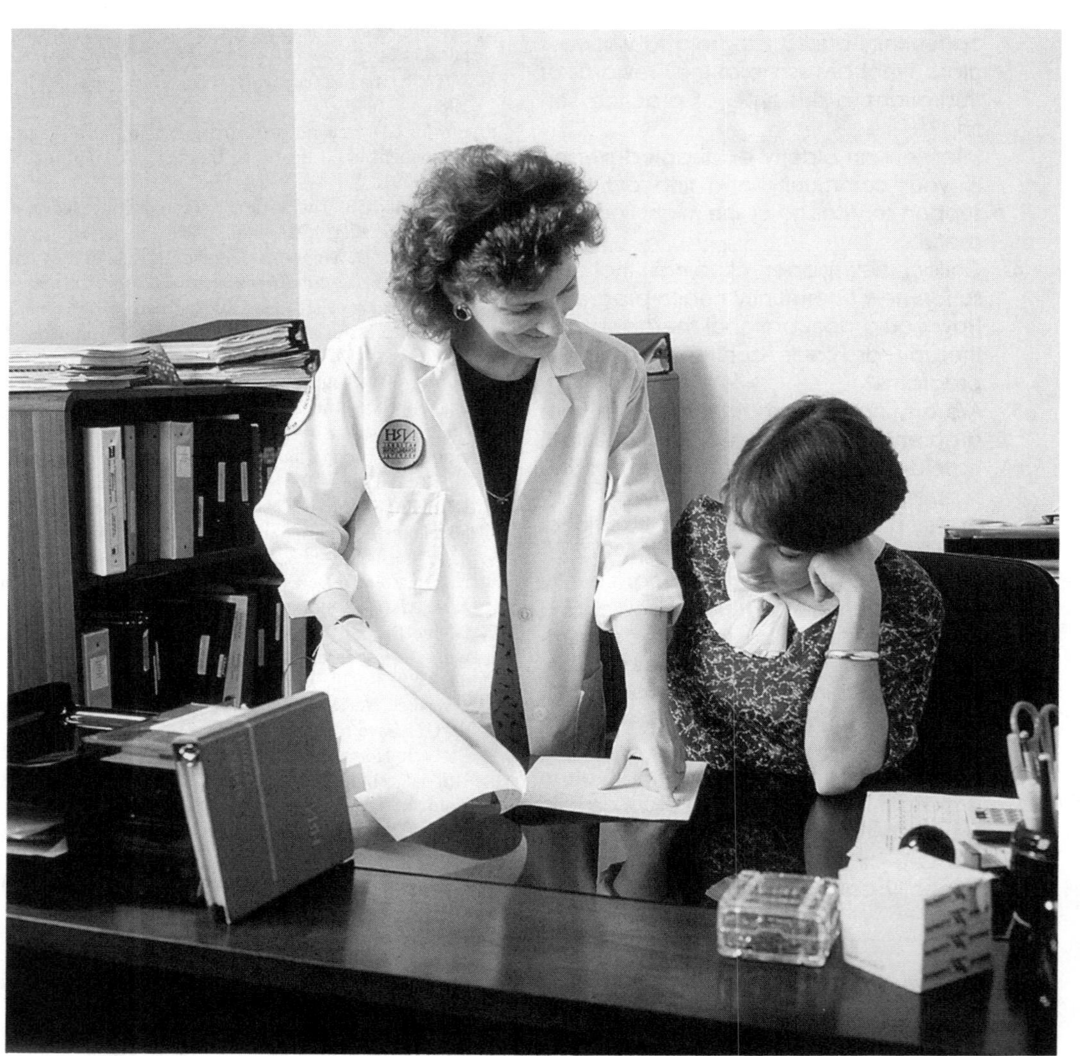

17 Indirect Service Careers in Occupational Therapy

The preceding chapters discuss careers in occupational therapy that involve providing direct service to clients. There are a number of occupational therapy careers, however, that do not involve direct client service. People in these careers provide supportive or supplementary services that meet a variety of professional or client-related needs. These careers can be grouped under the general heading of indirect service careers. The beginning student in occupational therapy should be aware of these additional career options, even though they demand either advanced clinical expertise, advanced levels of education, or both. In 1990, 27% of OTRs and 10.8% of COTAs reported that their primary job function was in indirect service (1).

Most OTRs and COTAs begin their careers as clinicians in a direct service role. As they gain experience and add to their knowledge and skills through continuing education programs or graduate study, they often move on to jobs that involve higher levels of responsibility. Figure 17.1 shows potential career paths for COTAs and Figure 17.2 shows career paths that are possible for OTRs. In this chapter we explore some of the career options in indirect service roles and discuss trends that are being seen in the 1990s.

MANAGEMENT

The occupational therapy manager directs the activities of an occupational therapy department or service program. As administrator of the program, the manager is responsible for mobilizing the human and material resources of the program in order to meet the goals of the organization in which it is housed. The manager has a variety of roles to fulfill. As chief liaison between the staff members and the administration of the organization, the manager interprets the organization's policies to the staff and implements the service program in accordance with those policies. The manager represents the needs of the program to the organization's administration. Good communication and interpersonal skills are essential tools for the program manager. Because the manager is accountable for the overall operation of the occupational therapy program, he or she must lead the staff in developing long-range plans and must think far ahead of present needs. Together the program manager and staff develop program goals and policies and procedures and establish standards of care. The manager is responsible for staffing the program, organizing the staffing patterns, and establishing lines of responsibility. The manager supervises the work of program staff and deals with any personnel problems that may arise. If the service program provides student education, the manager may also be responsible for developing and implementing a student program and supervising student performance. Supervision of related personnel (COTAs, aides, clerical staff, or volunteers) may also be part of the manager's responsibility.

Occupational therapy managers are accountable for the fiscal management of their programs and must provide the kind of documentation of service that is demanded by the administration for cost accounting and fiscal control. The manager participates in the development of the program budget and monitors expenditures. A knowledge of cost ac-

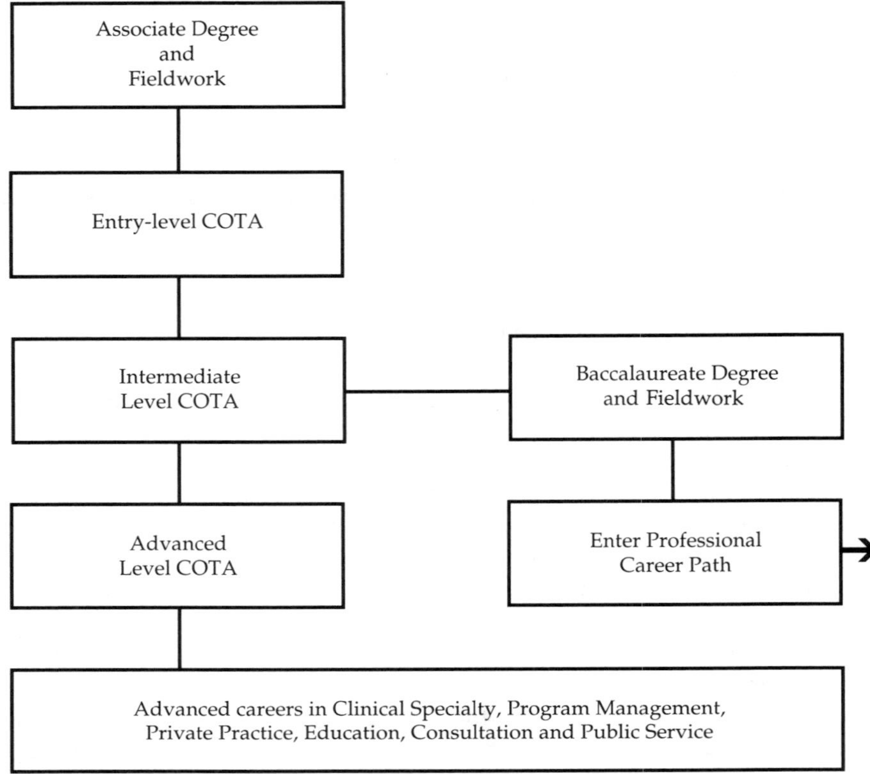

Figure 17.1. Career paths in technical occupational therapy.

counting and financial analysis is important for today's program managers (2). The manager also oversees the clinical service program and directs quality assurance studies to determine whether the service program is functioning effectively (3). The program manager may also serve a coordinating role, ensuring that the occupational therapy program does not duplicate services offered by other departments and works cooperatively with them.

Most occupational therapy managers rise to that position through years of experience working in their institution or organization. Beginning as staff therapists, they may later accept additional responsibilities as supervisors or take on limited administrative functions. As they gain experience in working within the organization, on-the-job training and continuing education may prepare them for higher level management responsibilities. Some managers seek additional education in health care management to do their jobs more effectively.

In 1991 AOTA's Special Interest Section in Administration had 3791 members. Some occupational therapy managers were beginning to assume the responsibility of managing multiple services (managing several related departments or coordinating interdisciplinary services). The chronic shortage of personnel was a major concern of occupational therapy managers as they tried to recruit personnel to fill vacant or new positions. Some managers were providing consultation to hospital and community agencies that were establishing new service programs, and others were providing consultation to insurance companies to review therapy services. Managers were increasingly collaborating with researchers to investigate the efficacy of occupational therapy

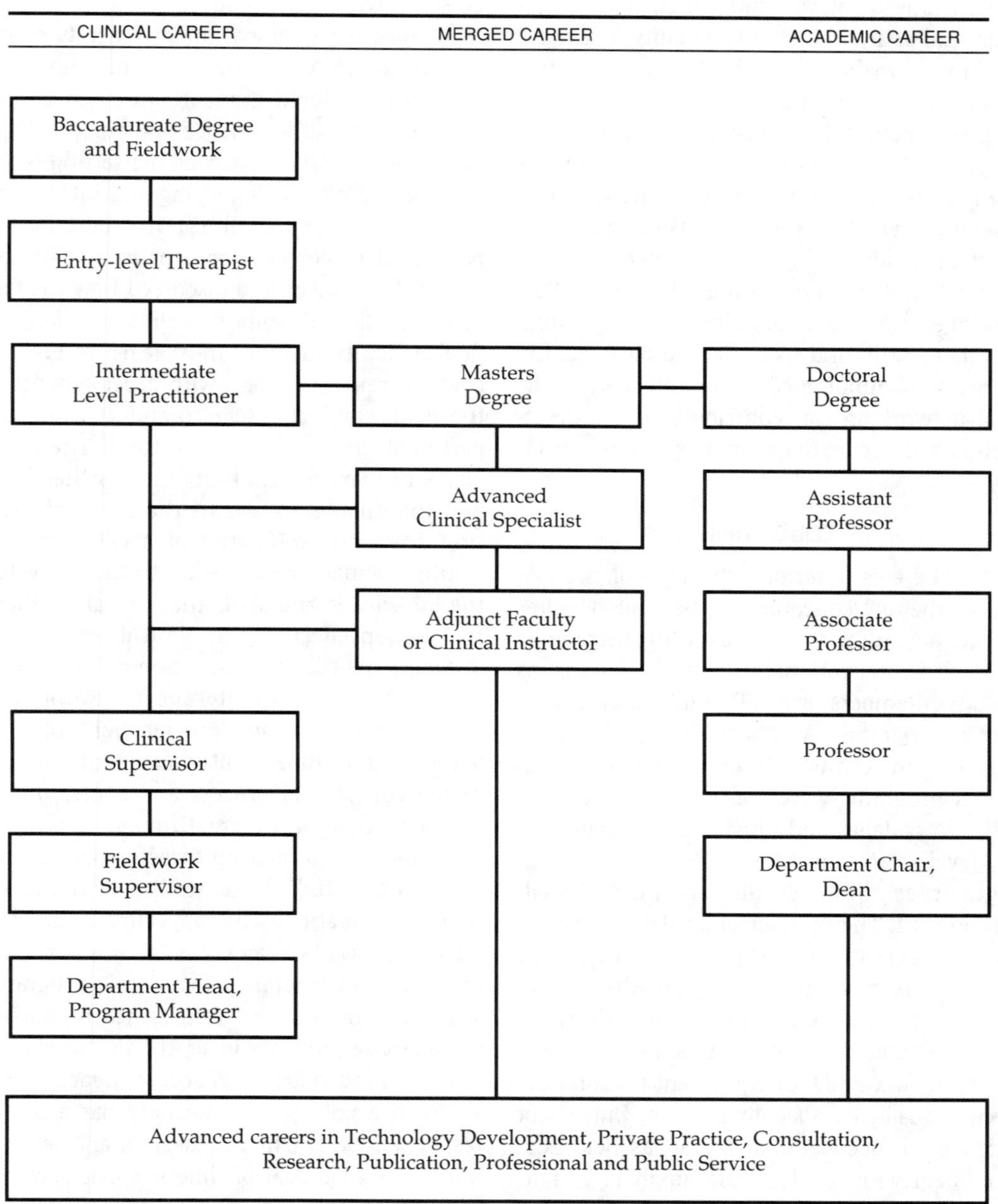

Figure 17.2. Career paths in professional occupational therapy.

methods. New technologies were being explored as occupational therapy managers sought ways of streamlining their data collection and analysis methods. Quality assurance continued to be emphasized in clinical programs, and the Deming method, developed to improve the quality of business operations, was being applied to health care management as well. Schell has suggested that occupational therapy managers should consider pursuing doctoral studies in order to sharpen their analytical and research skills. In the 1990s, management was a complex job, demanding advanced skills and specialized knowledge. Experience, continuing education, graduate study, and networking can contribute to the development of occupational therapy managers (4, 5).

EDUCATION

There is a serious shortage of occupational therapy educators in the United States today. According to 1991 data (6), there were only 864 occupational therapists serving as faculty members in OTR entry-level educational programs. Another 279 persons were teaching in technical level programs. Educational programs were continuing to develop, with 74 colleges and universities offering entry-level OTR education in 1991, and 72 colleges or technical institutes offering COTA education (6). The number of available full-time faculty has not increased proportionately. Part of the reason for this discrepancy is that in the 1980s many colleges and universities began to expect that potential faculty members would hold a Ph.D. or equivalent doctoral degree to qualify for a faculty position. Only about 0.8% of all occupational therapists held doctoral degrees in 1991, so the supply lagged far behind the demand. In COTA education the master's degree was considered the major qualification for faculty, and about 17% of OTRs and 0.7% of all COTAs held master's degrees in 1991, making a larger pool of prospective faculty available for COTA programs. The AOTA has actively encouraged graduate study for OTRs by offering graduate fellowships, but the pool of doctoral degree holders continues to be small within the field.

Most occupational therapy faculty members come from the ranks of clinicians. They have often entered graduate study to add to their professional knowledge and clinical skills, but some find that the academic setting is appealing and offers a satisfying and interesting career option. Mitchell (7) has described a pattern of career development from clinician to faculty member and discussed how the faculty role differs from the clinical role. The novice faculty member must learn to prepare courses, remain current with developments in the field, conduct research, and serve on department and college committees. The clinician's primary focus of attention is the client and the client's needs. In the academic setting, the focus is on student needs. The new faculty member must help students develop the knowledge and skills that will allow them to function effectively in clinical settings. In occupational therapy, education is a joint venture by academic faculty and fieldwork educators. Clinicians who provide fieldwork experiences for students play an important role in the educational process and contribute to the educational program through serving as role models and offering direct experience in subjects the student has studied in the classroom. Occupational therapy clinicians, both OTRs and COTAs, may serve as adjunct faculty or clinical instructors in academic programs and may provide guest lectures, teach courses, or supervise students in level I fieldwork.

The individual who accepts a faculty position in a college or university has a 3-fold responsibility: teaching, research, and service. Initially a good deal of time is spent developing courses, designing appropriate learning experiences for students, and assessing student progress. The faculty member must establish a research program and is expected to publish results that will add to the knowledge base of the field. Service on college and university committees, as well as professional and public service, is expected. The new faculty member must learn these new roles and master the art of teaching.

Career advancement takes place through promotion from assistant to associate professor, the rank at which tenure is awarded at most colleges and universities. Attainment of tenure depends on how well the faculty member fulfills his or her 3-fold responsibilities. Occupational therapy faculty have often found achieving tenured rank difficult for many reasons. As a service field, occupational therapy tends to encourage the development of clinical skills rather than research skills. The profession has not always valued research and scholarship as highly as have the more traditional academic disciplines. Only recently have occupational therapists in larger numbers begun to earn doctoral degrees. In 1991 it was estimated that 35.5% of faculty members teaching in professional educational programs were tenured at their institutions. There is also a fairly high turnover of faculty each year as faculty members change jobs or return to clinical practice. It will be critical to occupational therapy education for educators to earn tenure in greater numbers. Masagatani and Grant (8) have offered some helpful suggestions for faculty members to develop the necessary skills and accomplishments to qualify for tenured rank.

Once tenure is achieved, the occupational therapy faculty member may eventually be promoted to the rank of full professor. This is the highest academic rank and usually reflects national and international recognition in the field. Full professors are regarded as authorities in their discipline and are the senior members of an educational program's faculty. The tenured faculty member may fulfill the additional position of department chair or dean. The role of a chair of an academic department is comparable with that of a service program manager, but the goals and priorities of clinical and academic organizations are quite different. Colleges and universities are communities of scholars whose primary mission is the development and dissemination of knowledge. The department chair must recruit and hire new faculty members, develop and maintain a curriculum that is current with developments in the field, promote faculty research and engage in research activities, manage the finances and resources of the academic program, and participate in college and university committees. If the shortage of occupational therapy faculty members is serious, the shortage of chairs of academic departments is even more severe (9).

In 1991 the faculty of professional level programs had increased by only 9.6%, and at technical level programs, by 13%. Seven COTAs were teaching in professional education programs and 62 in technical education programs. A total of 946 persons belonged to AOTA's Education Special Interest Section in 1991 (6).

The educator shortage was continuing in the 1990s and was most critical at the professional education level. Clinicians were being urged to consider an academic career, but new funding sources needed to be developed to support graduate students. Better integration of the academic and clinical worlds would help to facilitate the transition of clinical therapists into faculty members. In the stagnant economy of the early 1990s, many colleges and universities were "downsizing" their staffs, and in some cases this meant cuts in faculty positions. Noncompetitive academic salaries were another problem, as they often lagged behind the salaries of clinicians (10, 11).

Approximately 10% of the OTRs and 20% of the COTAs were pursuing degrees beyond their entry level degree in 1990. AOTA was continuing to encourage the expansion of educational programs in those parts of the country that lacked occupational therapy personnel. Five new professional level programs opened in 1991 as well as four new technical level programs. Mitcham and Trickey have pointed out that, without adequate numbers of qualified faculty, educational programs cannot hope to meet the existing staff needs of the next decade. It may be that the financial stresses colleges and universities are facing are only temporary. If not, occupational therapy educational programs face a difficult future trying to produce enough graduates to fill available occupational therapy positions (6, 10, 11).

RESEARCH

Research has been a high priority in occupational therapy for the past three decades. The need to relate practice to theory and to show scientific evidence of the effectiveness of occupational therapy services has given rise to an increased demand for occupational therapy research. The problem again has been one of staffing. Researchers are highly educated individuals who have mastered the tools of scholarly inquiry. They are skilled in identifying researchable questions of significance to their field and in developing methods for studying these questions. This specialized skill can be gained only through a research-oriented doctoral degree program—but a very small number of occupational therapists have completed this level of education. There is a large gap between the number of researchers needed in occupational therapy and the number presently available. Students who have an interest in the scientific study of occupational therapy problems are strongly encouraged to continue their education to the doctoral level.

Although much of the research published in occupational therapy (and in other fields) is the product of university faculty members, there is a strong need for clinicians to take part in research activities as well. The OTRs and COTAs practicing in clinical settings can contribute to research efforts by participating in collaborative studies with faculty members, by collecting data on specific types of client problems and occupational therapy interventions, and by utilizing information gained from research reports in professional journals. Dunn (12) has emphasized the fact that clinicians can and do develop into researchers. They often face constraints from their administration, however, over the time spent in research activity that the administrator may feel should more properly be devoted to client service. Establishing a partnership between clinicians and faculty researchers may be the best solution to this dilemma. Dunn further suggests that clinicians can contribute to research by contributing money to research foundations, responding to research surveys, and supporting the efforts of their professional organizations to provide funding and resources for research in occupational therapy.

According to AOTA's 1990 Member Data Survey, 16.6% of the OTRs who were enrolled in an educational program in that year were pursuing doctoral degrees. Three universities currently offer doctoral degrees in occupational therapy: New York University, Boston University, and the University of Southern California (1, 6).

To be successful in a research career, an individual needs to have an inquiring mind and be able to look at problems critically and objectively. A good statistical background is necessary to analyze research data effectively, and computer skills are useful. Most importantly, the occupational therapy researcher must be familiar with the theories and basic principles of the field and able to identify research problems that will add to the knowledge of occupational therapy theory and practice. A career in research will bring professional recognition as well as personal satisfaction to the individual who is interested in solving problems that until now have remained unsolved.

CONSULTATION

Experienced occupational therapists who come from either a clinical or an academic background may be self-employed as consultants to organizations that request their services. An AOTA publication on private practice and consultation (13) defines consultation as giving advice, assistance, or an opinion based on professional knowledge, skill, or judgment. Consultation usually pertains to the application of occupational therapy treatment or to collaborative health programming. Thornton (14) emphasizes that consultants come from outside of organizations and that their purpose is to help the people within achieve the organizations' goals and purposes. The advice offered by consultants may be accepted or rejected by organizations. Consultants work, often on a contract basis, for the owners of organizations who hire them and share their expertise with the members of the organizations. The consultant's job is to listen and observe, identify the problems, and help the members of the organizations find ways to solve those problems. Consultants perform their role by working through other people. They consult about their discipline or area of expertise. Consultants are troubleshooters whose services may be sought for help with establishing, implementing, or evaluating occupational therapy services.

Occupational therapy consultants have pioneered in the development of new practice specialties in the field and have created jobs that were later filled by OTRs and COTAs. In some states consultants were used by school districts to help set up occupational therapy programs in public schools. Later these programs were operated by occupational therapy personnel employed by the school system. Some types of occupational therapy home health services were initiated in the same way. Occupational therapy consultants are often able to break new ground and develop new areas of practice (15). Consultants are agents of planned change and frequently function as educators or facilitators in order to make things happen. Consultants can only recommend change, however. It is up to the organization to decide whether to follow through on the suggestions.

Because of the varied environments in which consultation takes place, consultants must be creative and flexible. They must have broad clinical experience and a good knowledge of current trends and issues in health care. Maturity, a sense of humor, and good timing are also important characteristics for anyone who is considering a career as a consultant. Smith (16) has discussed some of the things to consider before becoming a consultant. She suggests that one should assess the depth of one's professional expertise, consider the ethical issues involved in consultation, and look for the reasons that underlie an organization's request for consultative services.

Consultation is considered an advanced career option in occupational therapy because of the broad range of experience and depth of knowledge that it requires. For the experienced occupational therapy clinician or faculty member, consultation offers opportunities to develop and implement innovative programming ideas.

During the early 1990s occupational therapists were consulting to schools that needed to serve larger numbers of disabled students, to long-term care facilities that wanted to maximize the independent functioning of their residents, and to businesses and industries that needed to comply with the Americans with Disabilities Act (ADA) regulations for accessibility and accommodations for disabled workers. Other therapists consulted to long-term care facilities about adaptive seating systems for residents, to an appliance manufacturer that wanted to design products that could be easily operated by elderly and disabled customers, and to architects who were designing barrier-free living environments. Consultation was increasingly being seen as a viable method of indirect service delivery, and occupational therapy personnel with specific areas of expertise were in demand for consultative services.

TECHNOLOGY DEVELOPMENT AND APPLICATION

The rapid development and proliferation of technology may revolutionize occupational therapy practice, just as it has already changed many other fields. Already technological advances are being put to work in occupational therapy clinics. Technology development differs from technology application in that it involves creating, testing, and modifying new pieces of equipment that will enable disabled persons to live and work with greater independence and personal control. Applying technology is the clinician's job, but creating new technology demands "what if" thinking. "What if there were a device that could make a paralyzed person walk again?" "What if an electrical mechanism could improve a person's coordination?" "What if . . .?"

Among the technologies already available is a robotic arm programmed by computer software to help people with high levels of quadriplegia feed themselves, use a telephone, and operate a computer (17). A new method based on functional electrical stimulation (FES) allows paralyzed persons to exercise their muscles, and a stored energy orthosis enables them to walk (18). A tongue-touch keypad that fits within the mouth enables quadriplegics to type, operate environmental controls, and maneuver their wheelchairs (19). Voice-activated workstations enable severely disabled persons to perform ordinary office operations independently (20).

Occupational therapy personnel who have advanced knowledge of computer and electronic technology could be in the forefront of this revolution. Because occupational therapists are skilled in activity analysis and adaptation, they are in a good position to work with technical specialists to develop new technological aids that can minimize many of the functional limitations imposed by handicapping conditions. Thus far, technology development has been a collaborative effort with ideas and know-how coming from occupational therapists, rehabilitation technologists, and biomedical engineers.

There are relatively few occupational therapists involved in technology development but more are involved in the testing and application of assistive technologies. An AOTA Special Interest Group on Technology was formed in 1991 with 886 members. This group hoped to address the growing development and use of assistive technology in occupational therapy practice. It planned to pay special attention to policy and legislative, theoretical, and clinical issues and to serve as an information disseminator about the new technologies.

In 1991 the AOTA's Representative Assembly approved a position paper on occupational therapy and assistive technology. The paper recognized occupational therapists' longstanding interest in technical aids and outlined some of the occupational therapy roles in the application of assistive technology (21). As an advanced career for occupational therapists, technology development and application will demand advanced education and technical skills. For those who wish to combine a desire to assist the disabled with a talent for invention and innovative thinking, technology development may be an ideal career.

OTHER INDIRECT SERVICE CAREERS

Some OTRs and COTAs have created their own indirect service careers by seeing an unmet need and setting out to fulfill it. One enterprising COTA became a travel consultant specializing in arranging tours for groups of disabled people (22). A group of OTRs surveyed handicapped, nonhandicapped, and elderly adults to determine their ability to open and use products that came in a variety of packaging modes. They found that the elderly especially had problems with certain types of packaging and notified the manufacturers of poorly designed packaging that made it hard for some consumers to use their products (23). An OTR who was a member of her hospital's safety committee developed and ran an injury prevention program for hospital personnel (24). Staff members of an adult day center developed a training program for the local police force, teaching them to recognize and appropriately deal with wandering Alzheimer's patients (25).

Therapists skilled in ergonomics were designing workstations in offices and industries that would prevent workplace injuries and increase worker productivity (26). Royeen has reminded OTRs and COTAs that they have many skills that can be applied in nontraditional settings (27). She encourages occupational therapy personnel not to be afraid of putting their knowledge to work in new ways. For many, indirect service careers provide interesting new challenges at the midpoint of their careers. Students should be aware of a variety of career options as they consider their own career path in occupational therapy.

SUMMARY

In all of the indirect service careers discussed in this chapter, additional education or experience beyond the entry level is needed. Occupational therapy personnel move through various stages in the course of their careers. Although all begin as practitioners, many move on fairly quickly to positions that require higher levels of skill and greater responsibility. Some individuals may prefer to remain in clinical practice, while others may move on to another type of occupational therapy career. Clinicians may enter a graduate program to gain more expertise in a specialized area of practice or to prepare themselves for a career in management, consultation, technology development, or research. Although it is often recommended that graduates of entry-level educational programs acquire some clinical experience before entering graduate study, it is also acceptable to enter a graduate program immediately after completing entry-level education. This choice must be made based on the individual's career goals and expectations. As knowledge and skills increase, the indirect service careers in occupational therapy open up new horizons to the practitioner. Students are advised to consider their long-range career goals even while they are enrolled in entry-level education and plan their career path in accordance with their personal interests and abilities.

Discussion Questions

1. Invite one or more OTRs who are employed in indirect service careers to your class. Ask them to share their experiences with you. How did they enter their advanced occupational therapy careers? What sort of rewards or satisfactions has it brought them?
2. Do any of the indirect service careers interest you? If so, how could you prepare yourself for this career?
3. Many COTAs and OTRs are reluctant to give up their clinical role in favor of an indirect service career. Would it be possible to combine a direct service role with an indirect service career? Suggest some ways of doing this.
4. Can you think of other indirect service careers that exist now or may develop in occupational therapy? Give some examples.
5. Why are indirect service careers usually an advanced career option?

References

1. AOTA: 1990 Member Data Survey, Special Insert. *OT Week* 5(22):1–8, 1991.
2. Laase S: Financial management. In Bair J, Gray M, eds. *The Occupational Therapy Manager*. Rockville, MD, AOTA, 1985, pp. 83–122.
3. Joe B: Quality assurance. In Bair J, Gray M, eds. *The Occupational Therapy Manager*. Rockville, MD, AOTA, 1985, pp. 251–265.
4. Schell BAB: Occupational therapy management: accepting the challenge. *AJOT* 43(4):215–217, 1989.
5. Lain DC: Deming method improves health care. *Adv Occup Ther* 8(15):18, 1992.
6. AOTA, Research Information and Evaluation Division: *1992 Education Data Survey, Final Report*, Rockville, MD, AOTA, 1992.
7. Mitchell M: Professional development: clinician to academician. *AJOT* 39:368–373, 1985.
8. Masagatani G, Grant H: Managing an academic career. *AJOT* 40:83–88, 1986.
9. Sieg K: Chairing the academic occupational therapy department: a job analysis. *AJOT* 40:89–95, 1986.
10. Mitcham MD, Trickey B: Faculty recruitment: addressing the needs today. *OT Week* 5(5):8–9, 1991.
11. Mastrangelo R: Budget ax threatening OT programs. *Adv Occup Ther* 8(34):9, 1992.
12. Dunn W: Occupational therapy's challenge: caregiving and research. *AJOT* 39:259–264, 1985.

13. The occupational therapist as a consultant. *Private Practice Information Packet*. Rockville, MD, AOTA, 1986, p. 37.
14. Thornton P: An approach to consultation. *Private Practice Information Packet*. Rockville, MD, AOTA, 1986, pp. 40–49.
15. Epstein C: Consultation: Communicating and facilitating. In Bair J, Gray M, eds. *The Occupational Therapy Manager*. Rockville, MD, AOTA, 1985, pp. 299–321.
16. Smith S: Private practice—home care—consultation for the occupational therapist. *Private Practice Information Packet*. Rockville, MD, AOTA, 1986, pp. 55–58.
17. Taylor B: Robotic arm helps individuals with mobility impairment to put their talent to work. *OT Week* 2(5):12–13, 1988.
18. Colan B: FES Pioneers plan to get people back to life. *Adv Occup Ther* 6(13):9, 1990.
19. Egan M: Technology on the tip of the tongue. *OT Week* 6(13):18, 1992.
20. Van Bronkhorst E: OTs help develop workstation. *OT Week* 3(31):4–5, 1989.
21. AOTA: Position Paper: Occupational Therapy and Assistive Technology. *AJOT* 45(12):1076, 1991.
22. Collobert B: Occupational therapy—helping the handicapped traveler. *Occup Ther Forum* IV(19):1–3, 1989.
23. Rider B, Akers B, Brashear R, Blasch D: Product packaging causes problems for the elderly. *Occup Ther News* 41(5):18, 1987.
24. Fox S: LaCrosse Lutheran OTs finding more work than they bargained for. *Adv Occup Ther* 6(41):18, 1990.
25. Marmer LA: Training police to help Alzheimer's patients. *Adv Occup Ther* 6(39):13, 1990.
26. Fox S: Ergonomics: designing jobs to fit the worker. *Adv Occup Ther* 6(31):1–2,1990.
27. Royeen CB: Employment of occupational therapists in non-traditional settings. *AJOT* 44(2):172–173,1990.

SUGGESTED READINGS

American Occupational Therapy Foundation: *Readings in Occupational Therapy Research*. Rockville, MD, AOTF, 1990.

Bair J, Gray M (eds): *The Occupational Therapy Manager*. Rockville, MD, AOTA, 1990.

Clark D (ed): *Technology Review '90: Perspectives on Occupational Therapy Practice*. Rockville, MD, AOTA, 1990.

SECTION III

CURRENT TRENDS AND FUTURE OUTLOOK

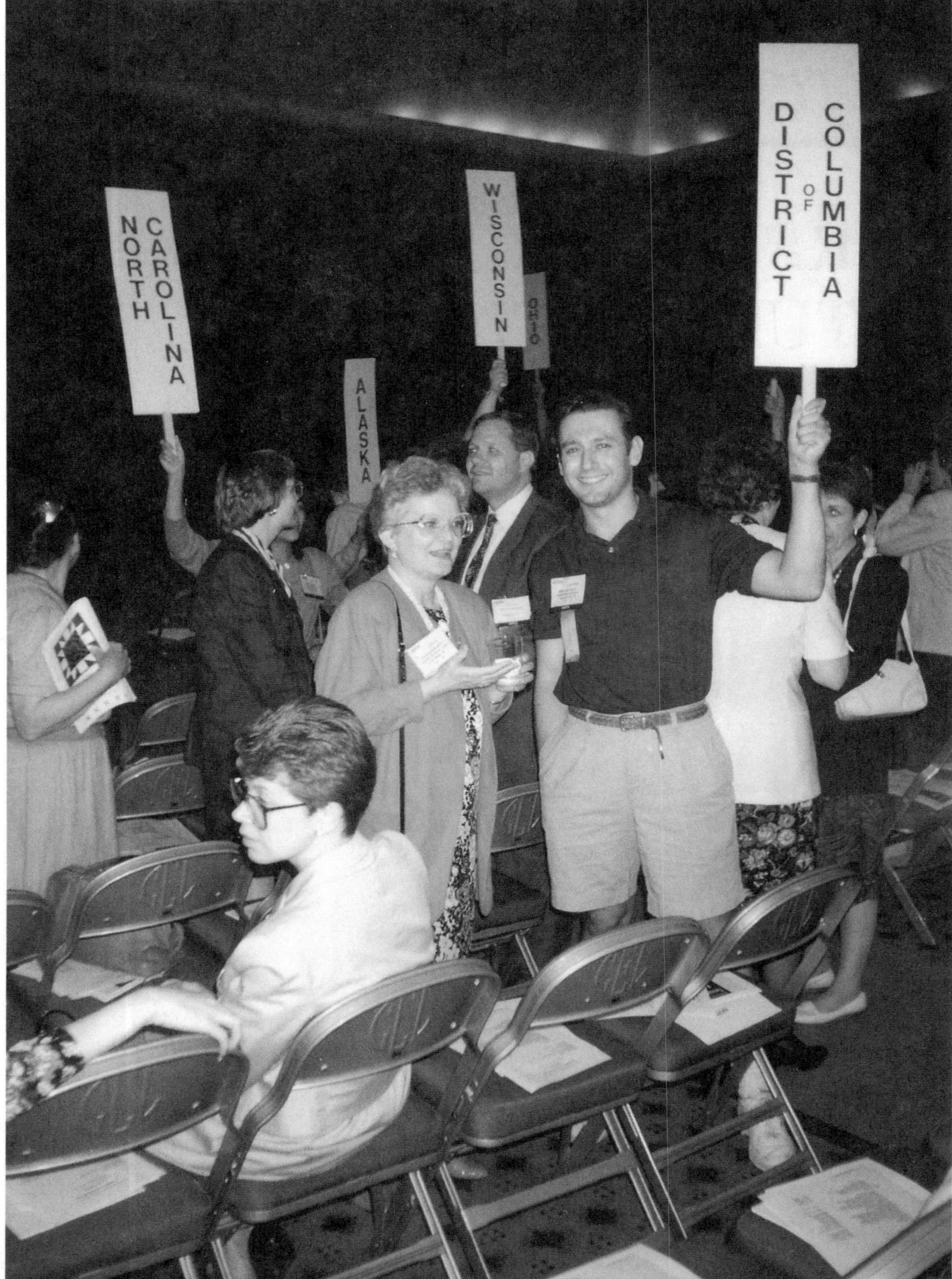
NORTH CAROLINA
WISCONSIN
OHIO
ALASKA
DISTRICT OF COLUMBIA

18 Professional Organizations

In any profession, practitioners inevitably feel the need to join forces with their colleagues in order to educate the public about the field, to achieve acceptance and recognition by outside groups, and to promote the advancement of the profession. Professional organizations help to achieve these goals and provide a variety of services that are helpful to their members. In occupational therapy, professional organizations have developed at the state, national, and international level. In this chapter we look at the professional organizations at each level to see what they contribute to the field and how they support the activities of their members.

AMERICAN OCCUPATIONAL THERAPY ASSOCIATION

In 1917 a small group of early pioneers in occupational therapy met to discuss forming a national organization that could unify the isolated occupational therapists then practicing and encourage the planned development of the new field. The founding members included George Barton, an architect who had suffered from tuberculosis and other health problems and who became convinced from personal experience that therapeutic activity could aid in recovery from physical and mental disorders. His secretary, Isabel Newton, also attended the planning meeting. Other founding members were: Susan Johnson, a craftsperson and early occupational therapy educator; Eleanor Clarke Slagle, an early student of curative occupations who later developed occupational therapy programs in Maryland and Illinois; Susan Tracy, a nurse who recognized the value of occupation for hospitalized patients and who taught an early course on that topic; Thomas Kidner, a British architect who developed a system of vocational rehabilitation for disabled Canadian veterans of World War I; and Dr. William Rush Dunton, Jr., a psychiatrist who promoted the use of occupation as part of the treatment program for the mentally ill. This diverse group of people shared a common interest in the use of occupation as a therapeutic tool, and they agreed to establish the National Society for the Promotion of Occupational Therapy on March 15, 1917. Barton was elected the first president of the society, with Slagle serving as vice president. The new organization took on the tasks of defining the field, expanding the practice of occupational therapy from the mental hospitals where it had originated into other areas of rehabilitation, and promoting the use of occupation as therapy.

In 1921 the name of the society was changed to the American Occupational Therapy Association (AOTA), and that name has endured to the present time. In the early 1920s, physicians and hospital administrators were beginning to seek occupational therapists to work in hospitals and urged the association to maintain a registry of qualified practitioners. Before doing so, however, the association undertook to establish minimum educational standards for occupational therapists. This was achieved in 1923, with a required minimum of 12 months of training, including 3 months of required hospital practice. The young association had also begun to publish a journal. The *Archives of Occupational Therapy*, first published in 1922, was owned and edited by Dr. Dunton. In 1925 its title was changed to *Occupational Therapy and Rehabilitation*, and subscription to the journal became a member benefit of the organization. In 1926 the organization's House of Delegates voted to establish a registry of qualified occupational therapists, and in 1932 the first registry was published with 318 names listed. In the same year the association moved from temporary quarters to rented office space in New York City and employed a secretary to help manage its affairs (1).

In 1931 the AOTA assumed another responsibility: accrediting occupational therapy educational programs. This function was shared with the American Medical Association. As a result of the initial visits to schools, new educational standards were developed that were adopted in 1935. In 1945 the association reconsidered the question of professional qualifications and undertook the development of a written essay examination that all potential occupational therapists were required to take and pass in order to qualify. The examination was revised in 1947 and was changed to a multiple-choice format. In the same year the association began to publish a new professional journal, the *American Journal of Occupational Therapy*, which eventually replaced *Occupational Therapy and Rehabilitation* as the official publication of the association.

By 1950 the association had begun to award honors and recognitions to those members who had made significant contributions to the field. In 1955 the association outgrew its office space and moved to a new location in New York City. During this period there was an increasing demand for occupational therapy personnel, and in an effort to meet this demand the AOTA developed educational standards for programs preparing occupational therapy assistants. In 1958 the association took on the additional function of reviewing and approving COTA educational programs. During the early 1960s the organization was restructured to improve its efficiency and ability to respond to member concerns. A major focus of the 1970s was the encouragement of state licensure for OTRs and COTAs. The association aided state organizations in writing licensure acts and provided consultation as state groups moved their practice acts through the legislative process. The AOTA was also becoming more active in legislative matters on the federal level and represented the interests of occupational therapists when bills concerning health care funding and programming were being considered by Congress. In 1972 the national office of the association was moved to the Washington, D.C. area, to facilitate participation in legislative matters. AOTA later purchased its own building for use as organizational headquarters (1).

GOALS AND FUNCTIONS OF AOTA

According to its current bylaws, the purpose of the AOTA is "to further the purposes set forth in the Articles of Incorporation through the enhancement of occupational therapy in order to enhance the health of the public in its medical, community, and educational environments through research, education, action, service, and the establishment and enforcement of standards" (2). In 1975 the organization's Delegate Assembly adopted a long range plan that was intended to guide the activities of the association in the years to come. The following are some of the goals identified in that document:

1. To provide opportunities for the expression of member concerns, to anticipate emerging issues, to facilitate decision making, and to expedite the translation of those decisions into action;
2. To support the development of research and knowledge bases for the practice of occupational therapy, and to promote the dissemination and sharing of such information;
3. To facilitate and support an educational system for occupational therapy that responds to current needs and anticipates, plans for, and accommodates to change;
4. To promote occupational therapy as a viable health profession;
5. To promote an understanding of occupational therapy that will have a strong

and significant impact on health policy and health care; and

6. To facilitate the formation of partnerships with consumers to promote optimal health conditions for the public (3).

STRUCTURE AND MEMBERSHIP

From an initial membership of 40 persons in 1917, the AOTA had grown to a membership of 43,911 in 1991 (4). Membership in AOTA is open to individuals (OTRs, COTAs, students) as voting members and to interested organizations and nonoccupational therapy personnel as nonvoting members. It should be noted that membership in AOTA is voluntary and is entirely separate from certification.

AOTA's current activities are the result of a partnership between a paid national office staff and occupational therapy personnel who volunteer to serve on committees and commissions or who hold elected office within the organization. Figure 18.1 shows the organization of the AOTA national office.

In 1992, 136 staff members were employed in the various divisions of the organization to carry out its day-to-day activities. An Executive Board is responsible for supervising the operations of the national office and for managing the affairs of the association. The elected president of AOTA and the executive director of the association office represent the association at the national level and serve as advocates for the organization to outside groups.

The voluntary sector of the organization consists of the individual members (OTRs, COTAs, and students) of the association. Elected officers guide the association's activities, with the president, vice president, secretary, and treasurer each serving for a 3-year term. Members are represented on the two major action bodies of the organization, the Representative Assembly and the Executive Board. Figure 18.2 shows the structure of the voluntary sector of AOTA.

The Representative Assembly is the legislative and policy-making body of the association and is composed of representatives and alternates who are elected from state organizations or election areas through a system of proportional representation. Those states with less than 5% of the association's total voting membership are entitled to one elected representative and one alternate. States that have

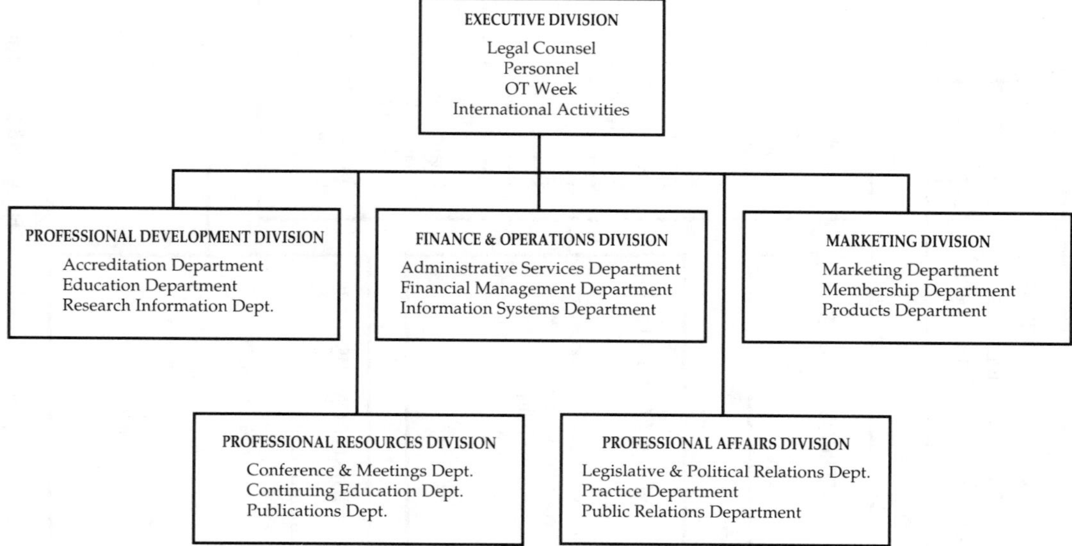

Figure 18.1. AOTA national office organization.

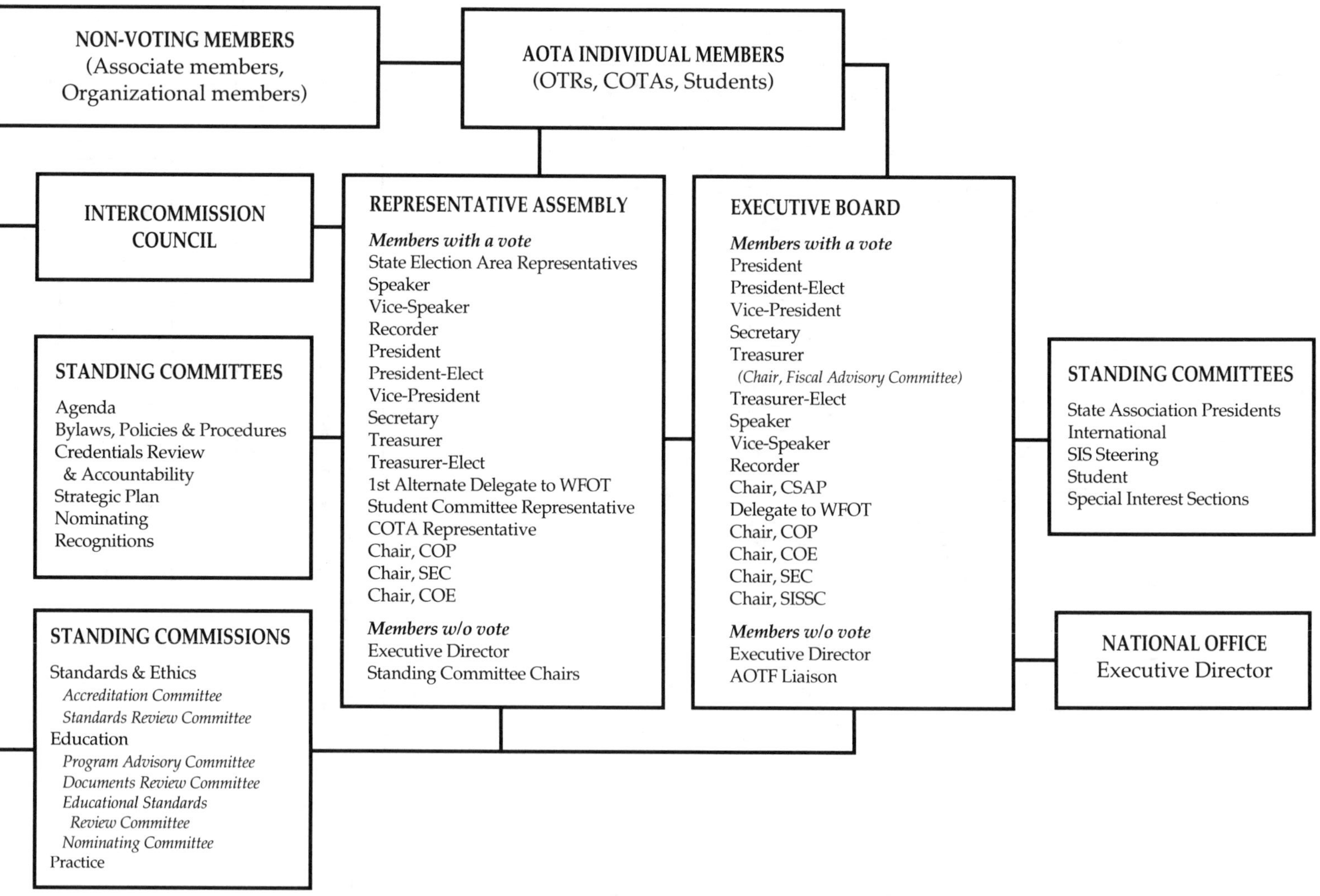

Figure 18.2. Organizational chart of the voluntary sector of the AOTA.

between 5 and 10% of the association's total membership may have two representatives and two alternates, and states with more than 10% may have three representatives and three alternates. Representatives and alternates each serve for a 3-year term or until successors have been elected. The Representative Assembly elects its own officers of speaker, vice speaker, and recorder. This body meets annually and formulates and approves policies for the association, approves its budget, fixes membership fees, and approves position statements on behalf of the association (2).

The Representative Assembly maintains three standing commissions and an intercommission council that promotes communication and interaction between the commissions. The three commissions have specific areas of function. The Commission on Standards and Ethics recommends the approval of necessary standards and ethics documents to the Representative Assembly. It reviews all standards and position papers for the association and enforces the standards and ethics of the organization. The Commission on Education promotes quality education and sets educational standards for programs preparing OTRs and COTAs relative to educator, student, and consumer needs. The Commission on Practice promotes quality occupational therapy practice and develops practice standards for OTRs and COTAs relative to practitioner and consumer needs. These commissions meet at least once a year to conduct their business and report back to the Representative Assembly. In addition to these bodies, the Representative Assembly maintains a group of standing committees that are charged with specific tasks related to the affairs of the association. In 1986, certification of qualified OTRs and COTAs was removed from the functions of AOTA and was placed under the jurisdiction of the American Occupational Therapy Certification Board (AOTCB). This group is separate from AOTA and monitors and controls the certification process.

The second action body of the organization is the Executive Board. This group is charged with managing the affairs of the association and consists of its elected officers, the officers of the Representative Assembly, the chair of the Committee of State Association Presidents, the association's delegate to the World Federation of Occupational Therapists, the chairs of the Representative Assembly's four commissions, and the chair of the Special Interest Section Steering Committee. The national office Executive Director and a liaison person from the American Occupational Therapy Foundation are nonvoting members of the Board. The Executive Board carries out the ongoing activities of the organization and implements the policies approved by the Representative Assembly. It monitors the finances of the association, prepares the budget, manages the national office, supervises grants and contracts, and prepares and approves plans of action. The Executive Board also maintains a number of standing committees that carry out specific functions.

Students may be interested to know that their interests are represented in AOTA by a standing committee of the Executive Board. This is the American Student Committee of the Occupational Therapy Association, or ASCOTA. The purpose of the committee is to provide student input into the decisions and actions of the association, to promote student well-being, and to enhance student understanding of the structure and function of the association. ASCOTA officers are elected from among the student members of AOTA, and student delegates serve on AOTA committees and provide student input to the Representative Assembly. ASCOTA publishes a student newsletter and a biannual journal (*Journal of Occupational Therapy Students,* or *JOTS*), sponsors student events at national conferences, and promotes student participation in state and national occupational therapy activities (2).

The AOTA has recognized the need to establish communication between OTRs,

COTAs, and students who share common interests in specific areas of practice. Nine special interest sections have been established in the practice areas of developmental disabilities, gerontology, mental health, physical disabilities, sensory integration, administration, work programs, technology, and education. Practitioners working in school systems, in home health, and in wellness and health promotion have petitioned for the establishment of special interest sections for those practice areas as well. The special interest sections publish newsletters for their members, sponsor educational events, hold meetings at annual conferences, and promote research in their practice areas. They provide a valuable communication link among practitioners working in the same specialty area and enable them to share information and identify new practice trends (2).

Members play an active role in the association. They may raise issues for discussion, formulate resolutions to be considered by the Representative Assembly, instruct their state delegates in voting on specific issues, and utilize the resources of the organization to obtain current information about occupational therapy education and practice. The national office staff provides the support services needed by members and now has an 800 number that members may call for information. Together, the members of the AOTA and its paid office staff work to achieve the goals of the association. In 1992, AOTA members celebrated the 75th year of the organization and looked forward to continued success in the future.

MEMBERSHIP BENEFITS

The American Occupational Therapy Association provides a variety of useful benefits to its members. AOTA members automatically receive the *American Journal of Occupational Therapy* each month as well as a weekly publication, *OT Week*, that provides news updates and employment information. A third publication, *Occupational Therapy News*, is published six times a year to give members information on AOTA elections and proposed bylaws changes. AOTA also publishes a variety of professional materials that are available to members at a reduced cost.

Information services are available from the association as well as access to the Wilma L. West Library of professional publications. A national conference is held annually, and AOTA also sponsors a number of continuing education programs for its members each year. Scholarship and fellowship programs as well as student loans and grants are available to AOTA members. A recognition program honors outstanding members of the association. A variety of insurance programs as well as a credit card program are open to AOTA members. In return for an annual membership fee, AOTA members receive the services of an active professional association that advocates for their interests and represents them in health care issues on the national scene (5).

AMERICAN OCCUPATIONAL THERAPY FOUNDATION

A second national organization in occupational therapy is the American Occupational Therapy Foundation. Created in 1965, the foundation was established for charitable, scientific, literary, and educational purposes. As a philanthropic organization, the foundation accepts donations and bequests from AOTA members and friends of occupational therapy. With these funds it supports a program of scholarship awards for OTR and COTA students in entry-level programs and graduate fellowships for students in advanced degree programs. Another major activity is the publication of monographs, public information materials, and the *Occupational Therapy Journal of Research* in order to increase public understanding of occupational therapy and to disseminate the results of scientific research conducted within the field. Promotion of occupational therapy research is a goal of the foundation, and it awards research grants to investigators who submit well-documented research proposals for review. A further interest of the foundation is the maintenance of an occupational therapy library. Donations to the library are actively encouraged, and the collection now numbers over 3600 volumes. Library materials are available to researchers and are now accessible by computer.

The American Occupational Therapy Foundation is entirely separate from the AOTA and has its own elected officers who administer its programs. In 1990 the AOTF celebrated its 25th year of service and plans to continue to expand its programs and activities (6).

STATE OCCUPATIONAL THERAPY ORGANIZATIONS

State occupational therapy associations are the grass roots level of the AOTA. The AOTA bylaws (2) provide for the recognition of state associations that have at least 10 voting members and that submit a set of bylaws for approval by the Committee of State Association Presidents of AOTA. State associations may elect delegates and alternates to the Representative Assembly and thus play a role in the development and implementation of policies at the national level. The purpose of state organizations is to collaborate with the AOTA and to carry out on the local level activities that advance the objectives of that organization. Once constituted, state associations may elect their own officers and carry out their own program of activities. Many state associations hold annual conferences, sponsor continuing education programs, provide information services to their members, and organize study groups and special interest groups. Today each of the 50 states has a state occupational therapy association, as do the District of Columbia and Puerto Rico. State associations may carry out AOTA projects on a local level and are active in communicating their concerns and needs to the national organization. A strong partnership has been established between state and national associations, with each level supporting the work of the other.

Most state occupational therapy associations encourage student membership in their organizations. Often OTR and COTA educational programs have their own student associations, and these may be combined into the state organization in order to share information, sponsor student events at state conferences, and aid in the establishment of professional identity among students. Students are encouraged to take an active part in local occupational therapy organizations, as they offer a way to meet and network with professional colleagues and can provide leadership training and professional development.

WORLD FEDERATION OF OCCUPATIONAL THERAPISTS

Discussions about the formation of an international occupational therapy organization began in 1951, and in 1952 delegates from nine countries met in Great Britain to hold a planning meeting. The organization that resulted from their efforts was named the World Federation of Occupational Therapists (WFOT). In 1992 it included 33 member countries or territories and 4 associate member countries. Another 6 countries were expected to become associate members later in 1992. Full membership requires that a country have a professional occupational therapy association of at least 12 members who are citizens of that country, have a constitution, and have an educational program in occupational therapy that meets WFOT standards. Associate membership requires a membership of four qualified occupational therapists who are citizens of the country. Figure 18.3 shows the structure of the WFOT.

WFOT has identified its major objectives as follows:

1. To act as the official international organization for the promotion of occupational therapy and to hold international congresses;
2. To promote international cooperation among occupational therapy associa-

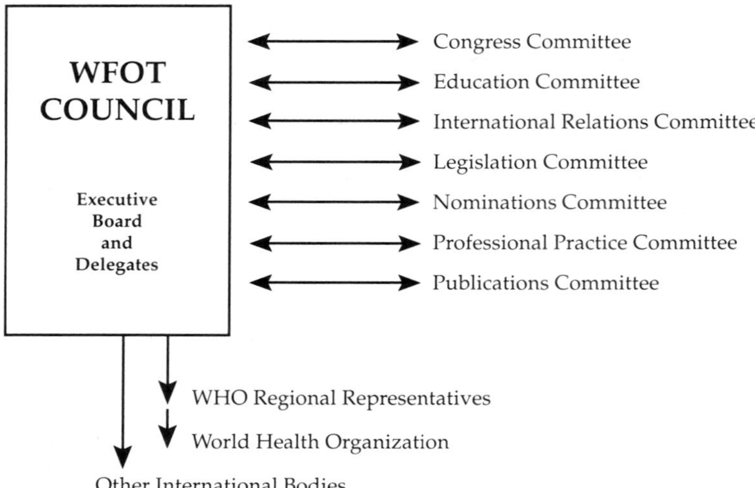

Figure 18.3. Organization of the World Federation of Occupational Therapists.

tions, occupational therapists, and between them and all other allied professional groups;

3. To maintain the ethics of the profession and to advance the practice and standards of occupational therapy;
4. To promote internationally recognized standards for education of occupational therapists;
5. To facilitate the international exchange and placement of therapists and students; and
6. To facilitate the exchange of information and publications, and to promote research (7).

Individual membership in the World Federation is open to any qualified occupational therapist who is a member in good standing of a full or an associate member organization. The ongoing business of the organization is carried on by a Council that meets every 2 years. A joint Congress and Council meeting are held every 4 years. In Council meetings, each member country is represented by a delegate and has one vote. A number of standing committees carry on specific tasks assigned by the Council and report on their work at the next Council meeting. Much of the committee work is conducted by correspondence, since members live and work in different parts of the world. The Congresses that are sponsored by the World Federation are international meetings at which papers are presented on topics relevant to occupational therapy. Professional and commercial exhibits are displayed, and film programs are shown. Social activities are included as well to promote friendship and communication between participants. Congresses are scheduled at different locations every 4 years and are planned and publicized well in advance. In 1990 an International Congress was held in Australia with the theme of "Focus '90: A Close-up, Wide-Angle, and Global View." The next Congress is scheduled for 1994 and will be held in London, England, with the overall theme of "Developing Opportunities."

Among the current activities of the World Federation are approving educational programs in occupational therapy that meet WFOT standards, creating opportunities for international experiences for occupational therapists and students, maintaining liaisons with international health organizations, encouraging the development of occupational therapy services in underserved areas of the world, and publishing monographs, bulletins, and Congress proceedings. The Federation has recently developed a foundation to receive funds that will be used to provide study and research opportunities for occupational therapists, enabling them to develop specialized skills and promoting professional development. The World Federation makes valuable contributions to occupational therapy practice and education on an international scale and provides a connecting link between the national associations of member countries.

SUMMARY

The professional organizations that have been described provide critical support and development services to their members and promote occupational therapy practice, education, and research on local, national, and international levels. These organizations are the voice of occupational therapy to people and organizations outside the field and represent the interests of OTRs, COTAs, students, and consumers of occupational therapy services. It is largely because of their efforts that occupational therapy has received positive recognition and acceptance by other health care professions, by legislators, and by the general public. Professional organizations have contributed substantially to the advancement of occupational therapy and will continue to do so. As new challenges arise, the professional organizations will be prepared to initiate policies and actions that will benefit occupational therapy personnel and the clients whom they serve.

Discussion Questions

1. Invite an officer or member of the Occupational Therapy Association in your state to visit your class. What are the issues that this organization is currently discussing? What actions is the organization taking?
2. How does the state organization relate to the AOTA?
3. Do professional organizations contribute to their members' sense of professional identity? How?
4. Does your curriculum have a student professional organization? If so, what activities is it involved in?
5. Many OTRs and COTAs belong to other organizations in addition to occupational therapy organizations. Interview some OTRs or COTAs and find out what non-OT organizations they belong to and why.
6. Are you a student member of the AOTA or your state occupational therapy association? What are some of the membership benefits for students?

References

1. Reed K, Sanderson S: Development of professional organizations. In *Concepts of Occupational Therapy*, ed 3. Baltimore, MD, Williams & Wilkins, 1992, pp. 247–261.
2. AOTA: *Bylaws*, 1981 Revision, Amended most recently in 1991. Rockville, MD, AOTA, 1981.
3. Long range plan. In *AOTA Member Handbook*. Rockville, MD, AOTA, 1980, pp. A3–A4.
4. AOTA Research Information and Evaluation Division: *Geographic Membership Data: 1992*. Rockville, MD, AOTA, 1992.
5. AOTA: *Benefits of AOTA Membership*. Rockville, MD, AOTA, 1990.
6. Devereaux EB: The American Occupational Therapy Foundation: Milestones of a quarter century. *AJOT* 44(4):295–297, 1990.
7. *World Federation of Occupational Therapists*. WFOT, Graphic Services, University of Western Ontario, London, Ontario, 1992.

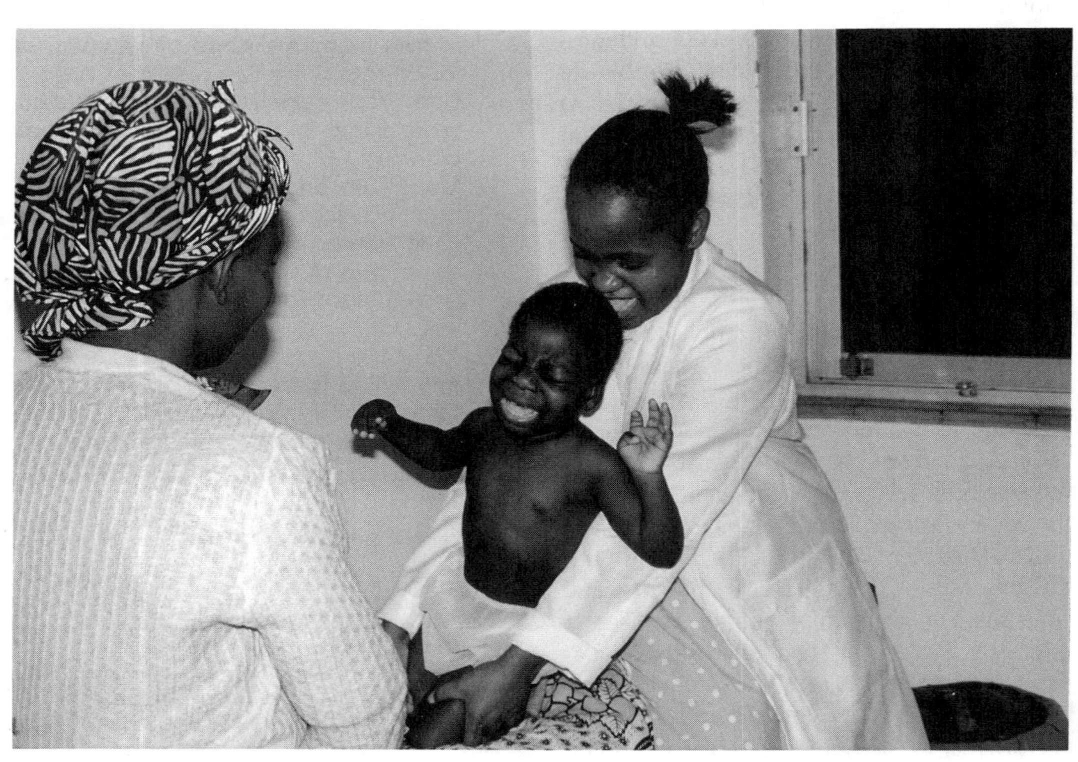

19 International Occupational Therapy

Although the United States has the largest number of practicing occupational therapists, occupational therapy is truly an international field. In 1992, 33 countries or territories had occupational therapy associations and were full members of the World Federation of Occupational Therapists (WFOT). Four additional countries held associate memberships in the WFOT, and negotiations were underway with six additional countries for associate membership. Occupational therapists are practicing their profession in many parts of the world and have been able to adapt occupational therapy concepts and therapeutic approaches to different cultures and environments. This chapter introduces the student to occupational therapy on an international scale and presents some examples of practice in countries outside the United States.

Table 19.1 provides information about some of the occupational therapy organizations around the world that are members or associate members of the WFOT (1). Many of these organizations publish a journal to keep their members informed of professional developments. A total of 256 schools were educating occupational therapists in 31 different countries in 1992 (2). Educational programs outside the United States must meet standards established by the WFOT in order to be approved by them. These educational standards are somewhat broader than those used in the United States and contain some content areas not required by the Educational Essentials of the American Occupational Therapy Association. In many foreign educational programs for the occupational therapist, the credentials awarded are different from those in the United States. Although some programs award a baccalaureate degree, others offer a diploma or certificate in occupational therapy or give a technician title. It appears that more programs are now moving toward the baccalaureate degree. Many educational programs abroad are located in technical schools or in hospital-based training schools. These institutions do not grant degrees but provide technical education in specialized fields. Most foreign occupational therapy educational programs are 3 or 4 years in length and provide concentrated education in occupational therapy theory and practice. Some countries also offer postgraduate educational programs.

HEALTH PROBLEMS WORLDWIDE

The World Health Organization (WHO) reported in 1992 that the decrease in infectious diseases has been counterbalanced by an increase in chronic degenerative diseases, and many countries are concerned about their increased aging populations. Polio has decreased by 70% in the last 10 years, but AIDs is spreading worldwide at a rapid rate (3). Along with AIDs has come an increase in the incidence of tuberculosis. Drug-resistant parasites and disease vectors have arisen in some parts of the world, while growing urban crime, ethnic conflicts, the nuclear threat, and natural disasters have combined to pose new health problems for the world's population.

The emphasis in international health care is shifting from treatment to prevention. There is increased recognition that lifestyle and environmental factors play major roles in disease prevention. The world's population has doubled since the middle of the century and

Table 19.1. Partial List of WFOT Member Organizations and Their Activities

Country or Territory	Organization	No. of Qualified Members[a]	No. of Schools	Journal	Recent Activities
Australia	Australian Assn. of Occupational Therapists	2646	5	Australian Occupational Therapy Journal	Will hold its 17th national conference in 1993; is celebrating 3 decades of OT education in Western Australia.
Austria	Verband der Diplomierten Ergotherapeuten Österreichs	338	3	ERGO	Health insurance has offered reimbursement of OT services; a 4th OT school opened in May.
Belgium	F.N.B.E.–N.B.F.E.	550	10		The Assn. hosted the 4th Eurpopean OT Congress in 1992 with speakers from over 20 countries.
Canada	Canadian Assn. of Occupational Therapists	5084	12	Canadian Journal of Occupational Therapy	Has developed an outcome performance measure; a new graduate program has recently opened.
Chile	Colegio de Terapeutas Ocupationales A.G.	250	1		
Republic of China	Occupational Therapy Assn. of the Republic of China	183	1	Chinese Journal of Occupational Therapy	In 1988, two educational programs were approved; an OT service rating scale was being designed.
Columbia	Asociation Columbiana de Terapia Ocupational	238	2	Accíon	Over 300 participants attended a 1990 conference on directions for OT.
Denmark	Danish Assn. of Occupational Therapists	2982	6	Ergoterapeuten	Research is being conducted on OT treatment of cerebrovascular accident patients.
Finland	Suomen toimentaterapeutiliitto ry	400	5	Toiminaterapeutti	In 1990 OT education celebrated its 20th year in Finland.
Germany	Verband der Beschäftiggungs und Arbietstherapeuten	3923	23	Beschäftigungstherapie und Rehabilitation	Assn. members are discussing whether OT education should be at the degree level.
Iceland	Icelandic Occupational Therapy Assn.	67	0	Blad-Id	The Assn. is pressing for the development of an OT educational program in Iceland.
India	All-India Occupational Therapists Assn.	57	5	Indian Journal of Occupational Therapy	New home care teams are being organized to help elderly clients.

Ireland	Assn. of Occupational Therapists of Ireland	146	1	O.T. Ireland	In 1992, a conference was held on OT Trends Worldwide.
Israel	Israeli Assn. of Occupational Therapy	800	3	Israel Journal of Occupational Therapy	Twenty Israeli OTs have completed advanced degree study at New York University
Italy	Associazone Italiana di Terapia Occupazionale	67	0	Notizie AITO	Held their 1992 conference on the theme of "The Sensory Dimension."
Japan	Japanese Assn. of Occupational Therapists	4455	33	Sagyo Ryoho	In 1990 over 1000 persons attended the national conference in Nagoya.
Luxembourg	A.L.E.D.	58	0		Held a conference on "Construire pour l'homme et ses capacities."
Malaysia	Malaysian Occupational Therapy Assn.	55	0		
Malta	Association of Occupational Therapists	9	0		The first OT course began in 1984 with 5 students; classes now accept 20 students.
Netherlands	Nederlandse Vereniging voor Ergotherapie	1163	2	Nederlandse Tijd-Schrift voor Ergo therapie	The Assn. celebrated its 20th year in 1992. National health service changes may improve reimbursement of OT services.
Norway	Norsk Ergoterapeutforbund	1206	3	Ergoterapeuten	Home care is increasing and institutional care is declining
Portugal	Associacao Portugesa de Terapia Ocupacional	351	2	Boletin de Assoc. Portugal de Terapia Ocupational	The Assn. hosted the 3rd European Congress of OTs in 1988
South Africa	South African Assn. of Occupational Therapists	688	7	South African Journal of Occupational Therapy	Courses to train support staff are expanding and the Assn. is building alliances with other health care groups to promote allied health services.
Spain	Asociacion Profesional Española de Terapeutas Ocupacionales	388	1	Boletin Ass. Española de Terapie Ocupacíon	

Table 19.1—*continued*

Country or Territory	Organization	No. of Qualified Members[a]	Number of Schools	Journal	Recent Activities
Sweden	Förbundet Sveriges Arbetsterapeuter	5587	8	Arbetsterapeuten	The Assn. celebrated its 10th anniversary in 1988.
Switzerland	Verband Schweizerischer Ergotherapeuten	782	3	Zeitschrifit fur Ergotherapie	The Assn. has joined with other health care Assns. to present a unified approach to health issues.
United Kingdom	British Assn. of Occupational Therapists	9494	26	British Journal of Occupational Therapy	National health insurance changes are changing OT services; community-based treatment is being emphasized.
USA	American Occupational Therapy Assn.	32,069	75	American Journal of Occupational Therapy	The Assn. celebrated its 75th year in 1992. A new, special interest group on technology was formed in 1991.
Zimbabwe	Zimbabwean Assn. of Occupational Therapists	20	1		Zimbabwe graduated the first student from its OT program in 1990.

[a]Registered occupational therapists only.

is expected to stabilize around 11 billion sometime during the next century. Most of the population will be concentrated in urban areas by then, and sustaining life and preventing disease and injury will be major challenges to health care professionals (4).

According to WHO, most deaths today are due to infectious and parasitic diseases (17,500,000 deaths), cardiovascular diseases (11,931,000 deaths), cancer (5,121,000 deaths), perinatal causes (3,116,000 deaths), chronic obstructive pulmonary disease (2,888,000 deaths), maternal causes (504,000 deaths), and other diseases—AIDS, diabetes, kidney failure—(5,431,000 deaths). WHO suggestions for lowering the death rate include immunizations for children to prevent childhood illnesses, better nutrition, clean water supplies, safe sewage disposal, air pollution control, better prenatal care, and access to medical services (5).

OCCUPATIONAL THERAPY TRENDS

The largest number of occupational therapists practicing abroad seems to be employed in institutional settings. In a growing number of countries (Australia, Canada, Belgium, Denmark, Israel, India, the United Kingdom, Norway, New Zealand, Sweden, Switzerland, and South Africa), however, there is a strong trend toward community-based practice, while hospital-based care seems to be declining. These countries are also experiencing an increased emphasis on geriatric care, are applying occupational therapy concepts to industrial settings, and are seeing more therapists engaged in private practice. The developing countries tend to have predominantly hospital-based practice and are more inclined to follow the medical model. Community-based rehabilitation programs are increasingly being used in developing countries to expand their rehabilitation services to rural areas and reach larger segments of the population.

Occupational therapists in other countries seem to be less specialized than those in the United States. Many of them practice in countries that have a form of national health care, so occupational therapy services must fit into the established health care system. In the early 1990s many countries were experiencing depressed economic conditions, and health care expenditures were being carefully monitored.

DEVELOPING OCCUPATIONAL THERAPY SERVICES

Laura Krefting, a Canadian occupational therapist who has been involved in prevention and early identification programs in several Asian countries, has noted that, when western occupational therapists try to help third world countries develop services, they usually transplant western service models to the developing country. This approach often fails because it may not fit the needs or the health care system of the developing country. In order to avoid this problem, Krefting suggests careful assessment of the country's morbidity and mortality patterns, the health care distribution system, and the potential for long-term sustainability of occupational therapy services.

Usually infectious diseases must be brought under control before the problems of chronic disease and disability can be addressed. The areas of greatest need are often in rural areas or urban slums. Developing occupational therapy services depend on an infrastructure of governmental and voluntary health agencies that contribute to health planning and establish program priorities. Krefting suggests that to encourage the development of occupational therapy services one must objectively document the observed rehabilitation needs, take part in developing a comprehensive plan for services, prioritize needs, and develop educational models to train rehabilitation professionals and aides. Only when programs are tailored to fit local needs and priorities do they take root and flourish (6).

SUPPORT PERSONNEL

There seems to be no exact equivalent to the certified occupational therapy assistant outside the United States. Technicians exist, but training is variable and these technicians may function only in specialized areas of practice, such as gerontology. Only 11 of the WFOT member organizations reported having trained support staff available in 1980. Of those who did, the support staff ranged from aides with minimal on-the-job training to technical assistants with over 3 years of training (7). It should be noted that several WFOT member countries are training community-based rehabilitation workers to expand rehabilitation services. These assistants are proving to be effective in providing basic care to larger numbers of disabled people, and since they are drawn from the native population, they have a good understanding of the language and culture of the people they serve.

AIDS SURVEY

In 1988 the World Federation of Occupational Therapists initiated a study of how many member organizations had members who were working with AIDS/human immunodeficiency virus (HIV) clients and what roles they were fulfilling with this population. Twelve member organizations reported that some of their members were seeing AIDS/HIV patients and four said that members were treating patients with drug addictions. The occupational therapy associations of Australia, Canada, and the United States had developed position papers describing occupational therapy roles with this disability group. Occupational therapy associations in Denmark, Ireland, Portugal, the United Kingdom, and the United States reported that services were rapidly developing to serve this group and that occupational therapists were involved in the programs in various ways. The World Federation expects to see large increases in this patient population as the disease spreads and will continue to monitor the use of occupational therapy in treatment programs (8).

OTHER INTERNATIONAL EFFORTS

Attempts are being made to increase contacts between occupational therapists in various parts of the world. The AOTA was planning to sponsor a WFOT-member therapist for a study tour of the United States in 1993. Up to 2 months of visits to occupational therapy programs would be permitted with transportation costs paid and local hospitality provided by AOTA members. This long-standing program has been most successful in enabling foreign therapists to see American programs firsthand and to study new treatment techniques and observe technological advances.

Another more recent development is a new occupational therapy journal entitled *Occupational Therapy International*. The first issue of the journal will appear in 1993 or 1994 and will include articles on clinical practice, research, education, professional issues, and trends in health care. The new journal should improve the communication of occupational therapists around the world and will enable them to learn more about practice and education trends in other countries.

EXAMPLES OF INTERNATIONAL OCCUPATIONAL THERAPY

To understand what occupational therapists are doing in other countries, let's look at brief summaries of articles that have appeared in WFOT publications in recent years.

South Africa

Lorenzo has described a training program for community rehabilitation workers to serve a rural population in the northeastern Transvaal. The district had an estimated disability rate of 5%, and the people's problems were compounded by poverty, lack of access to health care, maldistribution of health care resources, and negative attitudes on the part of the nondisabled population. Community education was believed to be necessary in order to reintegrate disabled persons back into the community. In 1989 a community-based rehabilitation trust was established, and this funded the training program as well as other projects. Community-based rehabilitation workers were trained in a 2-year curriculum that focused on disability and life skills development. It is hoped that the community rehabilitation workers will be able to provide basic therapy services and community education to enable more disabled people to live in the community and live a useful life (9).

Malaysia

The vocational integration of psychiatric patients is receiving more attention in Malaysia, and Yim has discussed some of the barriers to employment for these patients. The continuing stigma associated with mental illness is a major problem. The variable mental status of patients is another, along with side effects of medications and poorly controlled medication use. Inadequate support systems leave patients vulnerable to regression after being discharged from hospital care. A survey of 30 day-care patients found that unskilled or semiskilled workers had the most difficulty finding and keeping a job. Forty-three percent of the patients said that they could not cope with work tasks, and another 43% said that they had had interpersonal problems at work. Ninety percent were unwilling to inform prospective employers about their illness. As a result of the survey, greater family support and use of sheltered workshops to improve coping skills were recommended. More emphasis on building positive work habits, assertiveness skills, social skills, and communication skills was felt to be needed. A public education campaign to inform employers about the facts and myths of mental illness would be beneficial to change attitudes about the employment of the mentally ill (10).

Malta

There were in 1991 only 11 occupational therapists working on the island of Malta, but the field is gradually developing. An occupational therapy course was first conducted in 1984 for five students and was followed by another in 1985. The educational program now accepts 20 students per class. Graduates of the local program joined British-trained therapists to provide occupational therapy services on the island. Therapists were working in general hospitals, geriatric hospitals, and psychiatric hospitals. The Malta Occupational Therapy Association became an associate member of WFOT in 1988 (11).

Philippines

Because of staff shortages, traditional institutional rehabilitation is impractical in many developing countries. In the Philippines, a community-based rehabilitation approach (CBR) has been adopted. The program was initiated in 1989 and was intended to integrate rehabilitation services into primary health care settings. Sites are located in small communities and are staffed with a variety of primary health care and public health workers. The College of Allied Medical Professions of the University of the Philippines has made student training experiences available in the CBR programs, and occupational therapy students participate for 8 weeks of their senior year. Along with physical therapy and speech pathology students, they live in the community, staying with the family of a disabled person, and take part in the activities of the CBR program. A generalist approach is used, with students encouraged to consult with other disciplines and with health officials when needed. Students are supervised by a CBR coordinator and by an occupational therapy supervisor. This type of clinical experience is believed to provide a good foundation for later practice in rural areas and sensitizes students to the realities of community-based practice (12).

Norway

The city of Oslo developed a comprehensive plan for the care of its elderly citizens.

The plan included an accident prevention project that was organized and conducted by a multidisciplinary team that included two occupational therapists. The team decided to concentrate on the prevention of falls because during the preceding year there had been 300 fractures of the neck of the femur in elderly people. Home care workers were contacted and were given a half-day course in home accident prevention. Follow-up home visits were done, and talks were given at centers for the elderly. Norwegian occupational therapists also contribute to environmental health protection programs by adapting living environments and emphasizing preventive measures. They see such programs as a natural involvement for community-based therapists and give a high priority to preventive programs in their practice (13).

Scotland

In the United Kingdom, occupational therapists have long been aided by support staff members who have been trained in short courses or in-service education that followed College of Occupational Therapy guidelines. In Scotland it was decided to develop a training course for occupational therapy assistants using the vocational education system. The three Scottish occupational therapy schools joined forces with employers to design a 2-year in-service course for support staff that would result in a recognized qualification. A series of 12 study units was developed. Students continued to work at their facilities as they moved through the educational program and many assignments related to their own job situations. Graduates of the program may move directly into advanced levels of OTR educational programs, thus creating a career ladder for support personnel. In 1991 the program was jointly approved by the Scottish Vocational Education Council and the College of Occupational Therapists. Similar programs at four other vocational education colleges were approved, assuring a steady supply of trained occupational therapy assistants to work in Scottish programs (14).

Canada

Altman has described a comprehensive home care program located in the city of Vancouver, Canada. The program is part of the services offered by the Vancouver Health Department, which provides preventive services as well as continuing care to residents of the city. All health services are government funded. In home care the occupational therapist is part of a team that includes a physiotherapist, a home care nurse, a physician, and a long-term care case manager. The occupational therapist usually functions in a consultative role, recommending home modifications and adaptations where necessary. The client or caregiver is taught safe transfer techniques, joint protection, energy conservation, and alternative methods of personal care. The majority of clients are over 60 years of age with a variety of acute or chronic conditions. "At risk" clients are identified prior to hospital discharge, and referrals are made for home care services. The program provides a model for comprehensive public health services and is proving successful in maintaining elderly persons in their own homes (15).

Denmark

The World Health Organization has stated that by 1990 all member countries were to have quality assurance mechanisms in place to ensure the quality of health care services. In an effort to comply with this goal, the Danish National Health Service developed "reference programs" that provided guidelines for standard care in a number of diagnostic categories. Using a similar approach, the Danish occupational therapists developed occupational therapy reference programs that give a standard occupational therapy treatment protocol for many of the conditions treated by occupational therapists. These reference programs were based on research into activity, sensory integration, activity analysis, therapeutic media, work-related treatment, and treatment for special diagnostic groups. Frames of reference used in clinical practice were identified, and the occupational therapy process of service delivery was described. The occupational therapy reference programs will form the basis for a quality assurance program that is consistent with that of the National Health Service (16).

India

Like other countries, India is becoming more concerned about the problems of its growing population of elders. Kenkre has pointed out that in India the problems of the affluent elderly are quite different from those of the poor elderly. In the affluent group, degenerative diseases, cardiovascular problems, and neuromuscular disorders predominate, often complicated by hypertension, diabetes, and obesity. Among the poor, degenerative arthritis is frequently seen due to a lifetime of hard physical labor. Chronic diseases are common due to lack of access to medical care. Anemia is common because of low protein intake, and vitamin deficiencies are frequently seen. Tuberculosis incidence is very high among older people and is found at all social levels.

Indian occupational therapists use either preventive or restorative methods in dealing with the elderly and must analyze the social aspects of the patient's life as well as his or her physical limitations. Under the pressures of modern life, the traditional joint family system is breaking down, and elderly persons may no longer be cared for by younger family members. Help with self-care abilities is increasingly needed by elderly patients. More and more, preventive programs are being seen as the most useful approach to the problems of the elderly. Maintaining existing levels of function and enabling the elderly person to have some quality of life are seen as realistic goals of occupational therapy for this group of patients (17).

Zimbabwe

Zimbabwe gained its independence in 1980, and the new government began a drive to improve the health care of its black population. Part of the plan was aimed at upgrading the treatment of disabled children. A Children's Rehabilitation Unit was established at one of the two government hospitals, and there are plans to establish a second unit in another city. The unit serves high-risk newborns and children with developmental delays, neurological disorders, mental disability, and sensory disorders. The health care team of the unit includes an occupational therapist and provides family-centered services.

Since few health care professionals were available to provide care for a population of 9.4 million, a training program was begun in 1980 to train rehabilitation assistants who could provide basic rehabilitation services. These workers are supervised by a qualified therapist. Occupational therapy and physical therapy degree courses were established in 1987. It is important that therapists understand the culture and lifestyle of their client families so that the treatment suggestions are compatible with the family's living environment and way of life. In order to spread rehabilitation services into rural parts of the country, the Children's Rehabilitation Unit team travels to outlying areas and conducts 3- to 5-day workshops for families of disabled children. Therapists and rehabilitation assistants work together to try to solve problems of the children being seen. So far, the program is functioning well and appears well-adapted to local needs (18).

STUDY OPPORTUNITIES ABROAD

Students are often interested in the possibility of exchange programs or foreign study. The most recent revision of the educational standards for OTR education in the United States permits international fieldwork when the following conditions are met.

1. When the fieldwork is approved by the student's educational program,

2. When direct supervision is provided by an AOTCB-certified occupational therapist,
3. When there is no language barrier between the student, supervisor, and the client population, and
4. When the student's safety and rights are reasonably ensured (19).

In 1991 the World Federation of Occupational Therapists published a booklet that describes the conditions for student exchanges or fieldwork experiences in 12 of its member countries. This publication emphasizes that, before considering a foreign exchange or fieldwork program, students should consider their financial resources, their competency in the language of the host country, their emotional and physical health status, their knowledge and competencies in occupational therapy theory and methods, and their ability to complete all of the necessary paperwork for a foreign educational experience. As of 1991, exchange or fieldwork experiences were being offered in Australia, Austria, Belgium, Canada, Denmark, Germany, Ireland, Kenya, Norway, Portugal, Switzerland, and the United Kingdom (20).

WORKING ABROAD

Therapists and therapy assistants may also be interested in the possibility of working in a foreign country for a period of time. The World Federation of Occupational Therapists offers some practical advice to therapists who wish to work in a foreign country in their 1990 publication *Requirements for the Employment of Occupational Therapists in Member Countries of WFOT* (21). This publication points out that, although working abroad can be a uniquely enriching experience, one should ask the following basic questions of oneself before undertaking such a venture.

1. Do you have a speaking knowledge of the language of the host country? (This is essential for adequate communication with patients and staff in the workplace and also for daily living.)
2. Are you able to adapt to all kinds of conditions? (Although occupational therapy concepts are similar around the world, working conditions and equipment are not.)
3. How good is your emotional and physical health? (You must be able to adapt to changes in climate, nutrition, working hours, and attitudes.)
4. How good is your professional knowledge? (A therapist should have at least 1 year of clinical experience and preferably more before attempting to work abroad. You will be regarded as an expert and should be prepared to function as such.)
5. How well do you know your own country? (As a therapist working abroad you will unofficially represent your country. You should be prepared to answer questions on subjects such as your government, the educational system, cultural patterns, and political issues.)
6. How much do you know about sources of financial support for overseas assignments? (It is always best to seek financial support from resources within your own country. Are you familiar with the salary scale and the standard of living in the host country?)
7. Have you investigated the financial implications of taking money out of one country and into another? (Many countries have restrictions on the amount of money that can be brought in.)

The WFOT publication goes on to provide specific information on the immigration requirements and educational requirements to practice in each of its member countries.

A number of voluntary organizations that have an interest in rehabilitation offer opportunities for exchange programs between rehabilitation professionals. Partners of the Americas, the American Refugee Committee, and Rehabilitation International are examples of such organizations. The United States Department of Defense employs some occupational therapists to provide services to handicapped children who are military dependents and are stationed abroad. Some church groups offer missionary opportunities for those who wish to contribute their professional skills to church-sponsored hospitals and clinics abroad. Government agencies such as the Peace Corps recruit occupational therapists to serve 2-year terms of duty in countries that request assistance in developing rehabilitation services. Finally, private foundations offer some support for study or work abroad in professional fields. The student or therapist interested in such possibilities should thoroughly research potential funding sources before making a commitment to foreign study or employment. The American Occupational Therapy Association can provide a detailed listing of such sources on request (22, 23)

INTERNATIONAL AND REGIONAL CONFERENCES

The international congresses sponsored by the WFOT every 4 years offer occupational therapists and therapy assistants an opportunity to meet and talk with their colleagues from WFOT member countries. The next congress is scheduled for 1994 in London, England. Regional international meetings are also beginning to develop. In May of 1992 the Belgian National Federation of Ergotherapy hosted the fourth European Congress and Exhibition of Occupational Therapy in Ostende. Video presentations, papers, poster sessions, short courses, and visits to clinical programs were included in the program. The Nordic countries frequently sponsor regional seminars and conferences for members of their occupational therapy associations. Latin American associations have also joined forces to provide conferences and continuing education for occupational therapists in the South and Central American countries.

SUMMARY

Occupational therapy is growing and developing throughout the world, and therapists here and abroad are eager for communication and interchange with their colleagues in other countries. A variety of opportunities exist for travel, study, or employment in countries outside the United States. Therapists are advised to plan such experiences carefully so that maximum benefit will be obtained both by the individual and by the host country. The World Federation of Occupational Therapists provides a connecting link between occupational therapy organizations in its member countries and offers communication and exchange opportunities through its publications and international congresses. As the number of occupational therapists increases around the world, opportunities for exchange programs between schools and between occupational therapy organizations should expand.

Discussion Questions

1. Have you ever considered work or study outside the United States? If so, what countries interest you?
2. If you have the opportunity, invite a foreign-educated occupational therapist to attend your class. How was their education different from yours? What is practice like in their country?
3. Do you think that the development of rehabilitation services is a high priority of governments in developing countries? Why or why not?
4. Do you think that work, self-care, or leisure activities might vary with the culture and the country? How might they be different?
5. How might client attitudes toward rehabilitation and achievement of independent functioning vary from culture to culture?
6. Have any of your faculty members attended a WFOT World Congress? If so, ask them to share their experiences with you.
7. Could your student occupational therapy association contact and exchange

information with students of a foreign occupational therapy school?

8. **Could your curriculum host a foreign occupational therapy educator or clinician who wishes to visit the United States?**

References

1. *Annual Reports of Member Organizations*. World Federation of Occupational Therapists, 1991.
2. *List of WFOT-Approved Schools*. World Federation of Occupational Therapists, 1992.
3. Schwarz M: Mixed feelings in times of change. *WFOT Bulletin* 25:1–3, 1992.
4. Joe BE: Promoting a global perspective on health care. *OT Week* 6:(36):10, 1992.
5. Staff: Death toll around the world, from Health Notes. *OT Week* 6:(25):12, 1992.
6. Krefting L: The issue is: strategies for the development of occupational therapy in the third world. *AJOT* 46(8):758–760, 1992.
7. *Survey on Recognized Training of Support Staff*. World Federation of Occupational Therapists, 1980.
8. Valentin C: Results of survey of OTs treating AIDS patients. *WFOT Bulletin* 21:47–51, May 1990.
9. Lorenzo T: Strides in community rehabilitation worker training in a rural area of South Africa. *WFOT Bulletin* 24:2–5, Nov 1991.
10. Yim LS: Problems of employment of psychiatric patients. *WFOT Bulletin* 23:7–9, May 1991.
11. Briffa JZ: Recent developments in occupational therapy in Malta. *WFOT Bulletin* 23:16–18, May 1991.
12. Mendoza TC: Training occupational therapy students in the primary health care setting. *WFOT Bulletin* 24:12–15, Nov 1991.
13. Hanstveit S, Olufsen S: Accident prevention amongst the elderly. *WFOT Bulletin* 23:22–25, May 1991.
14. Stewart AM: A ladder of opportunities in Scotland—1991 higher national certificate—occupational therapy support. *WFOT Bulletin* 24:9–11, Nov 1991.
15. Altman G: Home care, occupational therapy in Vancouver, Canada. *WFOT Bulletin* 23:26–28, May 1991.
16. Voltelen T: Quality assurance in occupational therapy. *WFOT Bulletin* 22:25–35, Nov 1990.
17. Kenkre IR: Occupational therapy programme for the health and well-being of the elderly in India. *WFOT Bulletin* 22:47–50, Nov 1990.
18. Cortes D: The children's rehabilitation unit: a team approach to family rehabilitation in Zimbabwe. *WFOT Bulletin* 21:10–12, May 1990.
19. AOTA: Essentials and guidelines for an accredited program for the occupational therapist. *AJOT* 45(12):1077–1083, 1991.
20. Education Committee, WFOT: *Directory of Information for Student Exchange Within the Member Countries of WFOT*. 1991.
21. Publications Committee, WFOT: *Requirements for the Employment of Occupational Therapists in Member Countries of WFOT*. 1990.
22. Izutsu S: *Working Abroad: How to Get Started*. Rockville, MD, AOTA, 1991, pp. 1–14.
23. AOTA: *Opportunities for International Experiences*, Rockville, MD, AOTA, 1992, pp. 1–6.

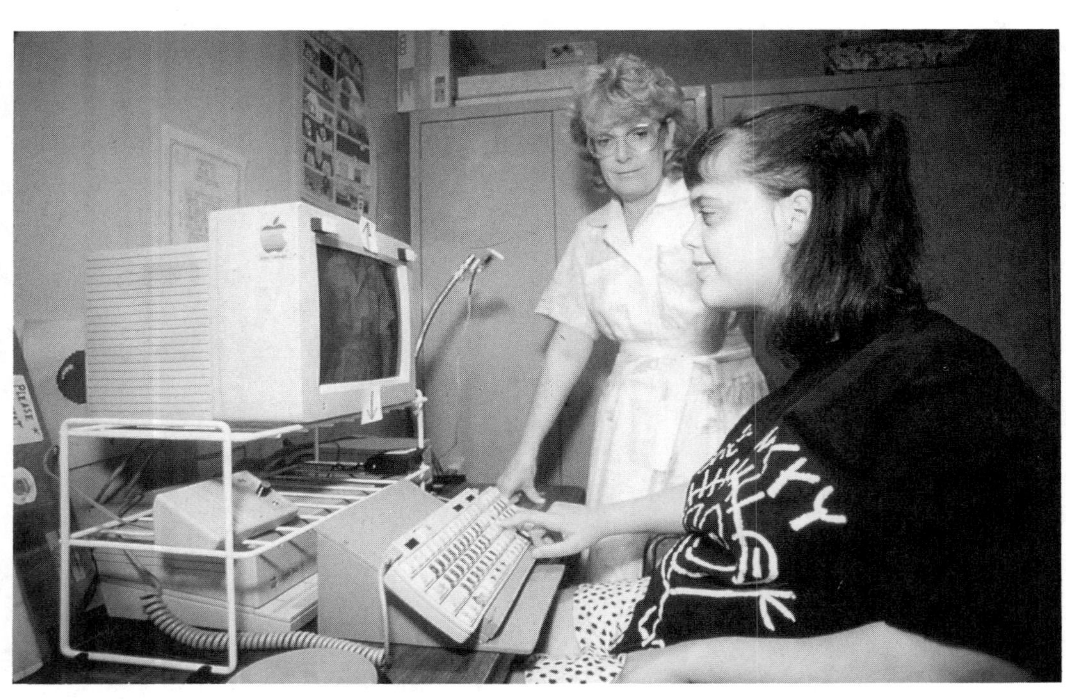
PLEASE

20 Current Trends and Future Outlook

Occupational therapy has grown and developed a great deal since its beginnings in the early years of the 20th century. Each succeeding generation of occupational therapists has faced new challenges and has adapted the traditions of the field to meet new needs and conditions. As we enter the 1990s, occupational therapy faces some landmark decisions, and the results of these decisions may well influence profound changes in the profession. In this final chapter we look at current trends in American society, in health care, and in occupational therapy. We will then look ahead to the future and examine some possibilities for future developments in health care and in the field of occupational therapy.

SOCIAL CHANGES

As the decade of the 1990s began, it was possible to observe a number of social changes in the United States that influenced the health of its citizens and made increased demands on health care providers and facilities. One important change was the aging of the U.S. population. The proportion of elderly people was increasing rapidly, particularly the over-75 age group. By the year 2000, this age group will have increased by almost 35%. The elderly are particularly heavy users of health and hospital services—from five to seven times that of the population as a whole. The growth of this segment of the population will be a major influence on health care patterns and funding arrangements. Largely because of this group of consumers, community-based care has become an important part of service delivery. The health needs of the elderly are expected to result in pressures to extend and expand both the Medicare and Medicaid programs. The use of technology to prolong life and the right to die are ethical issues particularly relevant to this consumer group.

Another recent trend is that consumers of health care are becoming more sophisticated. The baby boom generation tends to ask more questions about health care and demand better services. Consumers in this age group are taking more personal responsibility for their health and are well aware of the role of diet, exercise, stress, and lifestyle to their health. This knowledgeable attitude has spread to other groups of consumers as well. Consumers are beginning to change their image of the physician from that of a benevolent, paternalistic authority to that of a partner in maintaining one's health and dealing with illness. Consumers are likely to want to take a more active part in medical decisions that affect them and will be careful evaluators of new forms of health care delivery (1).

As we have seen in preceding chapters, the American population is becoming more culturally diverse. Health care in the United States is a patchwork of public and private institutions, agencies, state and regional consortia, and private entrepreneurs. It is difficult, if not impossible, for this kind of industry to be able to address the health needs of a large, diverse group of consumers. The public has become increasingly aware of large gaps in services for certain segments of the population: minority groups, the working poor, the elderly with only Social Security income, recent immigrant groups with little knowledge of how to gain access to health care, etc. The gap between health care services available to the wealthy and those available to the poor grows wider each year. These problems must be faced, and solutions must be found.

Economic conditions in the early 1990s were causing increased unemployment and homelessness among the population. Many people lacked health insurance and lacked access to health services. Increasing levels of crime and violence were resulting in more severe trauma cases and violent deaths. Particularly alarming was the increased use of weapons and violence among children and teenagers. The number of single parent families had increased dramatically due to a rising divorce rate. Nine-tenths of the single parents were women, many of whom had become impoverished following a divorce and who were struggling to raise their children under very difficult conditions. Lack of adequate day care for children of working parents compounded their problems (2).

The AIDS epidemic was sweeping through the country and the world. In 1991 alone there were 54,000 AIDS deaths in the United States. Along with AIDS came a resurgence of tuberculosis and other infectious diseases—rheumatic fever, cholera, and even the bubonic plague (3). The nation struggled to mobilize health care resources to deal with these problems, but in the absence of a unified health care system, government efforts tended to be piecemeal and inadequate.

The need for psychiatric care was increasing as problems of substance abuse, high stress levels, child abuse, suicide, and elder abuse increased. Many of the chronically mentally ill were either homeless and living on the streets or incarcerated in local jails because there weren't adequate treatment facilities for them.

It was increasingly being recognized that improvements in the general health of the population had more to do with sanitation, nutrition, education, lifestyle, and personal income levels than with medical treatment. Yet a large proportion of health care spending (as much as 30–40%) went toward the care of advanced illnesses rather than toward prevention and health maintenance (4).

Disability was emerging in the 1990s as the nation's greatest health problem, both in terms of cost and prevalence. In 1992 a National Center for Medical Rehabilitation Research was proposed, and if funded, would identify research priorities and develop a plan for investigating and solving some of the problems of chronic disability (5).

Government leaders and ordinary citizens recognized the magnitude of the problems facing the country, but few could agree on solutions. It was clear that many of the social changes being seen were affecting the health and well-being of large segments of the population. It is yet to be seen whether these problems will be addressed in a substantial way as we progress through the 1990s.

THE CHANGING HEALTH CARE SCENE

We have seen in previous chapters that health care facilities and services are undergoing rapid change in the United States. Escalating health care costs have forced changes in hospital utilization, making the hospital the location of care only for severe, acute illness and injury. Convalescent and restorative care must now be sought either from community-based services or from nursing homes. Whether the cost of such care is covered depends on an individual's health insurance or, in the case of the poor and the elderly, on the Medicaid and Medicare programs. Small community hospitals have been particularly hard hit by increasing costs and have found it difficult to compete with larger, better-funded hospitals. Mergers and closures have been the fate of many small hospitals, particularly in rural areas.

Reimbursement patterns are changing in health care. In the period from the 1960s to the 1980s, government and private insurance paid most health care costs. In the 1990s, as costs continued to rise, employers were finding that the health care costs for their employees were taking a larger share of their budget than were manufacturing costs. The federal government has made strong efforts to cut costs by reducing Medicare and Medicaid payments to doctors and hospitals for standard procedures. Both government and private insurers began to pass on more of the direct costs to consumers, but consumers were resisting. Whoever ends up paying the health care bills in the next decade is going to be very cost-conscious and will be looking for cost-effective health care services.

New technologies continued to develop that provided advanced treatment approaches to disease and disability. New drugs, new equipment, and new methods for diagnosis all contributed to advances in health care, but also contributed to rising costs. The new technologies were also giving rise to ethical dilemmas about who would be allowed to use them, under what conditions, and how they would be paid for.

Health care personnel has continued to increase to meet consumer needs. It has been predicted that the physician supply will soon exceed current needs. This excess may give rise to greater competition in medical practice or perhaps it may tend to even out the distribution of physicians geographically throughout the country (1).

The expansion of for-profit health care corporations has raised additional concerns about access to emergency care and hospital care for the indigent and the uninsured. The broad influence of the for-profit chains has caused changes in nonprofit institutions as well as they attempt to compete and keep up with the for-profits. Both groups were experiencing financial losses in the late 1980s, but after some restructuring appear to be holding their own.

The need for some type of comprehensive health care program for United States citizens is clear to many people, but there is little agreement on how it should be done. Many people are reluctant to give up their choice of a personal physician and control of their own medical care. Managed care as practiced in HMOs means that the primary physician serves as the gatekeeper to high-tech medical care and controls access to specialists and specialty services.

Many physicians now agree that health maintenance, patient education, and preventive services should receive a high priority within the total spectrum of health care. These programs are cost-effective and result in the greatest benefit for the greatest number of people. It is encouraging to note that the U.S. population appears to be responding positively to attempts to educate them on proper nutrition, the value of exercise, methods of stress reduction, the hazards of drug and alcohol use and smoking, and the need for prenatal care.

As economic conditions worsened in the United States, stress levels increased, and there was a perceived need for more mental health services. The existing services were unable to keep up with the demand, and most had long waiting lists. This is considered an area of shortage, and more personnel are needed to provide mental health services. Another area of shortage is in the care of the elderly. With the growing numbers of older persons, many more health care workers will be needed in this practice area. If some type of long-term care insurance is funded, geriatric services can be expected to expand rapidly.

Many challenges exist today for health care personnel. Caring for HIV/AIDS patients at various stages of their illness is a serious problem. Providing adequate living arrangements, supported work, and quality of life for severely disabled persons presents another challenge to health and social welfare personnel. Supportive services for the frail elderly will be increasingly needed, as will early intervention programs for at-risk and disabled children. Perhaps the greatest challenge of all is providing equity in access to health care services for all of our citizens.

OCCUPATIONAL THERAPY EMPLOYMENT TRENDS

The 1990 Member Data Survey conducted by the AOTA showed some interesting employment trends for OTRs and COTAs. Seventy percent of the OTRs who responded and 72% of the COTAs were employed full-time. Another 20% of the OTRs and 17% of the COTAs were working part-time. The total number who were actively employed was higher than in previous years, perhaps reflecting the depressed economy and/or the shortage of occupational therapy personnel. More OTRs were employed in urban areas, while the proportion of COTAs was greater in rural areas. More practitioners at both levels were becoming self-employed or were entering private practice. Ironically, while the public's need for mental health services was increasing, fewer OTRs and COTAs were working in this practice area. Salaries for both OTRs and COTAs were increasing at an average of 8% annually. New graduates' salaries have risen an average of 9% each year since 1986 (6).

The shortfall of occupational therapy personnel continued in 1990 with a 25% national shortage being documented. This shortage is expected to persist since occupational therapy educational programs are unable to produce enough graduates to meet current needs. A shortage of 50% has been predicted by the year 2000 (7). In 1992 the AOTA launched a full-scale recruitment drive to encourage students to consider a career in occupational therapy. Minority students are especially needed in order to provide services to the increasingly diverse client population. As new educational programs open in underserved areas of the country, the problem of maldistribution of occupational therapy personnel is expected to ease.

OCCUPATIONAL THERAPY PRACTICE TRENDS

During the 1990s, specialization was increasing in occupational therapy. The AOTA 1990 Member Data Survey reported that 58.2% of OTRs and 38.8% of COTAs considered themselves to be specialists in one particular area of practice (6). While specialization is desirable from many points of view, there are some types of practice (such as community-based practice) where a generalist approach may be preferable. When therapists are expected to deal with a variety of client problems, a broad range of knowledge and clinical experience is needed. Some observers have questioned the trend toward specialization, feeling that occupational therapy needs to be better defined as a profession before specialization should occur (8). Practitioners, however, appear to be moving in this direction.

Along with increasing specialization, many occupational therapists are earning advanced credentials in specialty areas. Examples include certification as a certified vocational evaluator, as a certified work capacity evaluator, or certifications in pediatrics, biofeedback, neurodevelopmental therapy, sensory integration, and hand therapy. Such qualifications imply that the individual has engaged in advanced study of a specific practice area and has developed a high level of skill. Advanced certifications must often be renewed after a period of time to insure that the practitioner has kept up with new developments (9).

In 1989 nearly one-fifth of the occupational therapy workforce was composed of COTAs. This group of staff members has been recognized for their important contribution to direct service programs in occupational therapy. With the current personnel shortage, COTAs are being relied upon to provide a great deal of client care, and COTA roles appear to be expanding. In 1992 AOTA was making a special effort to listen to the concerns of its COTA members and to identify their needs.

A strong trend is being seen in community-based care for those with chronic illnesses and disabilities and for the elderly. OTRs and COTAs are moving in greater numbers from hospital settings to community programs where follow-up and rehabilitation services are provided. As discussed in Chapter 16, this trend is very compatible with occupational therapy service delivery. Seeing clients in their own homes provides an opportunity to help them make practical adaptations that will make daily life easier. Students are likely to need better preparation for working in home care programs and will need to learn how to function as a consultant to nurses, aides, and families.

Technology in occupational therapy is becoming complex, and practitioners will need increased knowledge in order to apply existing technologies effectively and to aid in the development of new technologies. The increased use of technology is already leading to ethical questions. How appropriate is a given technology for a client? Does the use of elaborate equipment lead to a neglect of the client's psychosocial needs? Occupational therapy personnel will need to learn how to use technology as a treatment tool, recognizing its limitations and contraindications for its use.

Research into the effectiveness of occupational therapy treatment methods is urgently needed in order to justify the use of occupational therapy services and build an outcome-oriented profession. Clinical practitioners as well as faculty researchers will be expected to cooperate in research efforts so that a body of knowledge about human occupation and its use as a therapeutic agent can be generated.

In the late 1980s and early 1990s, industrial rehabilitation was emerging as a major practice trend in occupational therapy. King has shown that most therapists who were employed in work-hardening programs in the early 1990s had gained their knowledge of this practice area through work experience rather than through education (10). Educational programs will need to expand their coverage of this important practice area as work-related programs continue to develop and expand. Prevention of on-the-job injuries can be achieved through redesign of jobs, work stations, equipment, and changes in work habits and movement patterns.

The AIDS epidemic forced occupational therapists to think about their role in the treatment of this progressive disease. Pizzi pioneered this type of practice using the model of human occupation. He advised that in the early stages of the disease, psychosocial needs might take priority. Later when symptoms develop, performance of daily living tasks is affected, and patients are limited in their ability to work, participate in leisure activities, and care for themselves. As the disease progresses to terminal stages, issues relating to grief, loss of roles and functions, and dependency on others have to be confronted (11). Therapists are learning how to assess AIDS patients' needs as more of them are being seen in health care facilities. Physicians too are learning as they care for patients with this devastating disorder.

Reimbursement of occupational therapy services has been a continuing concern in the rapidly changing health care environment. It is increasingly necessary for OTRs to identify potential consumer markets, develop appropriate programs, and sell the services they have to offer. Occupational therapists have been slow to adapt to profit-oriented health care but have found it necessary to do so as hospitals and other facilities moved to a profit-making operating style. Target groups for occupational therapy services might include the frail elderly, young adults with sports injuries, persons with back injuries, injured workers, and children with developmental delays and learning disabilities. Occupational therapy services are still not as well-known and accepted as physical therapy services. In 1990, 99% of all HMO health plans covered physical therapy services, but only 87% covered occupational therapy services (12).

Wellness and prevention have become an important focus for occupational therapists. In 1986 the *American Journal of Occupational Therapy* published a special issue on health promotion that set the stage for occupational therapy involvement in this practice area. In 1988 AOTA published a resource guide on health promotion and wellness programs for members who were planning or participating in such programs. Holistic healing and alternative systems of medicine have received increased attention in recent years, and some methods such as acupuncture and chiropractic care are being added to the health care spectrum of services. Wellness depends in part on consumer education, and both OTRs and COTAs are participating in a variety of programs to teach people how to maintain their health, prevent injuries and illnesses, or to live with a chronic condition. The first International Health and Wellness Conference was held for allied health professionals in 1992 and reflected the growing interest in this aspect of practice.

EMERGING CAREER OPTIONS

As OTRs and COTAs enter new practice environments, new career options are emerging with occupational therapy concepts being applied in new ways. Some therapists have qualified as ergonomists and are redesigning work environments in order to prevent injuries and increase worker productivity. Others are working as case managers, coordinating all aspects of an individual client's care. Consultation on the accessibility of living and work environments for the disabled and the elderly is another unique application of occupational therapy skills. Some practitioners have developed new pieces of equipment or materials for patient education and market them privately. A few pioneers are working in vision therapy in collaboration with optometrists and ophthalmologists. Experienced therapists are often creating their own jobs in nontraditional settings, thus expanding occupational therapy practice and developing new sites for service delivery.

TOMORROW'S HEALTH CARE

As the nation's health care facilities face increasing pressure to serve underserved groups and at the same time cut their costs, they confront a real dilemma. Economists expect that the U.S. health care industry will continue to grow at a rate of 2–3% annually for the rest of the decade. If cost containment efforts are not successfull, consumers and third party payers will be spending considerably more in future years.

The effort to pass national health care legislation is likely to fail. The federal government will continue to be involved both in paying for services and in regulating them. The competitive health care environment encouraged by Presidents Reagan and Bush is expected to continue, but some regulation is likely at either the state or federal level. States appear to be taking a more active role in providing health care insurance to underserved groups. Private insurers will continue to define and limit what services they will pay for, and consumers may find themselves paying a larger share of the costs.

The hospital will continue to be used only for intense, high-tech care, and costs will continue to rise. Length of patient stays will continue to decline, and as many as 20% of all hospital beds may be taken out of service. As the aging population increases, hospital admissions may rise somewhat.

More and more health care services will move to outpatient and community settings. By the year 2000, these community health services are expected to provide up to 25% of the hospitals' total income. More physicians will be employed in salaried positions and will likely lose some of their autonomy and economic control of health care (1).

The use of managed care, such as provided by HMOs, is expected to nearly double during the 1990s. Even so, the cost of health insurance may rise by as much as 70% by the year 2000. Health care providers will have to compete aggressively for patients in an intensely competitive business environment (1).

Kaiser has predicted that, in tomorrow's health care system, outcome-based reimbursement will replace reimbursement by procedure. Growth areas will include rehabilitation, occupational health and wellness, primary care, home health, outpatient services, contract arrangements, and decentralized care. Cross-training may become common, with students being trained in more than one discipline in order to deliver multiple services. Lower-level technical staff will carry out many health care procedures to cut costs. There is likely to be more sharing of resources between facilities as costs increase. Patients will accept more responsibility for their own care, and health care personnel will adopt more of a "coaching" role rather than a direct intervention role. Prevention and community health will be important concepts in health care (5).

POTENTIAL CHANGES IN OCCUPATIONAL THERAPY PRACTICE

West has suggested that occupational therapy still needs to define and consolidate its practice, focusing on the use of occupation as therapy. She believes that outside forces have forced practitioners to define their field in terms that are not compatible with the profession. Increased specialization has served to fragment and divide occupational therapists, and West proposes that what is needed in the 1990s is greater unity and cohesion of the profession (13).

Baum has urged occupational therapy personnel to consider the costs of care, changing demographics, and changing health care needs when planning their services for the 1990s. Preventive services should be given high priority, she believes, as well as services that will help employers reduce their health care costs. Proving the cost-effectiveness of occupational therapy services is a first step in this direction. Participation in wellness and fitness programs and designing programs for people with chronic disabilities could aid in health maintenance and in improving employee productivity. Baum agrees that health services will be outcome-oriented in the 1990s, and occupational therapists will find it necessary to document the effectiveness of their interventions. They will also be expected to develop practice guidelines to ensure a high quality of care. Standards of care and performance measures, says Baum, will directly influence the patterns of service that will be reimbursed and will define the patient populations that will receive service. She also encourages occupational therapy personnel to take an active part in helping to solve the multiple problems that confront health care facilities today (14).

Apter and Kolodner have discussed the increasing problem of professional burnout among OTRs and COTAs. They note that work in health care settings is increasingly stressful, as therapists are working with more severely ill or injured patients and are at the same time expected to achieve higher levels of productivity. They urge occupational therapy personnel to recognize the signs of impending burnout and take steps to deal with it effectively. With the current shortage of personnel, we cannot afford to lose experienced workers because of job stresses (15).

Yerxa has pointed out that American society is just beginning to discover the capabilities of disabled people. She sees the population of people with chronic conditions as a primary target group for occupational therapy services in the years to come. She also urges practitioners to think about the relationship of occupational therapy to medical practice. Should the field continue its close association with the medical model or should it adopt a model more attuned to its focus on the development of individuals' potential within their natural environment? This issue has long been discussed in occupational therapy, but Yerxa suggests that the time is ripe for change in the profession's alliances (16).

POTENTIAL CHANGES IN EDUCATION

Yerxa has also graphically described the possibility that academic occupational therapy programs may not survive in the current academic climate. Occupational therapy programs are often small units within colleges or universities, and their faculty are often viewed as unproductive by administrators, since, until recently, few have held doctoral degrees and there has been little involvement in research and scholarly activity. In the current climate of downsizing and budget cuts, occupational therapy programs are vulnerable. Yerxa and others believe that they can be strengthened only by the development of an academic discipline that will study the principles of human occupation and the application of those principles to clinical practice. Larger numbers of occupational therapy faculty members will need to earn doctoral degrees, engage in meaningful research and publication, and participate fully in the mission of their institutions. Occupational therapy curricula may require major revision in order to provide students with an organized continuum of knowledge founded on a liberal arts base. More graduate programs must be developed to permit advanced study, and financial support must be found for graduate students (17).

West suggests that nonoccupational therapy faculty be used to add depth to educational programs and that occupational therapy curricula should teach principles rather than techniques. If occupational therapists are to become creative problem solvers rather than technicians, the knowledge of theory and principles of practice is more important than technical know-how (13).

Occupational therapy education is in a period of transition as it attempts to prepare students to enter the world of clinical practice while simultaneously trying to gear up to the demands of the academic environment. Progress is being made, but it will require more qualified occupational therapy faculty who are committed to an academic career and can meet the expectations of today's colleges and universities.

POTENTIAL CHANGES IN RESEARCH

West has emphasized the fact that increased research funding is needed to support investigations into high-priority questions that confront the profession. Another need is for outcome studies that document the effectiveness of occupational therapy intervention. Qualitative research methodology seems to hold promise as an appropriate method for occupational therapy researchers, and West urges its use by more investigators (13).

Gillette has provided some examples of occupational therapy questions that need to be explored through research. Among them are the following.

Can changes in underlying biological and neurophysiological mechanisms be documented after occupational therapy intervention?

How can improvements in client function be attributed to the effects of occupational therapy when clients are receiving multiple forms of treatment?

Can selected occupational therapy techniques (sensory integration, purposeful activity) be shown to directly influence neurochemical changes in schizophrenic patients?

How do individuals' activity choices influence the state of their health?

What characteristics make one person a good candidate for rehabilitation and another person a poor candidate?

What effect does meaningful activity have on mentally confused elderly persons?

What test instruments most effectively measure clinical and behavioral change? (18)

These are only a few of the questions occupational therapists need answers to. If the field is to progress and develop its full potential, it needs to produce researchers who can begin to investigate both basic and applied research questions.

DIRECTIONS FOR THE FUTURE

In 1990, 200 OTRs and COTAs met to discuss the future of the field. A wide range of ideas were presented and the participants developed a number of recommendations for actions that would lead to new directions for occupational therapy. Among the recommendations were the following.

Development of hierarchies of education and practice;

Increased faculty and student recruitment, especially among minorities;
Development of symposia to focus on graduate education, theory development, and research;
Study of where the control of fieldwork should be located and additional support for graduate education; and
Development of a professional focus statement (19).

These plans are already beginning to be implemented and incorporate some ideas that we discuss in this chapter. AOTA leaders and rank-and-file members are making an effort to create planned change in the profession in response to a changing social and professional environment. Ann Grady, then the AOTA president, pointed out that any major changes in a field's direction require input from many people. AOTA continues to seek advice from its members and from outside groups in planning for professional change. In planning for their future, occupational therapy personnel are strengthening the viability of the profession and guiding its development in a structured way. Nielson has recognized that for all of these plans to succeed it will be necessary for occupational therapy personnel to understand the concept of power and how to use the power they possess. She points out that occupational therapists' collective power comes from their professional base, whereas their individual power comes from their competence and ability to perform successfully in health care settings. She urges practitioners, educators, and researchers to develop their individual power and to unite in order to develop collective power. Only by mobilizing their power as a profession can occupational therapists hope to influence and exert some control over the systems they operate in, says Nielson (20).

MAINTAINING TRADITIONAL VALUES IN A CHANGING SOCIETY

Englehardt (21) notes that advances in technology invariably give rise to questions of ethics and values. Health care professionals, in particular, need to consider their traditional values in deciding how to apply technological advances. Will occupational therapy values and principles continue to be relevant? The answer given by occupational therapy leaders is a resounding "yes!" In 1986 Bing (22) reviewed some of the major concepts of the field as they were stated by its founders and pioneers and concluded that these ideas continue to express the basic philosophy of occupational therapy. "We will find comfort, safety, and stability . . . in those decades-old fundamentals and principles developed by our founders and practiced by our pioneers and each succeeding generation of therapists," said Bing, a former president of AOTA. "The belief system that has emerged . . . will continue to develop as time moves on" (22).

Another former president of AOTA agreed. Johnson (23) elaborated further on the impact of societal and health care changes on traditional occupational therapy values. She outlined six occupational therapy values that express basic beliefs about the field.

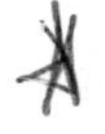

1. The value of the individual as a total person;
2. The value of purposeful activity and occupation in producing change and recovery;
3. The value of goal-oriented activity designed for a given individual's skills and abilities;
4. The value of permitting patients to choose meaningful activities . . . which parallel those they might normally engage in;
5. The value of seeing the individual interacting within the framework of the environment; and
6. The value we place on ourselves, our feelings, and our interactions with patients/clients as vital, integral, and caring components of the therapeutic process.

These values, which appear and reappear throughout the occupational therapy literature, continue to be meaningful to occupational therapists. Johnson notes that occupational therapists have been highly successful in adapting their tools, techniques, and values to new groups of clients. The repertoire of occupational therapists has expanded to include splinting and orthotics, use of self, prevocational exploration, and neurodevelopmental and kinesiological theories and techniques. Perhaps occupational therapists have overadapted, Johnson suggests. As a result, there is an increased demand for their services, but some of the new directions taken seem to be the result of external forces rather than the application of our traditional values.

Overadaptation to the changing health care scene has had some negative consequences, Johnson believes. Inadequate preparation for today's stressful clinical environments can lead to new therapists feeling overwhelmed by the demands being placed on them. Occupational therapy has not provided adequate nurturing or recognition for those of its members who work as administrators, clinical specialists, researchers, or curriculum directors. Practitioners have been so busy selling their clinical skills that they have neglected to do the work necessary to substantiate the effectiveness of those skills.

Finally, the field has become so concerned with personnel shortages that it has neglected its conceptual issues. The goal for the future, says Johnson, should be to "understand the cause of dysfunction; diagnose dysfunction as it affects performance and occupation; to identify and establish the appropriate program and process for specific individuals that will result in adaptation and . . . reintegration; and to bring about change in society and technology so that both share the responsibility for adapting to the needs of humans. . ." (23). Johnson sees occupational therapy as facing a conflict between a desire to retain traditional values and a recognition of the importance of science and research. Therapists, however, are worried about where an emphasis on science and research will take the field. Will occupational therapy continue to hold its humanistic values in a world where every fact must be proven and every method put to the test? Johnson concludes that the two points of view can be reconciled and that, by doing so, the profession will acquire new competence. "The process of adaptation will bring about change, but integration can provide us with a unity and a wholeness which we have not yet achieved" (23).

As occupational therapy prepares to enter its second century, it is readying itself to meet new challenges and expectations. Occupational therapists and therapy assistants will be able to successfully adapt to the changing health care scene. When questioning their contributions to the health care of the future, Dunn (24) suggests that occupational therapists ask themselves, "What business are we really in?" The answer is that occupational therapy is still in the business it has always been in—that of facilitating lifelong independence in individuals. Its methods have changed and will continue to change; its work sites may be different from those of the past, but the concerns of occupational therapists remain the same. Occupational therapy is in the business of helping people adapt to physical, psychosocial, and environmental changes in their lives, and it will be able to survive and grow in the health care environment of the 21st century.

Discussion Questions

1. What occupational therapy specialty areas may be most needed in the 1990s? Why?
2. Are the current trends in health care likely to improve the general health of the population?
3. Will the United States ever have guaranteed health care for all of its citizens?
4. The increasing cultural diversity in the United States poses real challenges to health care providers. How can occupational therapy personnel prepare themselves to work with more diverse client populations?

5. Many of the current health problems in the United States reflect social disorganization and the lack of preventive care for low-income and minority groups. What role can occupational therapists play in improving this situation?
6. Increasingly health care fields are experiencing a knowledge explosion as new information and technology develop rapidly. A commitment to lifelong learning is necessary to keep up with changes in practice. Are you ready to make this commitment?

References

1. Amara R: Health care tomorrow. *The Futurist* pp. 16–20, Nov–Dec, 1988.
2. Research Information and Evaluation Division, AOTA: *Trends in the Environment*. Rockville, MD, AOTA, pp. 1–9, 1989.
3. Staff: Ten health trends for 1992. *OT Week* 6(19):10, 1992.
4. Joe BE: Tomorrow's health care system? *OT Week* 6(20):10, 1992.
5. Egan M: Rehabilitation research plan prompts call to action. *OT Week* 6(19):8, 1992.
6. AOTA: 1990 Member Data Survey, Special Insert. *OT Week* 5(22):1–8, 1991.
7. Joe BE: AOTA recruitment efforts enlarge student pool. *OT Week* 6(16):8, 1992.
8. Heater SL: The issue is: specialization or uniformity within the profession. *AJOT* 46(2)172–173, 1992.
9. Mastrangelo R: OTs say credentialing adds practice options. *Adv Occup Ther* 6(12):1–2, 17, 1990.
10. King PM: Profiling the work-hardening therapist. *AJOT* 46(9):847–849, 1992.
11. Pizzi M: The model of human occupation and adults with HIV infections and AIDS. *AJOT* 44(3):257–264, 1990.
12. AOTA: HMO Industry Profile, Table 2, in *National Policy Forum*. Rockville, MD, AOTA, 1992, pp. 6.
13. West WL: Perspectives on the past and future, part 2. *AJOT* 44(1):9–10, 1990.
14. Baum CM: Nationally Speaking: The environment: providing opportunities for the future. *AJOT* 45(6):487–490, 1991.
15. Apter LC, Kolodner EL: Professional burnout: are you a candidate? *Occup Ther Forum* II(37):5, 1987.
16. Yerxa EJ: Some implications of occupational therapy's history for its epistemology, values, and relation to medicine. *AJOT* 46(1):79–83, 1992.
17. Yerxa EJ: Nationally Speaking: Occupational therapy: an endangered species or an academic discipline in the 21st century? *AJOT* 45(8):680–685, 1991.
18. Gillette NP: The Issue Is: Research directions for occupational therapy. *AJOT* 45(6):563–565, 1991.
19. Grady AP: Nationally Speaking: Directions for the future: opportunities for leadership. *AJOT* 45(1):7–9, 1991.
20. Nielson C: The Issue Is: Positioning for power. *AJOT* 45(9):853–854, 1991,
21. Englehardt T: The importance of values in shaping professional directions and behaviors. In *Proceedings. Target 2000: Occupational Therapy Education*. Rockville, MD, AOTA, 1986, pp. 39–44.
22. Bing R: Nationally Speaking: The subject is health: not of facts, but of values. *AJOT* 40:667–671, 1986.
23. Johnson J: Old values–new directions: competence, adaptation, integration. *AJOT* 35:589–598, 1981.
24. Dunn W: Keynote address: challenging our energies–a focus on the future. Annual Conference of the Wisconsin Occupational Therapy Association, September 19–20, 1986.

Suggested Readings

Amara R, Schmid G, Morrison JI: *Looking Ahead at American Health Care*. Washington DC, McGraw-Hill, 1988.

AOTA: Special Issue on Health Promotion. *AJOT* 40:11, Nov 1986.

AOTA: Special Issue on Technology. *AJOT* 41:11, Nov 1987.

AOTA: Special Issue on Ethics. *AJOT* 42:5, May 1988.

AOTA: Special Issue on AIDS. *AJOT* 44:3, March 1990.

AOTA: Special Issue on Cross-Cultural Perspectives in Occupational Therapy. *AJOT* 46:8, Aug 1992.

Rothman J, Levine R: *Prevention Practice: Strategies for Occupational Therapy and Physical Therapy*. Orlando, FL, WB Saunders, 1992.

SECTION IV

APPENDICES

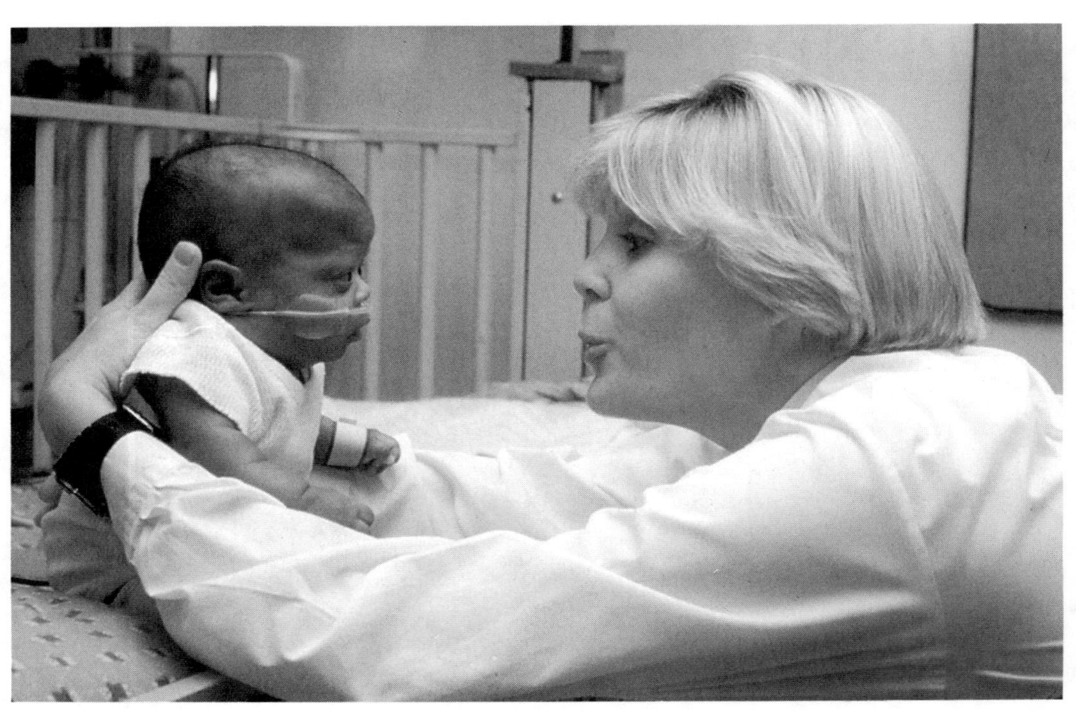

Appendix

1 Standards of Practice for Occupational Therapy[a]

PREFACE

These standards are intended as recommended guidelines to assist occupational therapy practitioners in the provision of occupational therapy services. These standards serve as a minimum standard for occupational therapy practice and are applicable to all individual populations and the programs in which these individuals are served.

These standards apply to those registered occupational therapists and certified occupational therapy assistants who are in compliance with regulation where it exists. The term *occupational therapy practitioner* refers to the registered occupational therapist and to the certified occupational therapy assistant, both of whom are in compliance with regulation where it exists.

The minimum educational requirements for the registered occupational therapist are described in the current *Essentials and Guidelines of an Accredited Educational Program for the Occupational Therapist* (American Occupational Therapy Association (AOTA), 1991a). The minimum educational requirements for the certified occupational therapy assistant are described in the current *Essentials and Guidelines of an Accredited Educational Program for the Occupational Therapy Asssistant* (AOTA, 1991b).

[a] AOTA Commission on Practice: Standards of Practice for Occupational Therapy. *AJOT 46(12):1082–1085, 1992.*

STANDARD I: PROFESSIONAL STANDING

1. An occupational therapy practitioner shall maintain a current license, registration, or certification as required by law.
2. An occupational therapy practitioner shall practice and manage occupational therapy programs in accordance with applicable federal and state laws and regulations.
3. An occupational therapy practitioner shall be familiar with and abide by AOTA's (1988) *Occupational Therapy Code of Ethics*.
4. An occupational therapy practitioner shall maintain and update professional knowledge, skills, and abilities through appropriate continuing education or in-service training or higher education. The nature and minimum amount of continuing education must be consistent with state law and regulation.
5. A certified occupational therapy assistant must receive supervision from a registered occupational therapist as defined by the current *Supervision Guidelines for Certified Occupational Therapy Assistants* (AOTA, 1990) and by official AOTA documents. The nature and amount of supervision must be provided in accordance with state law and regulation.
6. An occupational therapy practitioner shall provide direct and indirect services in accordance with AOTA's standards and policies. The nature and scope of occupational therapy services provided must

be in accordance with state law and regulation.

7. An occupational therapy practitioner shall maintain current knowledge of the legislative, political, social, and cultural issues that affect the profession.

STANDARD II: REFERRAL

1. A registered occupational therapist shall accept referrals in accordance with AOTA's *Statement of Occupational Therapy Referral* (AOTA, 1989) and in compliance with appropriate laws.
2. A registered occupational therapist may accept referrals for assessment or assessment with intervention in occupational performance areas or occupational performance components when individuals have or appear to have dysfunctions or potential for dysfunctions.
3. A registered occupational therapist, responding to requests for service, may accept cases within the parameters of the laws.
4. A registered occupational therapist shall assume responsibility for determining the appropriateness of the scope, frequency, and duration of services within the parameters of the law.
5. A registered occupational therapist shall refer individuals to other appropriate resources when the therapist determines that the knowledge and expertise of other professionals is indicated.
6. An occupational therapy practitioner shall educate current and potential referral sources about the process of initiating occupational therapy referrals.

STANDARD III: SCREENING

1. A registered occupational therapist, in accordance with state and federal guidelines, shall conduct screening to determine whether intervention or further assessment is necessary and to identify dysfunctions in occupational performance areas.
2. A registered occupational therapist shall screen independently or as a member of an interdisciplinary team. A certified occupational therapy assistant may contribute to the screening process under the supervision of a registered occupational therapist.
3. A registered occupational therapist shall select screening methods that are appropriate to the individual's age and development level; gender; education; cultural background; and socioeconomic, medical, and functional status. Screening methods may include, but are not limited to, interviews, structured observations, informal testing, and record reviews.
4. A registered occupational therapist shall communicate screening results and recommendations to appropriate individuals.

STANDARD IV: ASSESSMENT

1. A registered occupational therapist shall assess an individual's occupational performance components and occupational performance areas. A registered occupational therapist conducts assessments individually or as part of a team of professionals, as appropriate to the practice settings and the purposes of the assessments. A certified occupational therapy assistant may contribute to the assessment process under the supervision of a registered occupational therapist.
2. An occupational therapy practitioner shall educate the individual, or the individual's family or legal guardian, as appropriate, about the purposes and procedures of the occupational therapy assessment.
3. A registered occupational therapist shall select assessments to determine the in-

dividual's functional abilities and problems as related to occupational performance areas; occupational performance components; physical, social, and cultural environments; performance safety; and prevention of dysfunction.

4. Occupational therapy assessment methods shall be appropriate to the individual's age and developmental level; gender; education; socioeconomic, cultural, and ethnic background; medical status; and functional abilities. The assessment methods may include some combination of skilled observation, interview, record review, or the use of standardized or criterion-referenced tests. A certified occupational therapy assistant may contribute to the assessment process under the supervision of a registered occupational therapist.
5. An occupational therapy practitioner shall follow accepted protocols when standardized tests are used. Standardized tests are tests whose scores are based on accompanying normative data that may reflect age ranges, gender, ethnic groups, geographic regions, and socioeconomic status. If standardized tests are not available or appropriate, the results shall be expressed in descriptive reports, and standardized scales shall not be used.
6. A registered occupational therapist shall analyze and summarize collected evaluation data to indicate the individual's current functional status.
7. A registered occupational therapist shall document assessment results in the individual's records, noting the specific evaluation methods and tools used.
8. A registered occupational therapist shall complete and document results of occupational therapy assessments within the time frames established by practice settings, government agencies, accreditation programs, and third-party payers.
9. An occupational therapy practitioner shall communicate assessment results, within the boundaries of client confidentiality, to the appropriate persons.
10. A registered occupational therapist shall refer the individual to the appropriate services or request additional consultations if the results of the assessments indicate areas that require intervention by other professionals.

STANDARD V: INTERVENTION PLAN

1. A registered occupational therapist shall develop and document an intervention plan based on analysis of the occupational therapy assessment data and the individual's expected outcome after the intervention. A certified occupational therapy assistant may contribute to the intervention plan under the supervision of a registered occupational therapist.
2. The occupational therapy intervention plan shall be stated in goals that are clear, measurable, behavioral, functional, and appropriate to the individual's needs, personal goals, and expected outcome after intervention.
3. The occupational therapy intervention plan shall reflect the philosophical base of occupational therapy (AOTA, 1979) and be consistent with its established principles and concepts of theory and practice. The intervention planning processes shall include:
   a. Formulating a list of strengths and weaknesses.
   b. Estimating rehabilitation potential.
   c. Identifying measurable short-term and long-term goals.
   d. Collaborating with the individual, family members, other caregivers, professionals, and community resources.
   e. Selecting the media, methods, environment, and personnel needed to accomplish the intervention goals.

f. Determining the frequency and duration of occupational therapy services.
g. Identifying a plan for reevaluation.
h. Discharge planning.

4. A registered occupational therapist shall prepare and document the intervention plan within the time frames and according to the standards established by the employing practice settings, government agencies, accreditation programs, and third-party payers. The certified occupational therapy assistant may contribute to the formation of the intervention plan under the supervision of the registered occupational therapist.

STANDARD VI: INTERVENTION

1. An occupational therapy practitioner shall implement a program according to the developed intervention plan. The plan shall be appropriate to the individual's age and developmental level, gender, education, cultural and ethnic background, health status, functional ability, interests, and personal goals, and service provision setting. The certified occupational therapy assistant shall implement the intervention under the supervision of a registered occupational therapist.
2. An occupational therapy practitioner shall implement the intervention plan through the use of specified purposeful activities or therapeutic methods to enhance occupational performance and achieve stated goals.
3. An occupational therapy practitioner shall be knowledgeable about relevant research in the practitioner's areas of practice. A registered occupational therapist shall interpret research findings as appropriate for application to the intervention process.
4. An occupational therapy practitioner shall educate the individual, the individual's family or legal guardian, noncertified occupational therapy personnel, and nonoccupational therapy staff, as appropriate, in activities that support the established intervention plan. An occupational therapy practitioner shall communicate the risk and benefit of the intervention.
5. An occupational therapy practitioner shall maintain current information on community resources relevant to the practice area of the practitioner.
6. A registered occupational therapist shall periodically reassess and document the individual's levels of functioning and changes in levels of functioning in the occupational performance areas and occupational performance components. A certified occupational therapy assistant may contribute to the reassessment process under the supervision of a registered occupational therapist.
7. A registered occupational therapist shall formulate and implement program modifications consistent with changes in the individual's response to the intervention. A certified occupational therapy assistant may contribute to program modifications under the supervision of a registered occupational therapist.
8. An occupational therapy practitioner shall document the occupational therapy services provided, including the frequency and duration of the services within the time frames and according to the standards established by the employing facility, government agencies, accreditation programs, and third-party payers.

STANDARD VII: DISCONTINUATION

1. A registered occupational therapist shall discontinue service when the individual has achieved predetermined goals

or has achieved maximum benefit from occupational therapy services.

2. A registered occupational therapist, with input from a certified occupational therapy assistant where applicable, shall prepare and implement a discharge plan that is consistent with occupational therapy goals, individual goals, interdisciplinary team goals, family goals, and expected outcomes. The discharge plan shall address appropriate community resources for referral for psychosocial, cultural, and socioeconomic barriers and limitations that may need modification.
3. A registered occupational therapist shall document the changes between the initial and current states of functional ability and deficit in occupational performance areas and occupational performance components. A certified occupational therapy assistant may contribute to the process under the supervision of a registered occupational therapist.
4. An occupational therapy practitioner shall allow sufficient time for the coordination and effective implementation of the discharge plan.
5. A registered occupational therapist shall document recommendations for follow-up or reevaluation when applicable.

Standard VIII: Continuous Quality Improvement

1. An occupational therapy practitioner shall monitor and document the continuous quality improvement of practice, which may include outcomes of services, using predetermined practice criteria reflecting professional consensus, recent developments in research, and specific employing facility standards.
2. An occupational therapy practitioner shall monitor all aspects of individual occupational therapy services for effectiveness and timeliness. If actual care does not meet the prescribed standard, it must be justified by peer review or other appropriate means within the practice setting. Occupational therapy services shall be discontinued when no longer necessary.
3. A registered occupational therapist shall systematically assess the review process of patient care to determine the success or appropriateness of interventions. Certified occupational therapy assistants may contribute to the process in collaboration with the registered occupational therapist.

STANDARD IX: MANAGEMENT

1. A registered occupational therapist shall provide the management necessary for efficient organization and provision of occupational therapy services.
2. A certified occupational therapy assistant, under the supervision of a registered occupational therapist, may perform the following management functions:
   a. Education of members of other related professions and physicians about occupational therapy.
   b. Participation in (1) orientation, supervision, training, and evaluation of the performance of volunteers and other noncertified occupational therapy personnel, and (2) developing plans to remediate areas of skill deficit in the performance of job duties by volunteers and other noncertified occupational therapy personnel.
   c. Design and periodic review of all aspects of the occupational therapy program to determine its effectiveness, efficiency, and future directions.

d. Systematic review of the quality of service provided, using criteria established by professional consensus and current research, as well as established standards for state regulation; accreditation; American Occupational Therapy Certification Board (AOTCB) certification; and related laws, policies, guidelines, and regulations.
e. Incorporation of a fair and equitable system of admission, discharge, and charges for occupational therapy services.
f. Participation in crossdisciplinary activities to ensure that the total needs of the individual are met.
g. Provision of support (i.e, space, time, money as feasible) for clinical research or collaborative research when such projects have the approval of the appropriate governing bodies (e.g., institutional review board), and the results of which are deemed potentially beneficial to individuals of occupational therapy services now or in the future.

REFERENCES

American Occupational Therapy Association. (1979). The philosophical base of occupational therapy. *American Journal of Occupational Therapy*, 33, 785.

American Occupational Therapy Association. (1988). Occupational therapy code of ethics. *American Journal of Occupational Therapy*, 42, 795–796.

American Occupational Therapy Association. (1989). Statement of occupational therapy referral. In *Reference manual of the official documents of The American Occupational Therapy Association, Inc.* (AOTA) (p. VIII.1). Rockville, MD: Author (Original work published 1969, revised 1980).

American Occupational Therapy Association. (1990). Supervision guidelines for certified occupational therapy assistants. *American Journal of Occupational Therapy*, 44, 1089–1090.

American Occupational Therapy Association. (1991a). *Essentials and guidelines of an accredited educational program for the occupational therapist*. Rockville, MD: Author.

American Occupational Therapy Association. (1991b). *Essentials and guidelines of an accredited educational program for the occupational therapy assistant*. Rockville, MD: Author.

Prepared by the Commission on Practice (Jim Hinojosa, PhD, OTR, FAOTA, Chair).

Approved by the Representative Assembly March 1992.

*This document replaces the 1983 Standards of Practice for Occupational Therapy (*American Journal of Occupational Therapy*, 37, 802–804), which was rescinded by the 1992 Representative Assembly.*

Appendix

2 Occupational Therapy Code of Ethics[b]

The American Occupational Therapy Association and its component members are committed to furthering people's ability to function fully within their total environment. To this end the occupational therapist renders service to clients in all stages of health and illness, to institutions, to other professionals and colleagues, to students, and to the general public.

In furthering this commitment, the American Occupational Therapy Association has established the Occupational Therapy Code of Ethics. This code is intended to be used as a guide to promoting and maintaining the highest standards of ethical behavior.

This Code of Ethics shall apply to all occupational therapy personnel. The term *occupational therapy personnel* shall include individuals who are registered occupational therapists, certified occupational therapy assistants, and occupational therapy students. The roles of practitioner, educator, manager, researcher, and consultant are assumed.

PRINCIPLE 1 (Beneficence/Autonomy)

Occupational therapy personnel shall demonstrate a concern for the welfare and dignity of the recipient of their services.

A. The individual is responsible for providing services without regard to race, creed, national origin, sex, age, handicap, disease entity, social status, financiaı status, or religious affiliation.

B. The individual shall inform those people served of the nature and potential outcomes of treatment and shall respect the right of potential recipients of service to refuse treatment.

C. The individual shall inform subjects involved in education or research activities of the potential outcome of those activities.

D. The individual shall include those people served in the treatment planning process.

E. The individual shall maintain goal-directed and objective relationships with all people served.

F. The individual shall protect the confidential nature of information gained from educational, practice, and investigational activities unless sharing such information could be deemed necessary to protect the well-being of a third party.

G. The individual shall take all reasonable precautions to avoid harm to the recipient of services or detriment to the recipient's property.

H. The individual shall establish fees, based on cost analysis, that are commensurate with services rendered.

PRINCIPLE 2 (Competence)

Occupational therapy personnel shall actively maintain high standards of professional competence.

A. The individual shall hold the appropriate credential for providing service.

B. The individual shall recognize the need for competence and shall participate in continuing professional development.

[b] AOTA: Occupational Therapy Code of Ethics. *AJOT* 42(12):795–796, 1988.

C. The individual shall function within the parameters of his or her competence and the standards of the profession.
D. The individual shall refer clients to other service providers or consult with other service providers when additional knowledge and expertise is required.

PRINCIPLE 3 (Compliance with Laws and Regulations)

Occupational therapy personnel shall comply with laws and Association policies guiding the profession of occupational therapy.

A. The individual shall be acquainted with applicable local, state, federal, and institutional rules and Association policies and shall function accordingly.
B. The individual shall inform employers, employees, and colleagues about those laws and policies that apply to the profession of occupational therapy.
C. The individual shall require those whom they supervise to adhere to the Code of Ethics.
D. The individual shall accurately record and report information.

PRINCIPLE 4 (Public Information)

Occupational therapy personnel shall provide accurate information concerning occupational therapy services.

A. The individual shall accurately represent his or her competence and training.
B. The individual shall not use or participate in the use of any form of communication that contains a false, fraudulent, deceptive, or unfair statement or claim.

PRINCIPLE 5 (Professional Relationships)

Occupational therapy personnel shall function with discretion and integrity in relations with colleagues and other professionals and shall be concerned with the quality of their services.

A. The individual shall report illegal, incompetent, and/or unethical practice to the appropriate authority.
B. The individual shall not disclose privileged information when participating in reviews of peers, programs, or systems.
C. The individual who employs or supervises colleagues shall provide appropriate supervision, as defined in AOTA guidelines or state laws, regulations, and institutional policies.
D. The individual shall recognize the contributions of colleagues when disseminating professional information.

PRINCIPLE 6 (Professional Conduct)

Occupational therapy personnel shall not engage in any form of conduct that constitutes a conflict of interest or that adversely reflects on the profession.

This document was approved by the Representative Assembly in April 1988; it replaces the (1977/1979) "Principles of Occupational Therapy Ethics."

Appendix

3 Grounds for Discipline[c]

Incompetence. Engaging in conduct which evidences a lack of knowledge of, or lack of ability or failure to apply, the prevailing principles and/or skills of the profession for which the individual has been certified.

Unethical Behavior. Violating prevailing ethical standards of the profession relating to the safe, proficient and/or competent practice of occupational therapy, including:

a. Making false statements or providing false information in connection with an application for certification.
b. Misrepresentation of one's credentials (education, training, experience, competence).
c. Engaging in false, misleading or deceptive advertising.
d. Obtaining or attempting to obtain compensation by fraud or deceit.
e. Violating any federal or state statute or law which relates to the practice for which the individual has a certificate.
f. Engaging in assault and battery of patients or others with whom the practitioner has a professional relationship.
g. Engaging in sexual misconduct or abuse involving patients or others with whom the practitioner has a professional relationship.
h. Being convicted of a crime, the circumstances of which substantially relate to the practice of occupational therapy or indicate an inability to engage in the practice of occupational therapy safely, proficiently, and/or competently.
i. Otherwise violating the prevailing standards of the profession relating to the safe, proficient, and/or competent practice of occupational therapy.

Impairment. **The inability to engage in the practice of occupational therapy safely, proficiently, and/or competently as a result of substance abuse, or physical or psychological disability. This includes, but is not limited to:**

a. Engaging in professional practice while one's ability to practice is impaired by alcohol or other drugs.
b. Engaging in practice while one's ability to practice is impaired by reason of physical or mental disability or disease.
c. Being adjudicated mentally incompetent by a court.

For additional information contact: The American Occupational Therapy Certification Board, Inc.
4 Research Place, Suite 160,
Rockville, Maryland 20850-3226
(301)990-7979
FAX (301)869-8492

[c] AOTCB: *Disciplinary Action: A Process to Protect the Public.* Rockville, MD, AOATCB, 1991.

Appendix

4 Uniform Terminology for Occupational Therapy—Second Edition[d]

OUTLINE

Occupational Therapy Assessment
Occupational Therapy Intervention

I. **OCCUPATIONAL THERAPY PERFORMANCE AREAS**
   A. Activities of Daily Living
      1. Grooming
      2. Oral hygiene
      3. Bathing
      4. Toilet hygiene
      5. Dressing
      6. Feeding and eating
      7. Medication routine
      8. Socialization
      9. Functional communication
      10. Functional mobility
      11. Sexual expression
   B. Work Activities
      1. Home management
         a. Clothing care
         b. Cleaning
         c. Meal preparation and cleanup
         d. Shopping
         e. Money management
         f. Household maintenance
         g. Safety procedures
      2. Care of others
      3. Educational activities
      4. Vocational activities
         a. Vocational exploration
         b. Job acquisition
         c. Work or job performance
         d. Retirement planning
   C. Play or Leisure Activities
      1. Play or leisure exploration
      2. Play or leisure performance

II. **PERFORMANCE COMPONENTS**
   A. Sensory Motor Component
      1. Sensory integration
         a. Sensory awareness
         b. Sensory processing
            (1) Tactile
            (2) Proprioceptive
            (3) Vestibular
            (4) Visual
            (5) Auditory
            (6) Gustatory
            (7) Olfactory
         c. Perceptual skills
            (1) Stereognosis
            (2) Kinesthesia
            (3) Body scheme
            (4) Right-left discrimination
            (5) Form constancy
            (6) Position in space
            (7) Visual closure
            (8) Figure-ground
            (9) Depth perception
            (10) Topographical orientation
      2. Neuromuscular
         a. Reflex
         b. Range of motion
         c. Muscle tone

[d]AOTA: Uniform Terminology for Occupational Therapy, Second Edition. *AJOT* 43(12):808–814, 1989.

d. Strength
e. Endurance
f. Postural control
g. Soft tissue integrity

3. Motor
a. Activity tolerance
b. Gross motor coordination
c. Crossing the midline
d. Laterality
e. Bilateral integration
f. Praxis
g. Fine motor coordination/dexterity
h. Visual-motor integration
i. Oral-motor control

B. Cognitive Integration and Cognitive Components
1. Level of arousal
2. Orientation
3. Recognition
4. Attention span
5. Memory
a. Short-term
b. Long-term
c. Remote
d. Recent
6. Sequencing
7. Categorization
8. Concept formation
9. Intellectual operations in space
10. Problem solving
11. Generalization of learning
12. Integration of learning
13. Synthesis of learning

C. Psychosocial Skills and Psychological Components
1. Psychological
a. Roles
b. Values
c. Interests
d. Initiation of activity
e. Termination of activity
f. Self-concept
2. Social
a. Social conduct
b. Conversation
c. Self-expression
3. Self-management
a. Coping skills
b. Time management
c. Self-control

OCCUPATIONAL THERAPY ASSESSMENT

Assessment is the planned process of obtaining, interpreting, and documenting the functional status of the individual. The purpose of the assessment is to identify the individual's abilities and limitations, including deficits, delays, or maladaptive behavior that can be addressed in occupational therapy intervention. Data can be gathered through a review of records, observation, interview, and the administration of test procedures. Such procedures include, but are not limited to, the use of standardized tests, questionnaires, performance checklists, activities, and tasks designed to evaluate specific performance abilities.

OCCUPATIONAL THERAPY INTERVENTION

Occupational therapy addresses function and uses specific procedures and activities to (a) develop, maintain, improve, and/or restore the performance of necessary functions; (b) compensate for dysfunction; (c) minimize or prevent debilitation; and/or (d) promote health and wellness. Categories of function are defined as OCCUPATIONAL PERFORMANCE AREAS and PERFORMANCE COMPONENTS. OCCUPATIONAL PERFORMANCE AREAS include activities of daily living, work activities, and play/leisure activities. Performance components refer to the functional abilities required for occupational performance, including sensory motor, cognitive, and psychological components. Deficits or delays in these OCCUPATIONAL PERFORMANCE AREAS may be addressed by occupational therapy intervention.

I. OCCUPATIONAL PERFORMANCE AREAS

A. Activities of Daily Living

1. *Grooming*—Obtain and use supplies to shave; apply and remove cosmetics; wash, comb, style, and brush hair; care for nails; care for skin; and apply deodorant.
2. *Oral Hygiene*—Obtain and use supplies; clean mouth and teeth; remove, clean, and reinsert dentures.
3. *Bathing*—Obtain and use supplies; soap, rinse, and dry all body parts; maintain bathing position; transfer to and from bathing position.
4. *Toilet Hygiene*—Obtain and use supplies; clean self; transfer to and from, and maintain toileting position on bedpan, toilet, or commode.
5. *Dressing*—Select appropriate clothing; obtain clothing from storage area; dress and undress in a sequential fashion; and fasten and adjust clothing and shoes. Don and doff assistive or adaptive equipment, prostheses, or orthoses.
6. *Feeding and Eating*—Set up food; use appropriate utensils and tableware; bring food or drink to mouth; suck, masticate, cough, and swallow.
7. *Medication Routine*—Obtain medication; open and close containers; and take prescribed quantities as scheduled.
8. *Socialization*—Interact in appropriate contextual and cultural ways.
9. *Functional Communication*—Use equipment or systems to enhance or provide communication, such as writing equipment, telephones, typewriters, communication boards, call lights, emergency systems, Braille writers, augmentative communication systems, and computers.
10. *Functional Mobility*—Move from one position or place to another, such as in bed mobility, wheelchair mobility, transfers (bed, car, tub, toilet, chair), and functional ambulation, with or without adaptive aids, driving, and use of public transportation.
11. *Sexual Expression*—Recognize, communicate, and perform desired sexual activities.

B. Work Activities
   1. *Home Management*
      a. *Clothing Care*—Obtain and use supplies, launder, iron, store, and mend.
      b. *Cleaning*—Obtain and use supplies, pick up, vacuum, sweep, dust, scrub, mop, make bed, and remove trash.
      c. *Meal Preparation and Cleanup*—Plan nutritious meals and prepare food; open and close containers, cabinets, and drawers; use kitchen utensils and appliances; and clean up and store food.
      d. *Shopping*—Select and purchase items and perform money transactions.
      e. *Money Management*—Budget, pay bills, and use bank systems.
      f. *Household Maintenance*—Maintain home, yard, garden appliances, and household items, and/or obtain appropriate assistance.
      g. *Safety Procedures*—Know and perform prevention and emergency procedures to maintain a safe environment and prevent injuries.

2. *Care of Others*—Provide for children, spouse, parents, or others, such as the physical care, nurturance, communication, and use of age-appropriate activities.
3. *Educational Activities*—Participate in a school environment and school-sponsored activities (such as field trips, work-study, and extracurricular activities).
4. *Vocational Activities*
   a. *Vocational Exploration*—Determine aptitudes, interests, skills, and appropriate vocational pursuits.
   b. *Job Acquisition*—Identify and select work opportunities and complete application and interview processes.
   c. *Work or Job Performance*—Perform job tasks in a timely and effective manner, incorporating necessary work behaviors such as grooming, interpersonal skills, punctuality, and adherence to safety procedures.
   d. *Retirement Planning*—Determine aptitudes, interests, skills, and identify appropriate avocational pursuits.

C. Play or Leisure Activities
1. *Play or Leisure Exploration*—Identify interests, skills, opportunities, and appropriate play or leisure activities.
2. *Play or Leisure Performance*—Participate in play or leisure activities, using physical and psychosocial skills.
   a. Maintain a balance of play or leisure activities with work and activities of daily living.
   b. Obtain, utilize, and maintain equipment and supplies.

II. PERFORMANCE COMPONENTS

A. Sensory Motor Component
1. *Sensory Integration*
   a. *Sensory Awareness*—Receive and differentiate sensory stimuli.
   b. *Sensory Processing*—Interpret sensory stimuli.
      (1) *Tactile*—Interpret light touch, pressure, temperature, pain, vibration, and two-point stimuli through skin contact/receptors.
      (2) *Proprioceptive* — Interpret stimuli originating in muscles, joints, and other internal tissues to give information about the position of one body part in relationship to another.
      (3) *Vestibular* — Interpret stimuli from the inner ear receptors regarding head position and movement.
      (4) *Visual*—Interpret stimuli through the eyes, including peripheral vision and acuity, awareness of color, depth, and figure-ground.
      (5) *Auditory* — Interpret sounds, localize sounds, and discriminate background sounds.
      (6) *Gustatory* — Interpret tastes.
      (7) *Olfactory* — Interpret odors.
   c. *Perceptual Skills*
      (1) *Stereognosis* — Identify objects through the sense of touch.
      (2) *Kinesthesia*—Identify the excursion and direction of joint movement.

(3) *Body Scheme*—Acquire an internal awareness of the body and the relationship of body parts to each other.

(4) *Right-Left Discrimination*—Differentiate one side of the body from the other.

(5) *Form Constancy*—Recognize forms and objects as the same in various environments, positions, and sizes.

(6) *Position in Space*—Determine the spatial relationship of figures and objects to self or other forms and objects.

(7) *Visual Closure*—Identify forms or objects from incomplete presentations.

(8) *Figure-Ground*—Differentiate between foreground and background forms and objects.

(9) *Depth Perception*—Determine the relative distance between objects, figures, or landmarks and the observer.

(10) *Topographical Orientation*—Determine the location of objects and settings and the route to the location.

2. *Neuromuscular*
   a. *Reflex*—Present an involuntary muscle response elicited by sensory input.
   b. *Range of Motion*—Move body parts through an arc.
   c. *Muscle Tone*—Demonstrate a degree of tension or resistance in a muscle.
   d. *Strength*—Demonstrate a degree of muscle power when movement is resisted as with weight or gravity.
   e. *Endurance*—Sustain cardiac, pulmonary, and musculoskeletal exertion over time.
   f. *Postural Control*—Position and maintain head, neck, trunk, and limb alignment with appropriate weight shifting, midline orientation, and righting reactions for function.
   g. *Soft Tissue Integrity*—Maintain anatomical and physiological condition of interstitial tissue and skin.
3. *Motor*
   a. *Activity Tolerance*—Sustain a purposeful activity over time.
   b. *Gross Motor Coordination*—Use large muscle groups for controlled movements.
   c. *Crossing the Midline*—Move limbs and eyes across the sagittal plane of the body.
   d. *Laterality*—Use a preferred unilateral body part for activities requiring a high level of skill.
   e. *Bilateral Integration*—Interact with both body sides in a coordinated manner during activity.
   f. *Praxis*—Conceive and plan a new motor act in response to an environmental demand.
   g. *Fine Motor Coordination/Dexterity*—Use small muscle groups for controlled movements, particularly in object manipulation.
   h. *Visual-Motor Integration*—Coordinate the interaction of visual information with body movement during activity.
   i. *Oral-Motor Control*—Coordinate oropharyngeal muscula-

ture for controlled movements.

B. Cognitive Integration and Cognitive Components
   1. *Level of Arousal*—Demonstrate alertness and responsiveness to environmental stimuli.
   2. *Orientation*—Identify person, place, time, and situation.
   3. *Recognition*—Identify familiar faces, objects, and other previously presented materials.
   4. *Attention Span*—Focus on a task over time.
   5. *Memory*
      a. *Short-term*—Recall information for brief periods of time.
      b. *Long-term*—Recall information for long periods of time.
      c. *Remote*—Recall events from distant past.
      d. *Recent*—Recall events from immediate past.
   6. *Sequencing*—Place information, concepts, and actions in order.
   7. *Categorization*—Identify similarities of and difference between environmental information.
   8. *Concept Formation*—Organize a variety of information to form thoughts and ideas.
   9. *Intellectual Operations in Space*—Mentally manipulate spatial relationships.
   10. *Problem Solving*—Recognize a problem, define a problem, identify alternative plans, select a plan, organize steps in a plan, implement a plan, and evaluate the outcome.
   11. *Generalization of Learning*—Apply previously learned concepts and behaviors to similar situations.
   12. *Integration of Learning*—Incorporate previously acquired concepts and behavior into a variety of new situations.
   13. *Synthesis of Learning*—Restructure previously learned concepts and behaviors into new patterns.

C. Psychosocial Skills and Psychological Components
   1. *Psychological*
      a. *Roles*—Identify functions one assumes or acquires in society (e.g., worker, student, parent, church member).
      b. *Values*—Identify ideas or beliefs that are intrinsically important.
      c. *Interests*—Identify mental or physical activities that create pleasure and maintain attention.
      d. *Initiation of Activity*—Engage in a physical or mental activity.
      e. *Termination of Activity*—Stop an activity at an appropriate time.
      f. *Self-concept*—Develop value of physical and emotional self.
   2. *Social*
      a. *Social Conduct*—Interact using manners, personal space, eye contact, gestures, active listening, and self-expression appropriate to one's environment.
      b. *Conversation*—Use verbal and nonverbal communication to interact in a variety of settings.
      c. *Self-expression*—Use a variety of styles and skills to express thoughts, feelings, and needs.

3. *Self-management*
   a. *Coping Skills*—Identify and manage stress and related reactors.
   b. *Time Management*—Plan and participate in a balance of self-care, work, leisure, and rest activities to promote satisfaction and health.
   c. *Self-control*—Modulate and modify one's own behavior in response to environmental needs, demands, and constraints.

REFERENCES

American Medical Association. (1966–1988). *Physicians' current procedural terminology first–fourth editions (CPT 1-4).* Chicago: Author

American Occupational Therapy Association. (1979). *Occupational therapy output reporting system and uniform terminology for reporting occupational therapy services*. Rockville, MD: Author.

American Psychiatric Association. (1952–1987). *Diagnostic and statistical manual of mental disorders first–third editions (DSM-I-III-R).* Washington, D.C.: Author.

Medicare-Medicaid Anti-Fraud and Abuse Amendments (Public Law 95-142). (1977), 42 U.S.C. §1305.

Prepared by the Uniform Terminology Task Force (Linda Kohlman McGourty, MOT, OTR, Chair, and Mary Foto, OTR, Jane K. Marvin, MA, OTR, CIRS, Nancy Mahan Smith, MBA, OTR, and Rogert O. Smith, MOT, OTR, task force members) and members of the Commission on Practice, with contributions from Susan Kronsnoble, OTR, for the Commission on Practice (L. Randy Strickland, EdD, OTR, FAOTA, Chair).

Approved by the Representative Assembly April 1989.

Appendix

5 Sources of Information[e]

For further information about occupational therapy, contact the American Occupational Therapy Association, Inc., 1383 Piccard Drive, P.O. Box 1725, Rockville, MD 20849-1725. The general telephone number is (301)948-9626. Members may use a special toll-free information number: 1-800-THE AOTA. (You will need to give your AOTA membership number to use this line.)

The partial directory below shows which AOTA office to contact to obtain certain kinds of information.

For Information About:	Contact:
General information	Public Affairs Division
AOTA publications	AOTA Products
Membership benefits	Membership Information
Career Information	Public Affairs Division
Certification examination	American Occupational Therapy Certification Board
Student Loan Program	Membership Information
Current list of accredited educational programs	Education Division, Accreditation
Employment services	Member Services
Fellowships	American Occupational Therapy Foundation
Films	AOTA Products
Foreign graduate certification	American Occupational Therapy Certification Board
Graduate education	Education Division
Information packet, occupational therapy practice	AOTA Products
International issues	Executive Office
Job bulletins	*OT Week*
Job descriptions	Practice Division

[e] AOTA: Benefits of AOTA Membership. Rockville, MD, AOTA, 1990.

Legislation	Legislative and Political Affairs Division
Literature searches	Library
State regulation	Legislative and Political Affairs Division
OT personnel statistics	Research Information and Evaluation
Minority issues	Public Affairs Division
Position papers	Practice Division
Public information materials	Public Affairs Division
Recruitment materials	Public Affairs Division
Reimbursement issues	Legislative and Political Affairs Division
Research grants	American Occupational Therapy Foundation
Roles and functions of occupational therapy personnel	Practice Division
Salaries of occupational therapy personnel	Research Information and Evaluation
Speakers' network	Continuing Education, Practice Division
Standards of practice	Practice Division
State associations	Practice Division
Statistics	Research Information and Evaluation
Student newsletter	Education Division
Student scholarships	American Occupational Therapy Foundation
World Federation of Occupational Therapists	Executive Office

Appendix

6 Glossary

activity analysis the process of analyzing a given activity by breaking it down into its component parts

activity group a group of people engaged in a common activity or task

activity program a planned program of activities intended to promote the general health and well-being of residents in long-term care facilities

activity tolerance the ability to sustain a purposeful activity for a given period of time

activities of daily living (ADL) performance of self-care, work, and leisure activities

acute of short duration. Used to describe the first phase of an illness or diseases that run a rapid course

acute care the immediate treatment of life-threatening illnesses and injuries; the first stage of treatment

adaptation the act or process of adapting to changes in the external or internal environments

adapted equipment/environment specially designed equipment or surroundings that aid an individual in performing necessary daily tasks

adductor pads pads at the sides of a wheelchair to hold the hips and legs toward the midline of the body

affect emotional feeling, tone, or mood

AIDS acquired immunodeficiency syndrome

Alzheimer's disease degeneration of the medium and smaller blood vessels of the brain, resulting in cognitive and physical impairments

AMA American Medical Association

ambulate to walk about

ambulatory care medical care for patients who are able to get about

amputation the surgical removal of a body part

anorexia nervosa an eating disorder characterized by fear of becoming obese and refusal to eat

anxiety a state of worry or distress; apprehension

AOTA American Occupational Therapy Association

aphasia impaired spoken communication or poor comprehension of speech due to dysfunction of the language centers in the brain

arteriosclerosis a hardening or thickening of the walls of arteries, resulting in decreased blood flow to the heart, the brain, or the extremities

arthritis inflammation of the joints; may be seen in acute or chronic forms

arthroplasty the surgical reconstruction of a joint

assessment a method designed to evaluate or estimate a client's current functional status

athetoid relating to athetosis, a condition characterized by fluctuating muscle tone and slow, involuntary movements

attention span the length of time that a person is able to concentrate on a given task

auditory pertaining to the ability to hear and interpret sounds, localize sounds, and discriminate foreground from background sounds

augmentative communication communication through the use of mechanical devices that expand the individual's ability to communicate

autism, infantile a childhood syndrome characterized by solitary play, self-absorption, social inaccessibility, and language disturbances

avocational relating to activities outside of one's work; leisure pursuits

baseline information data on the patient's level of function when he or she is first seen by a health care worker

behaviorist theory a branch of psychology that attempts to explain human behavior in terms of learning principles and conditioning

bilateral on both sides of the body

bilateral integration the ability to coordinate both sides of the body during activity

biodevelopmental pertaining to both the biological and the developmental processes

biofeedback training the use of electronic devices to help an individual learn to gain voluntary control over autonomic body functions

biomechanics the science of the action of forces, internal or external, on the living body

biomedical the application of the natural sciences to the study of medicine, i.e., physics applications, etc.

body mechanics application of physics principles to avoid undue stress on joints or body parts

body scheme the awareness of the body and the relationship of body parts to one another

bone grafting transplanting bone tissue from one part of the body to another

brainstem the lower portion of the brain that connects the cerebral hemispheres with the spinal cord

bubonic plague an acute infectious disease with a high fatality rate; the Black Death of the Middle Ages

bulimia an eating disorder characterized by bouts of overeating followed by voluntary vomiting, fasting, or induced diarrhea

cardex information a card file at the nurses' station on a hospital unit that contains summarized information about the status of patients on the unit

case manager an individual who assumes responsibility for coordinating and following up on a given case, seeing that the needed services are obtained

categorization the identification of similarities and differences between environmental information

cerebral pertaining to the two hemispheres of the brain

cerebral arteriosclerosis narrowing of the blood vessels within the brain, which may result in headache, dizziness, insomnia, memory changes, or personality changes

cerebral palsy a group of nonprogressive disorders characterized by disturbances in muscle tone and motor control

cerebral vascular disease those diseases that result from changes in the blood vessels supplying the brain

certification a voluntary process whereby a nongovernmental agency documents that a person has qualified to practice a given profession

cervical pertaining to the neck

chart review the process of reading the patient's medical chart in order to better understand his or her condition

chart rounds meetings at which the health care team reviews the status of its patients and makes any necessary adjustments in the treatment program

cholera an acute infectious disease transmitted through contaminated water, milk, or food

chronic of long duration. Used to describe conditions that are long-standing

chronic brain syndrome permanent and generalized loss of cerebral function that may include disorientation, memory loss, confusion, and stereotyped behavior

clinical reasoning the process of reflective thinking that enables practitioners to make sound clinical judgments

closed-head injury a head injury in which there is little or no damage to the skull

co-dependency a psychological disorder resulting from living with or being raised by an addicted or disturbed family member

cognitive functions those mental processes that enable the brain to learn, remember, understand, form concepts, and solve problems

cognitive retraining a systematic method of helping a person to improve his or her understanding of concepts, ability to concentrate, memory, and orientation

collaborate, collaboration working cooperatively with others to achieve a mutual goal

coma, comatose a state of profound unconsciousness from which the patient cannot be aroused

commode a chair enclosing a chamber pot

competence the individual's adequacy or capability in a given task

concept formation the ability to organize a variety of information into thoughts and ideas

congenital anomalies structural abnormalities that are the result of birth defects or genetic disorders

consultation the act of providing expert advice, opinion, or information to other people

consult rounds the daily rounds of hospitalized patients conducted by the attending physician at which referrals for occupational therapy and other services may be made

continuum of care a series of services intended to meet different needs as the client goes through the life span

contracture a permanent muscular contraction that results in loss of function

conversation the use of verbal and nonverbal communication to interact with others

coordination the ability to use several groups of muscles in a combined way to smoothly execute complex movements

COPD chronic obstructive pulmonary disease such as emphysema

coping skills those abilities that enable an individual to identify and manage stress and related reactions

COTA certified occupational therapy assistant

CPR cardiopulmonary resuscitation; an emergency technique to restore breathing and heart rate following an injury

craniectomy the cutting out of a portion of the skull

craniotomy making a surgical opening in the skull

crossing the midline the ability to move the limbs and/or eyes across the sagittal plane of the body

cuing strategies methods of offering a patient cues in order to help him or her perform a given task

custodial institution one that provides the basic necessities of life but does not provide active treatment or training

CVA cerebrovascular accident; commonly known as a stroke. Bleeding, blockage of a vessel, or a blood clot in a vessel within the brain that results in paralysis, sensory loss, speech impairments, and other neurologic symptoms

daily living skills those abilities needed to function in daily life, i.e., grooming, dressing, eating, etc.

debridement the cutting out of dead tissue and foreign matter from a wound

deinstitutionalization the movement to shift treatment services from large governmental institutions to local community-based programs

dementia an irreversible deterioration of cognitive functions due to organic brain damage

depth perception the ability to determine the relative distance between objects, figures, or landmarks, and the observer

depression a clinical condition in which the patient feels dejected and hopeless and may withdraw from social contacts

detoxification unit a specialized treatment unit or program that helps addicted persons to recover from acute episodes and reduce their chemical dependencies

developmental pertaining to the process of human growth and development

developmental delay a condition in which a child is found to be functioning at a level below age or maturational expectations

developmental disability a severe, chronic disability that occurs before the age of 21 and results in functional limitations in at least three areas of life activity

developmental skills those abilities that children develop as they go through normal developmental stages, i.e., language, motor skills, etc.

diabetes a metabolic disorder characterized by a deficient supply of insulin and an inability to metabolize carbohydrates

diffuse brain damage widespread, generalized deficits in the brain

dilation enlargement or opening of a hollow structure

disability any restriction or lack of ability to perform an activity in the normal manner

discharge summary a written summary of the client's treatment and the results obtained prior to discharge from a service program

disease vector a carrier such as the mosquito that transmits disease to humans

documentation the written notes that describe the client's initial status and his or her progress during the treatment process

Down's syndrome a genetic disorder resulting in moderate-to-severe mental retardation and a typically mongoloid facial appearance

DRGs diagnostic-related groups, which are now the basis for reimbursement for hospitalized Medicare recipients

dysfunction disordered or impaired function

dyslexia an inability to learn to read or to interpret graphic symbols

efficacy the ability to achieve the desired result; effectiveness, efficiency

egalitarian equal; the idea that all members of a group have equal rights in the group

embolism an obstruction in a blood vessel, often by a blood clot

endurance the ability of the individual to sustain cardiac, pulmonary, and musculoskeletal exertion over time

energy conservation the application of energy-saving procedures to minimize energy output by the patient

entry level an OTR or COTA with less than 1 year of work experience

epilepsy a seizure disorder with brief, recurrent attacks that may include loss of consciousness, motor activity, and sensory phenomena

equilibrium balance

ergonomics the science of adapting jobs and work environments to human anatomical, physiological, and psychological characteristics in order to enhance workers' efficiency and well-being

ethics a system of moral principles or standards that govern personal or professional conduct

ethnography descriptive anthropology

evaluation the process of examining and judging the current status of an individual's health and ability to function in his or her daily life

existential pertaining to existence and individual experience

extensor muscles those muscles that extend or straighten a limb or a body part

eye tracking the ability to follow an object through the visual field using both eyes simultaneously

FES functional electrical stimulation

fieldwork supervised practical experience in clinical settings as a required part of the curriculum for occupational therapy students

figure-ground the differentiation between foreground and background forms and objects

flailing movements thrashing about wildly

focal brain damage localized injury to a specific part of the brain

forensic unit a specialized treatment unit or program that serves those who have been convicted of a crime and judged to be not guilty by reason of insanity

form constancy the recognition that forms and objects remain the same although their environments, positions, or sizes may change

fracture a broken bone or piece of cartilage

Freud's psychoanalytic theory a method of therapy developed by Freud that emphasizes bringing unconscious material to consciousness

function, functional performance a person's ability to perform those tasks necessary in their daily life

functional communication the ability to utilize equipment or systems to enhance or provide basic communication with others

functional mobility the ability to move from one position or place to another

gastric pertaining to the stomach

gastrointestinal referring to the stomach and the intestines; the digestive tract

gastrostomy the surgical creation of an artificial opening into the stomach

generalist one who practices general occupational therapy, dealing with a broad range of diagnoses and age groups

generalization of learning the ability to apply previously learned concepts and behaviors to new situations

generic relating to or descriptive of an entire group or class

geriatrics the branch of medicine that deals with the medical problems of the elderly

gerontic refers to working with the elderly

gerontology the study of old age

gestation the total length of a pregnancy

grooming the processes engaged in to care for the body, i.e., shaving, combing the hair, applying cosmetics, etc.

group practice the organization of a group of practitioners into a single health care unit such as a clinic or home health agency

gross motor coordination the use of large muscle groups for controlled movement

gustatory referring to the sense of taste

habilitation the acquisition of new skills that the client did not previously possess

handicap any disadvantage resulting from an impairment or a disability that limits or prevents individuals from fulfilling the normal role expectations for their age, sex, society, or culture.

health care corporation a business organization that owns and operates a number of health care facilities for profit

health insurance plans

indemnity benefit plan a type of health insurance in which the insurer pays the consumer for some of the costs of health care

service benefit plan a type of health insurance in which the insurer pays the hospital or physician for services rendered to the consumer

direct service plan a type of health insurance in which the insurer provides health care services directly to the consumer in return for prepayment

Medigap plans health insurance designed to cover some of the procedures that Medicare fails to cover for elderly people

pay-or-play plans a proposed type of health insurance in which employers would either provide health insurance to employees or would pay into a government program that would provide them with health insurance coverage

universal health insurance plan a proposed type of health insurance that would cover all U.S. citizens

hemiplegia paralysis of one side of the body

hierarchy a system that organizes things into successive ranks or grades

HIV human immunodeficiency virus

HMO health maintenance organization; a type of direct service health insurance plan

holistic, holism viewing something as a unified whole, i.e., the whole person

home health agency a public or private agency that provides nursing care and therapy services to clients in their homes for a fee

homonymous hemianopsia blindness for objects in one-half of the visual field, resulting from injury to one optic tract

hospice programs programs providing care for terminally ill patients and emotional support for them and their families

hospitals

voluntary nonprofit institutions sponsored by religious or charitable organizations

proprietary private, for-profit institutions

public government tax-supported institutions

hospital cooperative the combined unit formed when several small hospitals join together into a cooperative for the purchase of needed services and personnel

human occupation model a theoretical model of occupational therapy based on a description of the individual and his or her occupational roles

humanism, humanistic a philosophy concerned with human beings, their welfare and their achievements

hyaline membrane disease a respiratory distress syndrome of the newborn in which there is inadequate development of the lungs

hydrocephalus a condition in which excessive fluid accumulates in the ventricles of the brain, thinning the brain tissue and causing the skull to enlarge

hygiene caring for the body in order to maintain health, i.e., brushing teeth, bathing, toileting, etc.

hypertension high blood pressure

hyperventilate to overbreathe, taking rapid shallow breaths that can sometimes cause fainting

IEP individualized educational plan or program

impairment any loss or abnormality of psychological, physiological, or anatomic structure or function

independent living center a type of community program intended to provide services that support independent or assisted living for severely disabled people

indigent impoverished, needy

indirect service work that involves tasks other than direct services to clients

intensive care unit the hospital unit that provides extensive life support services for seriously ill and injured patients

interests those mental or physical activities that create pleasure and maintain attention

intervention the active process of treatment

intervention plan a written treatment plan that outlines the major goals of occupational therapy intervention and the methods to be used to achieve them

intracerebral contusion a bruising of the brain without rupture of the membranes surrounding it

intrinsic pertaining to the essential nature of a thing; inherent

intrinsic motivation motivation that comes from within the individual; self-motivation

itinerant traveling from one place to another in order to work

joint fusion a surgical procedure that fixes a joint in one position, rendering it immovable

joint manipulation passive movement of a joint by a therapist to increase range of motion and to reduce muscle tightness

kinesthesia the ability to identify the excursion and direction of joint movement

level of arousal the degree of alertness and responsiveness a patient shows to environmental stimuli

licensure official or legal permission from a governmental body to engage in a given occupation or to do or own a specified thing

life review group a type of group therapy that provides opportunities for elderly people to reminisce about their lives and share their memories and feelings with others

managed care a type of care in which a third party, usually an insurance company, determines what type of care will be covered and to what degree

manual muscle test a method of evaluating the strength of individual muscles or groups of muscles

Medicaid a federally funded program administered by the states that provides limited health care coverage for the poor

medical model the traditional model of medical practice that focuses on disease and its remediation or cure

Medicare a federally funded program to provide limited health care coverage to persons over the age of 65

medication routine the process of obtaining and taking medication on a regular basis as prescribed by a physician

memory

short-term ability to recall information for brief periods of time

long-term ability to recall information for long periods of time

remote ability to recall information from the distant past

recent ability to recall information from the immediate past

mentor an individual who counsels or teaches a younger or less experienced person

mentor relationship the relationship between an experienced OTR or COTA who offers support and advice to a less-experienced practitioner or student

monism a belief that a single factor or principle can be used to explain reality

moral treatment an 18th century approach to the treatment of mental illness that included the use of planned activities to help in normalizing patients' behavior

motor planning the ability to plan and execute purposeful movements

multiple sclerosis a chronic, progressive neurologic disease characterized by fluctuating periods of wellness and periods of serious impairment

muscle tone the amount of mild, continuous contraction that is present in normal living muscles

myoelectric prostheses artificial limbs that are operated electronically using the patient's remaining muscle function

nasogastric tube a tube inserted through the nose for feeding a patient who is unable to take food by mouth

national (universal) health care insurance a proposed plan under which all citizens would receive health care coverage

networking forming a set of contacts with colleagues for purposes of consultation and mutual support

neurasthenia, neurasthenic unexplained chronic fatigue and nervousness

neurodevelopmental referring to the gradual, progressive development of the nervous system

neuromuscular pertaining to the nerves and the muscles

neuromuscular facilitation and inhibition increasing or decreasing the activity of muscles through the specific application of sensory stimuli

neuromuscular functions performance of motor behaviors

neurophysiology the study of the functioning of the nervous system

neuropsychiatry, neuropsychiatric referring to nervous and mental diseases

neurosis a psychological or behavioral disorder characterized by anxiety

NICU neonatal intensive care unit

nonhuman environment the physical surroundings of an individual

noninvasive techniques methods that do not require entering the body of the patient

normalization the principle of allowing disabled persons to lead as normal a life as possible in community settings

obesity a condition in which there is an abnormal amount of fat in body tissues

occupation the active or "doing" process when one is engaged in goal-directed activity

occupation, therapeutic any purposeful activity used to prevent physical or mental dysfunction or to restore or improve function to a normal level

occupational behavior those behaviors or activities that an individual engages in in order to fulfill his or her occupational roles

occupational performance an individual's total pattern of activities, i.e., self-care, work, leisure, and organization of time

occupational science a scientific discipline that studies the human as an occupational being

occupational therapy the use of purposeful activity to achieve a functional outcome

occupational therapy process the method by which occupational therapy services are delivered to clients

olfactory pertaining to the sense of smell

oral hygiene the maintenance of a clean mouth and teeth

oral motor control the ability to coordinate the movements of the tongue and mouth

organic mental disorders those conditions that are believed to be the result of physiological or structural change or damage

orientation the ability to identify correctly persons, places, current date, time, and situation

orthopedics the branch of medicine concerned with restoring the function of the limbs and spine through medical, surgical, and physical methods

orthotics splints, braces, or slings used to relieve pain, maintain the alignment of joints, protect joints, improve function, or decrease deformity

OTR registered (certified) occupational therapist

palliative treatment treatment that reduces the symptoms but does not cure the disease

paradigm an example or model

Parkinson's disease a degenerative disease of the central nervous system characterized by increasing rigidity, tremors, and slowness of movement

pathology the anatomic or functional manifestations of disease

perception the brain's interpretation of information received through the senses

perceptual-motor skills those abilities that enable a person to interpret sensory cues and act upon the environment, i.e., kinesthesia, right-left discrimination, etc.

performance components the subskills necessary to perform daily life activities

perinatal pertaining to the period immediately preceding and following the birth of an infant

personality disorders a group of mental disorders characterized by long-standing patterns of maladaptive behavior

philanthropy charitable activities intended to increase the well-being of humankind

physiatrist a physician who specializes in physical medicine and rehabilitation

physiological insult a traumatic injury causing damage to one or more organ systems of the body

pluralism a belief that multiple factors or principles must be considered to explain reality

pneumonia inflammation of the lungs

polio poliomyelitis, an acute viral disease that may result in paralysis and atrophy of muscle groups

position in space the ability to determine the spatial relationship of figures and objects to the self, or to other forms or objects

postural control the ability to maintain the position of head, neck, trunk, and limbs with appropriate weight shifts, midline orientation, and righting reactions

practice models

medical model a practice model that emphasizes disease and its cure or remediation

child development model a practice model that employs normal development as its frame of reference in treating developmental disorders

educational model a practice model that focuses on educating children and helping them to achieve mastery of essential skills

human occupation model a practice model based on the individual and his or her occupational roles

social-ecological model a practice model that views clients in relation to their social background and environment

behavioral model a practice model that is based on learning theory and employs operant conditioning to systematically develop desired behaviors and extinguish undesirable ones

psychoeducational model a practice model that is based on identifying an individual's skill deficits and uses programmed instruction to achieve the target goals

praxis the ability to conceive and plan a new motor act in response to an environmental demand

prehension, prehensile related to the grasping and holding of an object

prevention minimizing the possibility of disease, dysfunction, or disability

prevocational evaluation assessment of work-related abilities and the potential for employment

primitive reflexes a group of automatic movement patterns seen in newborn infants that are controlled at the spinal and brainstem levels

private practice provision of occupational therapy services by an independent practitioner or group of practitioners

problem-solving ability the ability to recognize and define a problem, identify alternative plans, select a plan, implement it, and evaluate the outcome

professional philosophy the fundamental beliefs and values held by members of a given profession

program planning the process of designing an appropriate treatment program for a client

progressive resistive exercise exercise against an opposing force, in which the resistance is systematically increased in order to strengthen muscles

proprioception, proprioceptive the ability to interpret stimuli originating in muscles, joints, and other internal tissues to give information about the position of one body part in relation to another

prospective payment system a system of payment applied to Medicare billings in which specific costs are related to the patient's diagnosis or medical procedure and a set fee is paid

prosthetics artificial substitutes for missing body parts, such as artificial limbs

prototype an original form or model on which later refinements are based

psychoanalytic theory an approach to the treatment of neuroses that emphasizes unlocking long-repressed feelings and past experiences in order to allow the patient to better understand his or her behavior

psychodynamics the theory of human behavior that emphasizes the unconscious motivation and the functional significance of emotion

psychometric tests tests that measure psychological variables such as intelligence, aptitude, or emotional disturbance

psychosocial functions those mental functions that enable people to express their feelings, relate to others, and perceive themselves realistically

psychotropic drugs drugs that directly affect psychic functions, behavior, or experience, i.e., tranquilizers, mood-altering drugs, etc.

pulmonary pertaining to the lungs

purposeful activity meaningful occupation; an occupation with a goal

quality assurance systematic procedures designed to insure that quality standards are being met by employees

quality assurance program a method of studying the outcomes of therapy in order to assess the effectiveness of services being provided and to recommend changes in service delivery if necessary

quality of life considering a patient's satisfaction with life as well as his or her physical needs

range of motion a person's maximum span of joint movement

reality orientation a structured method for improving clients' alertness and cognitive functions

reconstruction aides civilian aides who were recruited to serve in U.S. army field hospitals as occupational workers during World War I

reductionism, reductionistic the philosophy of reducing the study of disease to its smallest biological unit of the cell; studying disease processes on the cellular level

referral an order or recommendation for specific health services

reflex an involuntary motor response elicited by a sensory stimulus

registry a listing of qualified practitioners

regression a return to more primitive patterns of behavior

rehabilitation restoration, after a disease or injury, of the ability to function in a normal or near-normal manner

rehabilitation agency a private or public organization providing outpatient rehabilitation services

reimbursement to pay back or compensate someone

reimbursement systems the various mechanisms by which health care is paid for, i.e., private insurance, Medicare, etc.

remedial intended to correct something

remotivation group a type of group therapy that helps clients become more interested in their surroundings and encourages the sharing of experiences

repertoire the range of skills, aptitudes, or abilities that an individual possesses

research scholarly or scientific investigation or inquiry

resection the surgical removal of a section or a part

respiratory pertaining to the lungs and the process of breathing

rheumatic fever a systemic inflammatory disease often followed by serious heart or kidney disease

rheumatoid arthritis a chronic inflammatory condition affecting the joints that results in pain and swelling of joints with increasing stiffness and disability

right-left discrimination the ability to differentiate one side of the body from the other

robotics the science of mechanical devices that work automatically or by remote control

roles those functions that one assumes or acquires in society, i.e., the roles of worker, parent, student, etc.

role delineation study a study of the various levels of a workforce that attempts to clarify the job functions of each level of worker

sacrum the last lumbar vertebra, or tailbone

schizophrenic disorders a group of mental disorders characterized by flat or inappropriate affect, social isolation, and delusions or hallucinations

screening the process of identifying those clients who may benefit from occupational therapy services

seizure disorder a condition in which there are periodic alterations in brain function, usually accompanied by motor, sensory, autonomic, or psychic symptoms

self-concept an individual's perceptions of self, both physically and emotionally

sensory referring to the senses

sensory aids devices to increase the efficiency of receiving sensory stimuli, e.g., hearing aids or eyeglasses

sensory awareness the ability to receive and differentiate between different forms of sensory stimuli

sensory deprivation lowering the amount of sensory signals from the environment, which may result in emotional, perceptual, and behavioral abnormalities in human beings

sensory integration the organization of sensory input for practical use; the ability to respond to sensory stimuli in a purposeful way

sensory processing the ability to interpret sensory signals

sensorimotor pertaining to both the sensory and the motor systems

sensory motor functions a group of performance components that depend on the ability of the central nervous system to organize and use sensory stimuli for interactions with the external environment

service competency the ability of a worker to meet defined job performance standards

service delivery the process of getting health care services to the people who need them

service management the administration of a service program

sexual expression the ability to recognize, communicate, and perform desired sexual activities

skilled nursing facility a nursing or convalescent home that provides skilled nursing care under the direction of a physician

socialization the ability to interact with people in appropriate contextual and cultural ways

soft tissue integrity the maintenance of anatomical and physiological normality of the interstitial tissue and the skin

spastic quadriplegia a nonprogressive condition in which the muscles are excessively tight and all four limbs are affected

specialization, specialist the trend of working with patients of a limited age range or diagnostic category

spinal cord injury damage to the spinal cord that may result in permanent paralysis and loss of sensation below the level of the injury

spinal meningitis inflammation of the membranes of the spinal cord

splint an appliance used to protect an injured body part or to immobilize or improve its function

standards of practice the minimum acceptable standards of service set by a professional body or a regulatory agency

standing tolerance the ability to stand for a given period of time

stereognosis the ability to identify objects through the sense of touch alone

strength the muscle power exerted when movement is resisted as with weights or gravity

stress management program a program designed to help people cope more effectively with stress in their daily lives

subdural hematoma a blood clot underneath the outer membrane that covers the brain and causes pressure on the brain, resulting in neurological symptoms

subtotal incomplete

supported employment the provision of supports and accommodations that enable physically or mentally disabled people to be employable

system consultation consultation that addresses the needs of a large system or agency

tactile pertaining to the sense of touch; the ability to interpret light touch, pressure, temperature, pain, vibration, and two-point stimuli through skin receptors

taxonomy a classification system

team models

interdisciplinary model a form of treatment in which a number of persons who represent different scientific or professional disciplines function as a team to provide client services

multidisciplinary model a form of treatment in which a number of disciplines contribute, but each functions fairly independently

transdisciplinary model a form of treatment in which various disciplines actually share one another's roles or function across disciplinary lines in order to provide efficient client service

technology the application of scientific knowledge to achieve specific objectives

technology transfer the transfer of technology from one field to another or from one application to another

temporal adaptation the ability to organize one's time in order to fulfill occupational roles and personal responsibilities

tenodesis splint a splint that allows pinch and grasp movements by using the wrist extensors

tenure a permanent position or appointment in an academic setting

time management the ability to plan and participate in a balance of self-care, work, leisure, and rest activities to promote personal satisfaction and health

topographical orientation the ability to determine the location of objects and settings and the route to the location

total hip arthroplasty a surgical procedure in which an artificial hip joint is created

tracheostomy surgical creation of an opening into the windpipe

traction pulling against resistance

trauma an injury caused by harsh contact with an object

trauma center a hospital that is especially equipped to care for severely injured patients

treatment any procedure used to cure a disease or pathological condition or to improve a person's health

treatment media, modalities the techniques and/or methods used by occupational therapists to treat patients

triage the screening and classification of patients to determine the priority of their needs

tuberculosis a bacterial disease most commonly affecting the lungs that results in fever and weight loss

ulcer a lesion on the surface of the skin or a mucous surface, usually with inflammation

upper extremities the hands, arms, and shoulders

use of self a therapist's planned use of his or her personality and perceptions as part of the therapeutic process

values those ideas or beliefs that are intrinsically important to an individual

valve incompetency inability of the valves in the veins to pump sufficient blood through the circulatory system

venous pertaining to the veins

ventricular hemorrhage bleeding within the ventricles of the brain

vestibular referring to the interpretation of stimuli received from inner ear receptors regarding head position and movement

visual referring to stimuli received through the eyes, including peripheral vision and acuity, awareness of color, depth, and figure-background differences

visual closure the ability to identify forms or objects from incomplete presentations

visual field cuts a patient's inability to see a part of the environment when looking straight ahead

visual motor integration coordination of visual information with body movement during activity

visual perceptual disorder impairment in the ability to analyze and interpret visual information

vocational pertaining to one's work

vocational evaluator a professional who evaluates peoples' capacity for productive employment

vocational rehabilitation a specialized field that is concerned with enabling disabled persons to resume productive employment

WFOT World Federation of Occupational Therapists

WHO World Health Organization

work simplification techniques methods that provide easier ways of accomplishing work tasks, minimizing stress on joints and avoiding fatigue

BIBLIOGRAPHY

Ayres AJ: *Sensory Integration and the Child*. Los Angeles, Western Psychological Services, 1979.

Bair J, Gray M (eds): *The Occupational Therapy Manager*. Rockville, MD, American Occupational Therapy Association, 1985.

Boyd W, Sheldon H: *Introduction to the Study of Disease*, ed. 8. Philadelphia, Lea & Febiger, 1980.

Chusid JG: *Correlative Neuroanatomy and Functional Neurology*, ed. 19. Los Altos, CA, Lange Medical Publications, 1985.

Clark PN, Allen AS: *Occupational Therapy for Children*. St. Louis, CV Mosby, 1985.

Clark RG: *Manter & Gatz's Essentials of Clinical Neuroanatomy and Neurophysiology*, ed. 5. Philadelphia, FA Davis, 1975.

Hensyl WR (ed): *Stedman's Medical Dictionary*, ed. 24. Baltimore, Williams & Wilkins, 1982.

Morris W (ed): *American Heritage Dictionary of the English Language*, New College Edition. Boston, Houghton Mifflin, 1981.

Occupational therapy definitions. In *Reference Manual of the Official Documents of the American Occupational Therapy Association, Inc*. Rockville, MD, American Occupational Therapy Association, 1985, pp. VII11–VII15.

Reed KL, Sanderson SR: *Concepts of Occupational Therapy*, ed. 2. Baltimore, Williams & Wilkins, 1983.

Trombly C: *Occupational Therapy for Physical Dysfunction*, ed. 2. Baltimore, Williams & Wilkins, 1983.

AOTA: Definition of Occupational Therapy Practice for State Regulation. *OT Week* 7(9):32–33, 1993.

Thomas CL (ed): *Taber's Cyclopedic Medical Dictionary*, ed. 15. Philadelphia, FA Davis 1985.

AOTA: Uniform terminology for occupational therapy, ed. 2. *AJOT* 43(12):808–815.

Figure and Table Credits

FIGURES

Figure 2.1. Clark PN: Human development through occupation: a philosophy and conceptual model for practice, part 2. *AJOT* 33(9):578, 1979.
Figure 4.1. Modified from Mosey A: *Occupational Therapy: Configuration of a Profession.* New York, Raven Press, p. 75, 1981.
Figure 9.1. OATA Member Data, 1991, and U.S. Bureau of the Census, Research Information and Evaluation, AOTA.
Figure 9.2. AOTA Member Data, 1991, and U.S. Bureau of the Census, Research Information and Evaluation, AOTA.
Figure 12.1. Designed by the occupational therapy staff of San Francisco General Hospital. From Dillard M, Andonian L, Flores O, Lai L, MacRae A, Shakir M. Culturally competent occupational therapy in a diversely populated mental health setting. *AJOT* 46(8):725, 1992.
Figure 18.1. Courtesy of AOTA. Provided by Jeanette Bair, Executive Director.
Figure 18.2. Courtesy of AOTA. Provided by Jeanette Bair, Executive Director.
Figure 18.3. From World Federation of Occupational Therapists brochure. Provided by Prof. Barbara Posthuma, Honorary Secretary.

TABLES

Tables 4.1. *Uniform Terminology for Occupational Therapy,* ed. 2. AOTA, *AJOT* 43(12):808–814, 1989.
Table 4.2. *Uniform Terminology for Occupational Therapy,* ed. 2. AOTA, *AJOT* 43(12):808–814, 1989.
Table 5.1. Data from *Education Data Survey: Final Report.* Research Information and Evaluation Department, Rockville, MD, AOTA, 1992, pp. 6, 11.
Table 6.1. Modified from Schell BA: Guide to occupational therapy personnel. *AJOT* 39:803–810, 1985.
Table 6.2. Modified from Schell BA: Guide to occupational therapy personnel. *AJOT* 39:803–810, 1985.
Table 6.3. AOTA: 1990 Member data survey. *OT Week;* 5(22):6, 1991.
Table 6.4. AOTA: 1990 Member data survey. *OT Week* 5(22):6, 1991.
Table 9.1. Data from Tables 17 and 18, AOTA 1990 member data survey. *OT Week* 5(22):4–5, 1991.
Table 9.2. Data from Table 28, AOTA 1990 member data survey. *OT Week* 5(22):6, 1991.
Table 9.3. Data from Table 24, AOTA 1990 member data survey. *OT Week* 5(22):6, 1991.
Table 9.4. Data from Table 39, AOTA 1990 member data survey. *OT Week* 5(22):8, 1991.
Table 10.1. Data from *American Hospital Association Statistics, 1991–1992.*
Table 10.2. Data from *American Hospital Association Statistics 1991–1992.*
Table 16.1. Data from Table 17, AOTA 1990 Member Data Survey, Summary Report, Special Insert. *OT Week* 5(22):4–5, 1991.
Table 16.2. Data from Table 29, AOTA 1990 Member Data Survey, Summary Report, Special Insert. *OT Week* 5(22):6, 1991.
Table 16.3. From Tulanian M, Hammond S, Tulanian S: *The Business Management of Private Practice: Occupational Therapy, Physical Therapy.* Middletown, CA, Applied Educational Systems, 1985, pp. 11–12.
Table 19.1. Unpublished data from 1991 reports of member countries. World Federation of Occupational Therapists.

Cover Photograph Courtesy of the American Occupational Therapy Association, Rockville, MD.
Pages 2, 6, 20, 34, 48, 58, 82, 92, 108, 116, 126, 138, 150, 160, 172, 184, 220, and 234. Courtesy of AOTA.
Page 70. Courtesy of Good Samaritan Hospital, Cincinnati, OH.
Page 196. By Bruce E. Tapper. Courtesy of *OT Week.*
Page 206. Courtesy of Barbara E. Joe.

Index